Dogs, Zoonoses and Public Health

Dogs, Zoonoses and Public Health

Edited by

Calum N.L. Macpherson

Windward Islands Research and Education Foundation
St George's University
St Georges
Grenada
West Indies

Francois X. Meslin

Animal and Food-Related Public Health Risks Team
Department of Communicable Diseases Surveillance and Response
World Health Organization
Geneva
Switzerland

and

Alexander I. Wandeler

WHO Collaborating Centre for Rabies Control, Pathogenesis and Epidemiology
in Carnivores
OIE Reference Laboratory for Rabies
Animal Diseases Research Institute
Nepean
Ontario
Canada

CABI *Publishing*

CABI *Publishing* is a division of CAB *International*

CABI Publishing
CAB International
Wallingford
Oxon OX10 8DE
UK

CABI Publishing
10 E. 40th Street
Suite 3203
New York, NY 10016
USA

Tel: +44 (0)1491 832111
Fax: +44 (0)149 833508
Email: cabi@cabi.org
Web site: http://www.cabi.org

Tel: +1 212 481 7018
Fax: +1 212 686 7993
Email: cabi-nao@cabi.org

A catalogue record for this book is available from the British Library, London, UK.

Library of Congress Cataloging-in-Publication Data
Dogs, zoonoses, and public health / edited by Calum N.L. Macpherson, Francois X. Meslin, Alexander I. Wandeler.
    p. cm.
  Includes bibliographical references (p.).
  ISBN 0-85199-436-9 (alk. paper)
    1. Zoonoses. 2. Communicable diseases in animals. 3. Animals as carriers of disease. 4. Dogs--Diseases. 5. Public health. I. Macpherson, C. N. L. (Calum N. L.) II. Meslin, F.-X. (Francois-X.) III. Wandeler, Alexander I.

RA639 .D645 2000
614.4'3--dc21

                                                                              00-057966

ISBN 0 85199 436 9

Printed and bound by Cromwell Press, Trowbridge, from copy supplied by the author.

Contents

Contributors

J.J. Arzt, DVM, MPVM
WHO/PAHO Collaborating Center
on New and Emerging Zoonoses,
Department of Population Health
and Reproduction,
School of Veterinary Medicine,
University of California, Davis,
CA 95616
USA

R.W. Ashford, PhD, DSc, DIC
Liverpool School of Tropical
Medicine, Pembroke Place,
Liverpool, L3 5QA
UK

A.M. Beck, ScD
Center for the Human Animal
Bond,
School of Veterinary Medicine,
Purdue University,
West Lafayatte,
IN 47907-1243
USA

J. Bingham, BVSc, Dphil
OIE Reference Laboratory for
Rabies,
Onderstepoort Veterinary Institute,
Private Bag XO5,
Onderstepoort, 0110
South Africa

B.B. Chomel DVM, PhD
WHO/PAHO Collaborating Center
on New and Emerging Zoonoses,
Department of Population
Health and Reproduction,
School of Veterinary Medicine,
University of California,
Davis, CA 95616
USA

P.S. Craig, MSc, PhD
Department of Biological Sciences,
The University of Salford,
Salford, M5 4WT
UK

C.F. Curtis, BvetMed, DVD
MRCVS, 7 Chadwell, Ware,
Hertfordshire, SG12 9JX
UK

T.J. Daniels, PhD
Vector Ecology Laboratory,
Louis Calder Center,
Fordham University,
PO Box K,
53 Whippoorwill Road,
Armonk, NY 10504
USA

M.A. Gemmell, BVSc
Sudbury House,
1 Purfleet Place, King's Lynn,
Norfolk, PE30 1JH
UK

J. Leney, MSc
World Society for the Prevention
of Cruelty to Animals,
2 Langley Lane,
London, SW8 1TJ
UK

C.N.L. Macpherson, PhD, DIC
Windward Islands Research and
Education Foundation, St George's
University, PO Box 7,
St Georges, Grenada
West Indies

H.C. Matter, Dr.phil.nat
Swiss Federal Office of Public
Health,
CH-3003 Bern
Switzerland

F.X. Meslin, DVM
Animal and Food-Related Public
Health Risks Team,   .
Department of Communicable
Diseases Surveillance and
Response,
World Health Organisation,
CH-1211 Geneva 27
Switzerland

M.A. Miles, MSc, PhD, DSc
FRCPath
Pathogen Molecular Biology and
Biochemistry Unit, Department of
Infectious and Tropical
Diseases, London School of
Hygiene and Tropical Medicine,
Keppel Street, London,
WC1E 7HT
UK

R. Muller, DSc, FIBiol
St. Albans,
Hertfordshire, AL4 0SS
UK

P.A.M. Overgaauw, DVM, PhD
Department of Regulatory Affairs
and Technical Services,
Virbac Netherlands,
Barneveld
The Netherlands

J. Remfry, PhD, VETMB, MRCVS
Animal Protection Consultancies
and Projects,
19 Moxon Street, Barnet,
Hertfordshire, EN5 5TS
UK

R.A. Robinson, BVSc, MPH, PhD
College of Veterinary Medicine,
Western University of Health
Sciences,
309 E. Second St/College Plaza,
Pomona, CA 91766-1854
USA

K.F. Snowden, DVM, PhD
College of Veterinary Medicine,
Department of Veterinary
Pathobiology,
College Station,
TX 77843-4467
USA

F. van Knapen, DVM, PhD
Department of the Science of Food
of Animal Origin,
Faculty of Veterinary Medicine,
Utrecht University,
Utrecht
The Netherlands

J.A. Vexenat, MSc, PhD
Laboratorio de Microbiologia,
Faculdade de Agronomia e
Medicina Veterinaria, Campus
Universitaria UNB, CP 04508 CEP
70910/970, Brasilia, DF
Brazil

A.I. Wandeler, PhD
WHO Collaborating Centre for
Rabies Control, Pathogenesis and
Epidemiology in Carnivores,
OIE Reference Laboratory for
Rabies,
Animal Diseases Research
Institute, Nepean,
Ontario, K2H 8P9
Canada

Preface

Dogs were domesticated by humans approximately 14,000 years ago and became associated very closely with human activities, including, hunting, guarding, and herding and for food. This association was strengthened over time in many cultures, with dogs entering dwellings and sharing human space and time, and acting as social partners and companions. Today, there are hundreds of different breeds of dog, which are divided into sporting dogs, hounds, working dogs, terriers, toys and non-sporting dogs. These breeds are used for various purposes in different parts of the world. Dogs are used ubiquitously for guarding and this role is appreciated and utilized even by those peoples whose religious beliefs deem them as impure. Dogs are used for law enforcement, detecting people being smuggled across international borders, for sniffing out drugs and other illegal substances and for crowd and individual control. Dogs have numerous roles in the medical field and are increasingly used as "the eyes" for blind people and "ears" for deaf people. To the vast majority of people dogs serve as companion animals and companion animal medicine is increasingly being recognized as an important area of human health. Dogs may permit people to live healthier, happier lives, and recent studies have shown the benefits dogs impart to many diverse groups, such as children, elderly people and those isolated by stigmatizing diseases, such as AIDS. Globally diverse groups of people use dogs for sport and for hunting. They are valued for their ability to find prey in rain forests, great grassland areas and in the frozen lands of the Arctic and Antarctic. In this area dogs are also used for transport. In the extensive sheep rearing areas of the world, such as in North and South America, northern and southern Africa, Australia, New Zealand, northwest China, Mongolia and in much of Europe dogs play an essential role in herding.

Attitudes regarding dogs vary greatly according to socio-cultural and religious backgrounds. In cities and towns, many people regard dogs as a serious public health nuisance, with their fouling of pavements and public parks, dog bites, their persistent barking, particularly at night, and their movements which may cause traffic accidents. In much of the developing world, stray dogs usually outnumber owned dogs and this cohort presents its own problems from scavenging from garbage sites, indiscriminate defecation, barking and pack behaviour. All of these negative attributes polarize people's opinions about dogs in general. Because of the strong views held by both dog lovers and haters it is difficult to get a balanced view, but whatever one's opinion, dogs are now an important part of our society, in every corner of the world.

The number of dogs in the world today is estimated to be around 500 million and dogs are the most widespread and abundant of all carnivores. The size of the overall dog population is related to that of the human population and increases as the human population increases. The number of dogs per human being and dog population densities vary greatly from area to area. Many studies conducted in both developed and developing countries have shown that in most instances dogs are highly dependent on humans or human activities. This association exists even in countries where the human-dog relationship seems to be loose. In most countries there invariably exists a close physical contact between dogs and children.

Dogs are unwittingly reservoirs, carriers and transmitters of many zoonotic infections, including viruses, bacteria and protozoan and helminth parasites. These pathogens are transmitted accidentally to humans either directly, through close contact, or indirectly through environmental contamination or via an arthropod vector. Some of these infections such as rabies, leishmaniasis and hydatidosis are widespread and result in significant economic and public health problems. People with impaired immune systems are at special risk and should therefore take greater precautions to avoid infection with a number of bacterial and parasitic zoonoses, as well as emerging diseases which have a zoonotic potential.

The objectives of this book are to review the anthropological aspects of the human-dog relationship and identify the benefits which may be derived from and attitudes *vis- à-vis* this association in different parts of the world, where cultural attitudes towards dogs differ greatly. This section is followed by a review of the current knowledge on dog population biology and ecology, also in the context of human populations, settlements and activities. Attention is paid to the basis of the human-dog dependency, components within a dog population and providing methods for calculating data, such as population size and turnover: important criteria for designing disease prevention and control programs. The next sections compile recent data on all the major viral, bacterial and parasitic zoonoses shared by humans and dogs. The final chapters deal with dog and disease control and prevention aspects, including current and future methods for dog population management.

It is the aim of this book to provide those interested in dogs and the world we share with them, a comprehensive account of the public health aspects of this encounter. It also aims to examine how our interaction with dogs in different cultures and socioeconomic conditions facilitates both beneficial and harmful processes and how the zoonotic diseases are currently being controlled.

Calum N.L. Macpherson
Francois X. Meslin
Alexander I. Wandeler

23 May 2000

Chapter One

The Human-Dog Relationship: a Tale of Two Species

Alan M. Beck

Animals have generally played a great role in human ecological adjustment. Just as credible a reason as any for the domestication of animals is their use as pets. In other words, there is as much reason to believe that man's psychological needs were the primary cause for domestication of animals as that man needed to use animals for such material purposes as the saving of human labor and the satisfaction of a hunger for food.

Boris M. Levinson (1969)

It is common that different species of animals may share the same environment and often benefit from each other's presence. They may follow one another for food, or flee together even when only one senses the danger. In natural symbiotic relationships, one participant does not significantly alter the physiology of the other. This is not what has happened with people and their domesticated animals and especially the human relationship with companion animals.

Domestication

Domestication is a biological process; the artificial selection (by people not nature) of an animal's characteristics by breeding animals with the desired characteristics and discouraging, or prohibiting, the propagation of those animals without the desired characteristics (Darwin, 1859). This selective breeding alters the frequency of certain genes in the breeding population. The genes themselves are not altered (mutated), only their frequency of occurrence. The desired attributes will now occur more often than expected.

Physiological processes and patterns of behavior are much less changed by selective breeding. Hence, the gestation period, size of the genital organs and social behavioral patterns of modern domesticated animals are basically the same as those of their wild ancestors.

Many of the economic, social and even aesthetic characteristics sought by people for their domesticated animals are more commonly observed in the younger individuals of the wild type. Breeding food animals like pigs and cows that retain their more juvenile form means having animals that do not expend energy on bone elongation, but more efficiently deposit more meat and fat on shorter bodies, which is, of course, what is desired. Initially, most domesticated animals were smaller than their wild ancestors, but later the domesticated forms were further manipulated to produce animals that were much smaller or even larger; examples include Shetland ponies and Shire horses, who are smaller and larger than their progenitors, and the toy breeds of dogs, like the Chihuahua or the Newfoundland or Saint Bernard, who are actually larger than any wild canid. Domesticated animals often have other attributes associated with the retention of juvenile characteristics. In the sexually mature adult this is known as neoteny or pedomorphosis (Campbell, 1966). Neoteny is either early sexual maturation or retarded development of adult features although the organism becomes sexually mature while retaining immature morphology, like thinner hair, shorter horns and smaller teeth (Price, 1984, 1998; Coppinger and Schneider, 1995).

Interestingly, neoteny is one of the ways living forms can evolve relatively quickly, for many inherited characteristics can be selected at the same time and the species can change with greater rapidity. It has been noted that human beings, *Homo sapiens*, have more in common with juvenile great apes, e.g. gorillas and chimpanzees, than with full grown ones. The ability to stand erect, relative hairlessness, lack of heavy brow and relatively short arms are characteristics of very young apes and people. As the ape matures, the pelvis rotates and forces the animal to stand and walk using its arms as well as its legs; the animal becomes hairier, a heavy brow ridge develops and the face, arms and body grow to the proportions recognized as the adult form. Human beings, however, never outgrow their infantile characteristics (De Beer, 1958; Montagu, 1962; Campbell, 1966, 1972).

In addition to infantile physical characteristics, humans possess many juvenile behavioral characteristics including staying with parents longer than the total longevity of most animals, and a need for touch and bonding more like what most animals exhibit only during their immature stage of development. The need to be part of a family even extends to a family oriented social structure that may persist for the individual's whole life. The fact that the great apes outgrow these juvenile behaviors and physical characteristics is in part why none have been particularly successful as pets, despite their genetic relationship to us. Apes and all the larger monkeys are trainable and can be conditioned to tolerate the human way of life, but none thrive in it. Apes and the larger monkeys cannot remain house pets once they mature. In contrast, dogs thrive with people.

Promoting the breeding of carnivores that retain their juvenile attributes would encourage playfulness, and less aggressiveness, making them better companions and easier to handle. In addition, such a breeding program would also promote other juvenile traits usually considered more attractive. Most people find animals with wide eyes and short snouts pleasing. These are typically, features of the young. Many of the animals that are particularly enjoyed by our culture are those that retain some of the physical attributes of the young, like the seal, dolphin, and squirrel.

Animals were domesticated, for one reason or another, because we liked them. Therefore, many of today's domestic animals were created by selectively breeding animals that retained the traits of the young, e.g. cattle, pigs, dogs and to a somewhat lesser extent, cats. All of these retain many body characteristics and behaviors of the juvenile throughout their lives.

Perhaps a naturally occurring neoteny permitted humans to evolve rapidly away from their primate ancestors thus avoiding competition with them that we humans may not have survived. In many ways, cultures evolve by a natural selection process as well. Humans, with their juvenile qualities, maintain behaviors more typical of the young. Hence, they extend parenthood and closeness with each other, i.e. human social order and culture. Man, not dog, is man's first domesticated animal.

The ancestor of the dog

It is now generally accepted that dogs, *Canis familiaris*, were first tamed then domesticated from the wolf, probably one of the smaller subspecies of *Canis lupus pallipes* or the now extinct *C. lupus variabilis* (Clutton-Brock, 1995). The relationship between humans and dogs began in prehistoric times, some 12,000 years ago, about the time people started living in villages. Sheep and goats are traced back approximately 10,000 years, cats about 5000 (Morey, 1994).

As prehistoric peoples traveled from place to place in search of game and fertile lands, wild wolves undoubtedly followed, attracted by the prospect of an easy meal on the bones, uneaten food and even the human waste people left behind. At this stage the wolf was not so much loved as tolerated. An uneasy symbiosis must have developed. Wolves warned humans of approaching danger and may have even led early hunters to animals that both could eat. Taming occurred as individual animals were rewarded with food when they approached. Tamed animals could be captured and bred. Keeping the offspring of those animals, particularly those with the juvenile qualities people wanted, began the domestication process.

Dogs that accepted people as an innate response were bred, but they still retained much of the behaviors of the pack oriented animal. In time, dogs responded to humans as members of their pack and treated them more as their conspecifics (members of the same species). The conventional definition of a pack implies members of the same species, as the conventional definition of aggression implies a conspecific interaction. If we extend both these concepts to include ecological and social "conspecifics", if not necessarily genetic conspecifics, we can explain a great deal of our interactions with domesticated dogs.

The first extension of the dog-human pack hypothesis would be that a dog and its owner (master) are a true social group. From the human's point of view, the dog is a "member" of the family, indeed, most people who are dog owners specifically refer to their animals as a member of the family (Beck and Katcher, 1996). Most people intuitively respond to a dog's "play-soliciting bow" or growl in much the same way another dog would. It is this preference to exist in a pack, dominated by a leader that forms the basis for many successful human-dog relationships. When there is a lack of a clear hierarchy or when the animal, not human, is the leader, we see problems in the family, including animal bite and inappropriate behaviors.

The rate and range of changes that distinguish the dog from wolf or even from one dog breed to another has been increased by selective breeding within relatively small populations. Dogs were bred to meet the demands of differing climates and roles (Coppinger and Coppinger, 1996, 1998). There is no one reason for the domestication or even keeping of dogs. Nevertheless, dog keeping is common around the world.

The dog population

The dog population in urban and suburban areas is composed of three interacting, and at times interchangeable, subpopulations: (1) pets that never roam without human supervision; (2) straying pets that roam continuously or sporadically; and (3) ownerless animals usually referred to as strays (see Chapter 2). Social attitude towards strays is ambivalent. On one hand, they are protected because society is unwilling to either socially or financially support animal control and, on the other hand, they are unfairly blamed by popular literature as the major cause of dog bite injuries (Beck, 1980).

Estimates of the total dog population come from local, regional, or national surveys and there is considerable variation in methods used. Most rely on surveys of consumer panels and estimate about 52 million owned dogs in the USA (Patronek and Glickman, 1994). The data from the only true statistical probability sample indicated that about 28% of USA households have at least one dog, with an average of 1.5 dogs, per household for a total estimated population of 41 million dogs (Crispell, 1994). In the USA, all estimates indicate that the owned dog population is decreasing (Patronek and Glickman, 1994). This may not be true in developing countries where the owned and stray dog population is believed to be increasing. This may be because more people are moving in urban areas and resources may be more available.

Today, more than 61% of USA households have some companion animal, 39% have dogs - 31% have more than one (American Pet Products Manufacturers Association, 1999). In Australia, approximately 60% of the 6.2 million households have one or more pets; 53% of the households have either a dog or a cat (McHarg *et al.*, 1995). Dog, cat, and/or bird ownership in European households are 71% in Belgium, 63% in France, 60% in The Netherlands, 55% in Britain, 61% in Italy, 37% in the GDR, 70% in Ireland, averaging 52% for all the 17 European countries surveyed (Reader's Digest Association, Inc., 1991).

By contrast, there are relatively few studies of urban stray or feral dogs. Specific populations have been studied in Baltimore, Maryland, USA (Beck, 1973, 1975), St Louis, Missouri, USA (Fox *et al.*, 1975), New York City (Rubin and Beck, 1982), Berkeley, California, USA (Berman and Dunbar, 1983), Italy (Hansen, 1983), Newark, New Jersey, USA (Daniels, 1983a, b) and some areas in Mexico and the American southwest (Daniels and Bekoff, 1989).

As a general rule, straying pets are more common in high human density, low- to middle-income areas, especially where people have direct access to the streets (e.g. areas of low- to middle-income private housing or row houses). Ownerless strays are more common in low-density, low-income areas where there is shelter and fewer requests for animal control, such as around parks, dumps or abandoned parts of the inner city (Beck, 1973; Scott and Causey, 1973; Fox *et al.*, 1975; Nesbitt, 1975).

It is important to distinguish straying pets from ownerless strays, because they cause different problems for society and are managed or controlled by different means (Beck, 1974). Straying pets are best managed by encouraging and enforcing responsible ownership, while strays are controlled by capture and alterations of the environment, e.g. the boarding-up of vacant buildings and clearing dumps and urban lots (Beck, 1981).

One adaptation of unowned stray dogs in an urban environment is to behave like socialized pet dogs (Rubin and Beck, 1982). In that way they are indistinguishable from owned stray dogs and are tolerated as loose pets and not wild dogs - a form of "cultural camouflage". Therefore the differences between owned and unowned stray dogs are not easily observed without extensive study.

No country has an official census of their pet or feral dog population, although methods exist for those interested in animal control or public health (Beck, 1982; Bögel, 1990). There are also no precise figures as to the number of animals killed in animal shelters. In the USA, estimates range between 2 and 6 million for dogs and cats killed in animal shelters each year (Rowan, 1992). The popular press often quotes in excess of 12 million.

As the urban stray dog population comes mostly from the pet population, we assume the population of stray dogs is also decreasing. By domesticating the dog, people assumed responsibility for its survival, and like other domestic animals, the dog does not do well without the intervention of humans. In urban areas stray dogs do not reproduce well enough to establish a wild population and so soon disappear if people do not abandon pets (Beck, 1973). One indication that urban stray dogs appear to be recruited from the pet population is the great variation of breeds, often like the owned population. In rural areas of developed countries and developing countries the dog population develops some uniformity (Perry and Giles, 1970; Scott and Causey, 1973; Nesbitt, 1975).

Social conflicts of dog-human contact

Most of the problems associated with animals in populated areas concerns dogs. The major issues associated with dogs in cities include animal bite, environmental damage, potential disease, and humane considerations for the animals themselves. These are real issues but there are also real solutions.

Dog bites

One concern about dogs in cities is that they may bite people, especially children. All of the USA studies using reported bite-rate data show the same pattern; people ages 4-19 receive about 20% of all dog bites (Harris *et al.*, 1974; Beck *et al.*, 1975; Hanna and Selby, 1981; Lauer *et al.*, 1982; Beck, 1991).

Contrary to the public's perception, in the USA the owned pet dog, not strays, leads the pack in bite rate. Dogs owned by the neighbor of the victim have the highest rate, followed by those owned by the family of the victim. Strays had the lowest rate. However, bites from strays are more commonly reported than bites from owned animals. Where there is good reporting of all bites, like in population based surveys or on military bases, non-owned or stray dogs account for less than 10% of all bites (Beck, 1991). One reason for the disproportionate "over-reporting" of strays is the perception that strays cause more disease, like rabies. Stray dogs may be perceived to be less healthy because they are ownerless or have less responsible owners because they let their animals run free. In either case, these dogs may indeed get less veterinary care, including appropriate vaccinations against disease, like rabies. Therefore, people tend to seek medical care and report the bite more frequently when bitten by an animal whose owner is not known; 50% of people bitten by dogs without known owners sought medical treatment compared to only 29% of people bitten by family owned dogs and 39% when the dog was owned by a neighbor (Beck and Jones, 1985).

Considering the patterns of dog bite injury, it is not surprising that a leash law, in one form or another, is common in many cities around the world. This simple regulation is a way of reducing animal bite and many of the problems associated with dogs. The law should set a maximum length of leash - about 1.8 m (6 ft) or less. People should not tether their dogs on ropes too much longer as longer leads can endanger the animals by being entangled.

Dog bite can be serious, as many infectious agents have been identified at the site of a bite (Talan *et al.*, 1999) and death from trauma has been reported (Pinckney and Kennedy, 1982; Borchelt *et al.*, 1983; Sacks *et al.*, 1989). Nevertheless, serious infection and fatal injury is rare. With the exception of the potential of rabies, the vast majority of bites are no more serious than the slips and falls associated with childhood - indeed, the injuries associated with routine child play are more common (Weiss *et al.*, 1998). But we should always try to minimize bite injury. The safest and most humane way to reduce bites from dogs is a public health policy that encourages having dogs that are well socialized to people and keeping dogs on a leash or always having them supervised when on public property.

In the USA, stray dogs continue to have little impact on human public heath, be it from animal bites (Beck, 1991) or rabies (Beck *et al.*, 1987; Torrence *et al.*, 1995). For some people, ownerless dogs are part of the urban scene who live out their lives as wild canids. For others, strays are animals that must be captured as pests and removed from life on the streets, after which, they are usually killed, although some are adopted and become owned pets.

Owned dogs with undesirable behaviors, like biting, are more likely to be relinquished to an animal shelter. Compared with dogs having no unwanted behavior, dogs that exhibit unwanted behaviors daily, e.g. barking, chewing, hyperactivity, inappropriate elimination, aggressiveness toward other pets, and aggressiveness toward people, have a higher risk to be relinquished to an animal shelter, 1.3 versus 8.5 (Patronek *et al.*, 1996). Controlling the conflicts between the owner's expectations and the dog's nature is one of the important issues in public health and animal welfare. Avoiding owner-dog conflicts is one of the most efficient ways to lessen relinquishment of dogs to animal shelters and reduce dog bites.

Dogs and disease

With the exception of rabies, most of the diseases transmitted from dogs to humans do not attract much public attention in North America and Europe. However, dog waste, a perennial nuisance in cities, is more than just an esthetic problem. Dog feces in public areas allows parasite transmission from dog to dog and is also a human public health issue (see Chapters 4-10).

There are numerous studies establishing that dogs are frequently parasitized by *Toxocara canis* and failure to clean up after dogs seeds the environment with *Toxocara* eggs and it is now widely recognized that the ingestion of embryonated *Toxocara* eggs can cause human illness, i.e. toxocariasis or visceral larva migrans. The disease has two forms, an intestinal migration or ocular involvement (Glickman and Shofer, 1987; Chapter 8).

The best way to lessen the occurrence of parasite contamination is routine veterinary care. Animals that are routinely "de-wormed" do not pass contaminated feces, which is particularly important for those dog owners with young children.

Dog waste, apart from being a source of parasites is viewed as a kind of environmental pollution. To address this problem, most large metropolitan areas in North America and Europe have laws that restrict the activity of animals, especially dogs, in public areas. Most cities in the USA prohibit pets from entering restaurants or food stores or going on public transportation except for animals in enclosed carriers or service dogs assisting people with special needs.

One of the most common regulations to reduce dog waste in public areas is to encourage or require dog owners to have their dogs use the street, rather than sidewalk for defecation, the so-called "curb your dog laws". In this way people do not step into waste and the waste is carried to storm drains during street washing or rain. In addition, most cosmopolitan centers encourage or enforce clean-up after your dog when in public, "scoop laws" (Beck, 1979). Basic courtesy permits dogs and people to share the cities in ways that benefit both.

The social and health benefits of dogs in society

Dogs are present in almost all human settings and many share the human home as well. For some, they replace the children who have grown and moved away or perhaps were never born, and for others, they are playmates for the children still at home. In the USA, more than half of the families that have a dog also have children at home. At the very least, for some people, dogs afford increased opportunities to meet other people. We are beginning to understand this complex bond between pets and people; two species with the common goal of surviving and enjoying life together (Beck and Meyers, 1996).

People with good human contact are healthier than those who are isolated from others (Lynch, 1977; House *et al.*, 1988; Schone and Weinick, 1998). Because pet animals, especially dogs, are perceived as members of the family, pet ownership is one way people can be protected from the ravages of loneliness (Katcher and Beck, 1986; Beck and Katcher, 1996). Unlike talking to other humans, people experience a decrease of blood pressure talking to pets, indicating that they are more relaxed with them than with people (Katcher *et al.*, 1983; Baun *et al.*, 1984; Wilson, 1991). Even in the presence of unfamiliar dogs, people experience a temporary decrease in blood pressure (Friedmann *et al.*, 1983).

The psychological and physiological responses to association with animals appear to manifest themselves when people are asked to describe the perceived benefits for having a dog. More than 95% of dog owners list "companionship" and nearly half list "good for the family health" as their reasons for ownership. Nearly three-quarters include "fun to watch" and "like a child or family member" and 64% report the dog is a source of "security" (American Pet Products Manufacturers Association, 1999). Dogs providing a sense of security or safety appears to be especially appreciated for older adults (Erikson, 1985; Norris *et al.*, 1999). But this person's subjective perception appears to be founded in objective findings. In 1980, there was the first epidemiological report documenting the value of pet ownership. A study of 92 people hospitalized after a heart attack found that 94% of those who happened to own pets were alive after the first year compared with 72% of those who did not own any animal. The ownership of any animal correlated with improved survival. A discriminate analysis demonstrated that pet ownership accounted for 2-3% of the variance (Friedmann *et al.*, 1980). While 2-3% may seem small, the impact, considering the frequency of heart disease, is significant and cost effective. A more recent and extensive follow-up with 369 patients also demonstrated that dog owners had a significantly improved one-year survival after an acute myocardial infarction than non-owners (Friedmann and Thomas, 1995).

A more recent study of the benefits of interactions with animals found that pet owners had reductions in some common risk factors for cardiovascular disease when compared with non-owners (Anderson *et al.*, 1992). Pet owners had lower systolic blood pressures, plasma cholesterol and triglyceride values. While pet owners engaged in more exercise, they also ate more meat and "take-out" foods than non-owners and the socioeconomic profiles of the two groups were very similar. It appears that pet ownership may reduce the risk factors associated with cardiovascular disease, possibly for reasons that go beyond simply an association with risk behaviors.

Serpell (1991) reported that dog owners experienced fewer minor health problems and increased the number and duration of their recreational walks. The effects persisted over the 10-month study period and there was no clear explanation for the results. Naturally occurring events in people's lives are enhanced because of animal companionship. For instance, people walking with their dog experience more social contact and longer conversations than when walking alone (Messent, 1983; McNicholas and Collis, 2000).

In one study, nearly 1000 non-institutionalized older adult Medicare patients were evaluated prospectively. Those subjects who owned pets appeared to experience less distress and required fewer visits to their physicians than non-owners. While animal ownership generally had value, the most remarkable benefits to health were for those who owned dogs (Siegel, 1990). Most of the people noted that the pets provided them with companionship and a sense of security and the opportunity for fun/play and relaxation. Animals allowed people to experience bonding. Siegel (1993) suggested that pets have a stress-reducing effect. The elderly often benefit the most from the companionship of animals (Dembicki and Anderson, 1996). Many indicators of life's satisfactions, including health and personal safety, decline after retirement but the decrease is significantly less among pet dog owners compared to non-owners (Norris *et al.*, 1999). Consequently, support has grown for protecting the right of pet ownership for older adults living in the community and encouraging animal contact for those in long-term nursing home settings.

The use of animals in therapeutic settings

Long before there was any evidence that animal contact enhanced physical and mental health, animals were being used in therapeutic settings, referred to as "animal-facilitated therapy" or AFT. Much of the early literature documents nothing more than fortuitous interactions with animals that happen to be present in a therapeutic setting (Beck, 1985; Beck and Katcher, 1996). The animals, mostly dogs, were originally included in the setting to provide the expected comfort traditionally associated with pet care. Often the best "medicines" are appropriate concentrations of what is generally beneficial (Beck and Katcher, 1984). From the very beginning AFT has paralleled the use of animals as pets and many of the therapeutic uses are extensions of the health benefits now recognized for those who own or interact with companion animals. The most common kinds of AFT programmes are: (1) institutionally based programs where animals either reside in the facility or are brought by visitors; (2) non-institutional programs for older adults where animal contact is facilitated in people's homes; (3) service animals for the disabled in the home setting using specially trained animals, usually dogs; and (4) horseback riding (equine) programs providing riding directed towards physical therapy. The most common therapeutic animal is the dog. Today, AFT programs occur throughout the developing world.

A survey of 150 selected US and 74 Canadian humane societies found that 49 (46%) of the US and 49 (66%) of the Canadian society programs ran AFT programs. More than 94% used dogs and/or cats, 28% rabbits, 15% small mammals, 10% birds (excluding poultry) in their programs. More than 48% of US and 43% of Canadian programs consulted health professionals about zoonotic prevention. Nearly 10% of community-based and 74% of hospital-based programs had printed guidelines. Potential problems involve rabies, *Salmonella* and *Campylobacter* infections, allergy, and ringworm (Walter-Toews, 1993). Other zoonotic infections include *Cryptosporidium* and other protozoan (see Chapter 5) and cestode (see Chapter 7) infections.

While AFT has a good safety record, there are greater risks as programs involve more people. The potential exists for zoonotic infectious or parasitic disease, bite injury, accident, or allergy. Prevention can be addressed by: (1) proper selection of animals; (2) not including people who are allergic to animals; (3) having comprehensive infection-control programs in the setting; (4) having pet policies with advice from public health veterinarians; and (5) developing a surveillance and response program (Schantz, 1990). Future research will improve both the safety and efficacy of the use of animals in therapeutic settings.

Conclusions

Dogs have been part of human households ever since people began living in villages, some 12,000-15,000 years ago. Interactions with dogs may very well be one of our more successful strategies for survival. Today, dogs continue to play a major role in the lives of people around the world. While the medical history of our relationship with animals, including dogs, documents mostly the detrimental effects of animal contact, including zoonoses and injury from bites, there is a long history of healthy interaction. While animal contact carries risks, the frequency of most zoonotic diseases can be lessened, perhaps even eliminated, with animal management practices that would serve both humans and the animals themselves. Veterinary care to manage bacterial, viral and parasitic infections; mechanical restraints, like leashes and cages; selective breeding, responsible legislation, and owner education have made animal ownership a safe, healthy, and rewarding experience for many. Modern and sensitive public health policy would also help many enjoy dogs while protecting the public's health. There is substantial evidence to support the positive benefits of animal companionship for various segments of the population, especially children, the elderly, socially isolated, and the handicapped. More research needs to be directed to establish both the scope of these benefits and ways to channel the information more effectively to improve the public health of the community. In addition, more research is needed on how to better incorporate dogs for those in urban centers so both the animals and people can enjoy improved physical and psychological health.

References

American Pet Products Manufacturers Association (APPMA) (1999) *1997 National Pet Owners Survey*. APPMA, Greenwich, Connecticut, pp. 359.

Anderson, W.P., Reid, C.M. and Jennings, G.L. (1992) Pet ownership and risk factors for cardiovascular disease. *Medical Journal of Australia* 157, 298-301.

Baun, M.M., Bergstrom, N., Langston, N.F. and Thoma, L. (1984) Physiological effects of petting dogs: influences of attachment. In: Anderson, R.K., Hart, B.L. and Hart, L.A. (eds) *The Pet Connection*. University of Minnesota, Minneapolis, pp. 162-170.

Beck, A.M. (1973) *The Ecology of Stray Dogs: a Study of Free-ranging Urban Animals*. York Press, Baltimore, pp. 98.

Beck, A.M. (1974) Ecology of unwanted and uncontrolled pets. In: Proceedings. *National Conference on the Ecology of the Surplus Dog and Cat Problem*. American Veterinary Medical Association, Chicago, pp. 31-39.

Beck, A.M. (1975) The ecology of "feral" and free-roving dogs in Baltimore. In: Fox, M.W. (ed.) *The Wild Canids*. Van Nostrand Reinhold Co., New York, pp. 380-390.

Beck, A.M. (1979) The impact of the canine-waste law. *Environment* 21, 29-31.

Beck, A.M. (1980) Ecological aspects of urban stray dogs. *Compendium on Continuing Education* 2, 721-724, 727.

Beck, A.M. (1981) Guidelines for planning for pets in urban areas. In: Fogle, B. (ed.) *Interrelations between People and Pets*. Charles C Thomas, Springfield, Illinois, pp. 231-240.

Beck, A.M. (1982) Free-ranging dogs. In: Davis, D.E. (ed.) *CRC Handbook of Census Methods for Terrestrial Vertebrates*. CRC Press, Boca Raton, Florida, pp. 232-234.

Beck, A.M. (1985) The therapeutic use of animals. *Veterinary Clinics of North America, Small Animal Practice* 15, 365-375.

Beck, A.M. (1991) The epidemiology and prevention of animal bites. *Seminars in Veterinary Medicine and Surgery (Small Animal)* 6, 185-191.

Beck, A.M. (1996) Ecological aspects of urban stray dogs-update. In: Voith, V.L. and Borchelt, P.L. (eds) *Readings in Companion Animal Behavior*. Veterinary Learning Systems, Trenton, New Jersey, pp. 259-263.

Beck, A.M. and Jones, B. (1985) Unreported dog bite in children. *Public Health Reports* 100, 315-321.

Beck, A.M. and Katcher, A.H. (1984) A new look at pet-facilitated therapy. *Journal of the American Veterinary Medical Association* 184, 414-421.

Beck, A.M. and Katcher, A.H. (1996) *Between Pets and People: the Importance of Animal Companionship*. Purdue University Press, West Lafayette, Indiana, pp. 316.

Beck, A.M. and Meyers, N.M. (1996) Health enhancement and companion animal ownership. *Annual Review of Public Health* 17, 247-257.

Beck, A.M., Loring, H. and Lockwood, R. (1975) The ecology of dog bite injury in St. Louis, Mo. *Public Health Reports* 90, 262-269.

Beck, A.M., Felser, S.R. and Glickman, L.T. (1987) An epizootic of rabies in Maryland, 1982-1984. *American Journal of Public Health* 77, 42-44.

Berman, M. and Dunbar, I. (1983) The social behaviour of free-ranging surburban dogs. *Applied Animal Ethology* 10, 5-17.

Bögel, K. (ed.) (1990) *Guidelines for Dog Population Management*. WHO and WSPA, Geneva, Switzerland, pp. 116.

Borchelt, P.L., Lockwood, R., Beck, A.M. and Voith, V.L. (1983) Attacks by packs of dogs involving predation on human beings. *Public Health Reports* 98, 57-66.

Campbell, B. (1966) *Human Evolution*, 2nd edn. Aldine Publishing, Chicago, pp. 469.

Campbell, B. (1972) *Sexual Selection and the Descent of Man 1871-1971*. Aldine Publishing, Chicago, pp. 378.

Clutton-Brock, J. (1995) Origins of the dog: domestication and early history. In: Serpell, J. (ed.) *The Domestic Dog*. Cambridge University Press, Cambridge, pp. 7-20.

Coppinger, R. and Coppinger, L. (1996) Biologic bases of behavior of domestic dog breeds. In: Voith, V.L. and Borchelt, P.L. (eds) *Readings in Companion Animal Behavior*. Veterinary Learning Systems, Trenton, New Jersey, pp. 9-18.

Coppinger, R. and Coppinger, L. (1998) Differences in the behavior of dog breeds. In: Grandin, T. (ed.) *Genetics and the Behavior of Domestic Animals*. Academic Press, San Diego, pp. 167-202.

Coppinger, R. and Schneider, R. (1995) Evolution of working dogs. In: Serpell, J. (ed.) *The Domestic Dog*. Cambridge University Press, Cambridge, pp. 21-47.

Crispell, D. (1994) Pet projections. *American Demographics* Sept, 59.

Daniels, T.J. (1983a) The social organization of free-ranging urban dogs, I. Non-estrous social behavior. *Applied Animal Ethology* 10, 341-363.

Daniels, T.J. (1983b) The social organization of free-ranging urban dogs, II. Estrous groups and the mating system. *Applied Animal Ethology* 10, 365-373.

Daniels, T.J. and Bekoff, M. (1989) Populations and social biology of free-ranging dogs, *Canis familiaris. Journal of Mammalogy* 70, 754-762.

Darwin, C. (1859) *The Origin of Species*. New York, Mentor Books, [1958] pp. 479.

De Beer, G.R. (1958) *Embryos and Ancestors Revised*, 3rd edn. Oxford University Press, Oxford, pp. 197.

Dembicki, D. and Anderson, J. (1996) Pet ownership may be a factor in improving health for the elderly. *Journal of Nutrition for the Elderly* 15, 15-31.

Erikson, R. (1985) Companion animals and the elderly. *Geriatric Nursing* March/April, 92-96.

Fox, M.W., Beck, A.M. and Blackman, E. (1975) Behavior and ecology of a small group of urban dogs (*Canis familiaris*). *Applied Animal Ethology* 1, 119-137.

Friedmann, E. and Thomas, S.A. (1995) Pet ownership, social support, and one-year survival after acute myocardial infarction in the Cardiac Arrhythmia Suppression Trial (CAST). *The American Journal of Cardiology* 76, 1213-1217.

Friedmann, E., Katcher, A.H., Lynch, J.J. and Thomas, S.S. (1980) Animal companions and one-year survival of patients after discharge from a coronary care unit. *Public Health Reports* 95, 307-312.

Friedmann, E., Katcher, A.H., Thomas, S.A., Lynch, J.J. and Messent, P.R. (1983) Social interaction and blood pressure: influence of animal companions. *Journal Nervous and Mental Diseases* 171, 461-65.

Glickman, L.T. and Shofer, F.S. (1987) Zoonotic visceral and ocular larva migrans. *Veterinary Clinics of North America, Small Animal Practice* 1, 39-52.

Hanna, T.L. and Selby, L.A. (1981) Characteristics of the human and pet populations in animal bite incidents recorded at two Air Force bases. *Public Health Reports* 96, 580-584.

Hansen, J. (1983) The wild dogs-Italy. *New Scientist* 3(March), 590-591.

Harris, D., Imperato, P.J. and Oken, B. (1974) Dog bites - an unrecognized epidemic. *Bulletin of the New York Academy of Medicine* 50, 980-1000.

House, J.S., Landis, K.R. and Umberson, D. (1988) Social relationships and health. *Science* 241, 540-545.

Katcher, A.H. and Beck, A.M. (1986) Dialogue with animals. *Transactions and Studies of the College of Physicians Philadelphia* 8, 105-112.

Katcher, A.H., Friedmann, E., Beck, A.M. and Lynch, J.J. (1983) Looking, talking and blood pressure: The physiological consequences of interaction with the living environment. In: Katcher, A.H. and Beck, A.M. (eds.) *New Perspectives on Our Lives with Companion Animals*. University of Pennsylvania Press, Philadelphia, pp. 351-359.

Lauer, E.A., White, W.C. and Lauer, B.A. (1982) Dog bites: a neglected problem in accident prevention. *American Journal of Diseases Children* 136, 202-204.

Levinson, B.M. (1969) *Pet-Oriented Child Psychotherapy*. Charles C. Thomas, Springfield, Illinois.

Lynch, J.J. (1977) *The Broken Heart: the Medical Consequences of Loneliness*. Basic Books, New York, pp. 271.

McHarg, M., Baldock, C., Headey, B. and Robinson, A. (1995) *National People and Pets Survey*. Urban Animal Management Coalition, Australia, pp. 27.

McNicholas, J. and Collis, G.M. (2000) Dogs as catalysts for social interactions: Robustness of the effect. *British Journal of Psychology* 91(Part 1), 61-70 [Feb].

Messent, P.R. (1983) Social facilitation of contact with other people by pet dogs. In: Katcher, A.H. and Beck, A.M. (eds) *New Perspectives on Our Lives with Companion Animals*. University of Pennsylvania Press, Philadelphia, pp. 37-46.

Montagu, M.F.A (1962) Time, morphology and neoteny in the evolution of man. In: Montagu, M.F.A. (ed.) *Culture and the Evolution of Man*. Oxford University Press, New York, pp. 324-342.

Morey, D.F. (1994) The early evolution of the domestic dog. *Scientific American* 82, 336-347.

Nesbitt, W.H. (1975) Ecology of a feral dog pack on a wildlife refuge. In: Fox, M.W. (ed.) *The Wild Canids*. Van Nostrand Reinhold Co., New York, pp. 381-396.

Norris, P.A., Shinew, K.J., Chick, G. and Beck, A.M. (1999) Retirement, Life Satisfaction and Leisure Services: The Pet Connection. *Journal of Park and Recreation Administration* 17, 65-83.

Patronek, G.J. and Glickman, L.T. (1994) Development of a model for estimating the size and dynamics of the pet dog population. *Anthrozoös* 7, 25-41.

Patronek, G.J., Glickman, L.T., Beck, A.M., McCabe, G. and Ecker, C. (1996) Risk factors for relinquishment of dogs to an animal shelter. *Journal American of the Veterinary Medical Association* 209, 572-581.

Perry, M.C. and Giles, R.H., Jr. (1970) Studies of deer-related dog activities in Virginia. *Proceedings 24th Annual Conference of the Southeastern Association of Game and Fish Commissioners,* pp. 64-73.

Pinckney, L.E. and Kennedy, L.A. (1982) Traumatic deaths from dog attacks in the United States. *Pediatrics* 39, 193-196.

Price, E.O. (1984) Behavioral aspects of animal domestication. *Quarterly Review of Biology* 59, 1-32.

Price, E.O. (1998) Behavioral genetics and the process of animal domestication. In: Grandin, T. (ed.) *Genetics and the Behavior of Domestic Animals.* Academic Press, San Diego, pp. 31-65.

Reader's Digest Association, Inc. (1991) *Reader's Digest Eurodata - a Consumer Survey of 17 European Countries.* London, pp. 267-269.

Rowan, A.N. (1992) Shelters and pet overpopulation, a statistical black hole. *Anthrozoös* 5, 140-143.

Rubin, H.D. and Beck, A.M. (1982) Ecological behavior of free-ranging urban dogs. *Applied Animal Ethology* 8, 161-168.

Sacks, J.J., Sattin, R.W. and Bonzo, S.E. (1989) Dog bite-related fatalities from 1979 through 1988. *Journal of the American Medical Association* 262, 1489-1492.

Schantz, P.M. (1990) Preventing potential health hazards incidental to the use of pets in therapy. *Anthrozoös* 4, 14-23.

Schone, B.S. and Weinick, R.M. (1998) Health-related behaviors and the benefits of marriage for elderly persons. *The Gerontologist* 38, 618-627.

Scott, M.D. and Causey, K. (1973) Ecology of feral dogs in Alabama. *Journal of Wildlife Management* 37, 252-265.

Serpell, J. (1991) Beneficial effects of pet ownership on some aspects of human health and behavior. *Journal of the Royal Society of Medicine* 84, 717-20.

Siegel, J.M. (1990) Stressful life events and use of physician services among the elderly: the moderating role of pet ownership. *Journal of Personality and Social Psychology* 58, 1081-1086.

Siegel, J.M. (1993) Companion animals: in sickness and in health. *Journal of Social Issues* 49, 157-167.

Talan, D.A., Citron, D.M., Abrahamian, F.M., Moran, G.J. and Goldstein, E.J.C. (1999) Bacteriologic analysis of infected dog and cat bites. *New England Journal of Medicine* 340, 85-92.

Torrence, M.E., Beck, A.M., Glickman, L.T., Pérez, C.M. and Samuels, M.L. (1995) Raccoon rabies in the mid-Atlantic (epidemic) and southeastern states (endemic) 1970-1986, an evaluation of reporting methods. *Preventive Veterinary Medicine* 22, 197-211.

Walter-Toews, D. (1993) Zoonotic disease concerns in animal assisted therapy and animal visitation programs. *Canadian Veterinary Journal* 34, 549-551.

Weiss, H.B., Friedman, D.I. and Cohen, J.H. (1998) Incidence of dog bite injuries treated in emergency departments. *Journal of the American Medical Association* 279, 51-53.

Wilson, C.C. (1991) The pet as an anxiolytic intervention. *Journal Nervous and Mental Disease* 179, 482-489.

Chapter Two

Dog Ecology and Population Biology

Hans C. Matter and Thomas J. Daniels

This chapter reviews studies of dog ecology with special reference to developing countries. After a few general considerations regarding the past and present role of dogs in human society and some ecological issues, methodological aspects of the analysis of dog population data is discussed. This section is followed by a review of dogs in the Americas, Asia (including data on dingoes in Australia), and Africa. Particular emphasis is given to aspects of social organization, spatial and temporal resource use, as well as predation and food resources. Finally, a few recommendations are made regarding future work and the need for continued attention to ecological issues as a means of addressing public health problems associated with the presence of dogs in society.

Dogs: partners and pests

Initial contacts between humans and semi-docile wolves (*Canis lupus*), based on mutual benefit and tolerance, marked the origin of a co-evolutionary process that created the archetypal domestic animal, *Canis familiaris*, some 10,000-14,000 years BP (before present). Populations of dogs that were closely associated with humans probably became well established in the early village-farming communities of the Near East (Lawrence, 1967). Both the combination of a hunting symbiosis and a more sedentary lifestyle resulting from the development of agriculture may have been important factors promoting the domestication process (Eaton, 1969). However, the reasons for the close human-dog relationship are not always obvious and may, in some instances, be totally obscure (Meggitt, 1965). Dogs subsequently spread to virtually all areas colonized by humans and today domestic dogs outnumber all other domesticated or wildlife carnivore species on earth (Lawrence, 1967; Clutton-Brock, 1977; Davis, 1978; Wandeler *et al.*, 1993). Estimates of worldwide dog abundance have been placed at a number as high as 500 million or more, with factors such as geography, climate, availability of vital resources (food and shelter), and human attitudes toward dogs dictating local abundance (Wandeler *et al.*, 1993). Of these, the single most important influence on dog numbers is the attitude of humans. A review of the literature on dogs and their role in African cultures by Frank (Frank, 1965), and a similar review in native South America by Latocha (cited in Wandeler *et al.*, 1993), demonstrate how attitudes toward dogs and the reasons for keeping them vary according to the culture, status, social interests, religious conviction, and economic activities of the people. In some cultures dogs are associated with the supernatural, either as divine beings, evil spirits, or demonic assistants (Serpell, 1998). In western societies people have the right to own dogs, but also the obligation to care for them. Dog owners are held responsible for the actions of their dogs and can be taken to court, e.g. if their dog has bitten somebody. In other cultures the obligations placed on dog owners are often considerably less restrictive (De Balogh *et al.*, 1993; WHO, 1984).

Since the first contacts between humans and cohabiting canids, this evolving relationship has become more and more diverse and complex. The variety of roles that dogs may play in human societies is truly impressive. Dogs may be kept or tolerated as social companions and pets, as something to care for, as a protector to make one feel safe, or as a social partner. The human-dog relationship is often similar to the one of parent and child in that it is asymmetrical and dependency-based (Topal and Csanyi, 1998). In addition, dogs are kept for commercial interest, for hunting, herding (livestock), or guarding, as sled animals, as bed-warmers or as a source of food. Dogs fulfill specific tasks in the domain of service and assistance (search-and-rescue, assistance for physically disabled people, bomb and drug detection, etc.) and they play an increasingly important role in animal-assisted therapy programs (Waltner-Toews, 1993). Pet ownership has been associated with survival after heart attack, dramatic reductions in the need for psychotropic medication, reduced risk for cardiovascular disease, and increased well-being for people with different syndromes and diseases (Allen, 1998). Finally, dogs may be used as laboratory animals, as models for studying diseases and testing vaccines, and as sentinels for infectious diseases and carcinogens (Hommel *et al.*, 1995; Bukowski and Wartenberg, 1997). In a study on the historical development of human relationships with companion animals, Collins identified nine detailed patterns of change by analyzing elegies and other comments on the death of companion animals published in English between 1500 and 1900 (Collins, 1998). He noted a general shift of emphasis away from an animal's utility and towards the pleasure and amusement of its company. Furthermore, he found an increasing tendency for the concept of love to appear as a central component of the relationship.

Despite the benefits, the relationship between human and pet populations also represents a source of concern at several levels. Dogs are rejected because of their lack of cleanliness (in both a religious and a hygienic sense), because they bite, because they are a nuisance, or because they are disease vectors. Breakdown in the pet-owner relationship produces millions of unwanted dogs annually (Kass and Hart, 1998). Economic impoverishment, war or civil conflict, high population growth, and migration and urban decay often result in the presence of high numbers of poorly supervised dogs. For example, respondents to a household survey conducted in Soweto, South Africa, noted that local dog problems included strays in the road and in their yards, fighting among dogs, killing chickens, making noise, biting children, fecal contamination of public places, bitches in heat, tearing open rubbish, and uncontrolled breeding (McCrindle *et al.*, 1998).

Public health problems caused by dogs impact us both directly (zoonoses, contact injuries) and indirectly (environmental pollution) (Carding, 1969; Feldmann and Carding, 1973; Baxter and Leck, 1984; Baxter, 1984a, b). Dogs harbor a great variety of macroparasites, microorganisms, and viruses (Coman, 1972; see also Chapters 3-9). They are associated with more than 60 zoonotic diseases, the most important being rabies, echinococcosis and toxocariasis (Robinson *et al.*, 1989; Meslin, 1995; Scrimgeour *et al.*, 1996; Ibrahim and Gusbi, 1997; Macpherson and Wachira, 1997; Ouhelli *et al.*, 1997; WHO, 1998). Dogs are the primary animal implicated in bite injuries, which are a source of significant morbidity because of scarring and wound infection caused by various agents (Goldstein, 1992; Matter, 1998a; Talan *et al.*, 1999). Other important effects of dog bites, aside from the accompanying pain, are anxiety, disfigurement, and the costs of medical care (Sacks *et al.*, 1989; Wright, 1991). Dogs are the principal reservoir of rabies and the main vector transmitting the disease to humans, other domestic animals, and wildlife (Laurenson *et al.*, 1997). As such, they are responsible for more than 90% of human rabies deaths worldwide (Meslin *et al.*, 1994).

The volume of dog urine and feces deposited on public or private property represents a significant health issue in many cities. In the USA alone, it is estimated that the daily production of dog feces amounts to several thousand tons while that of urine reaches several dozen million liters (Anvik *et al.*, 1974). As a consequence, public sites such as beaches, parks, and particularly playgrounds that are heavily fouled by dogs (and cats) may be an important source of infection (OLorcain, 1994; Abou-Eisha and Abdel-Aal, 1995; Hejny-Brandl, 1995; Schöttler, 1998). Horn *et al.* investigated sand pits in children's playgrounds in Hanover, Germany, for the presence of parasites and found that a large proportion, more than 60%, of these playgrounds were contaminated with parasite eggs, mainly from *Toxocara* spp. and other common helminth parasites (Horn *et al.*, 1990). In other European cities the proportion of *Toxocara* spp.-infected playgrounds was variable (Horn *et al.*, 1990; Grimason *et al.*, 1993). Even aerial pollutants from dogs (bacteria, fungi) may represent a health risk for dog owners (Hartung, 1997). The growing awareness of problems caused by free-ranging domestic dogs, i.e. those dogs with unrestrained access to public property, is reflected in the increasing number of articles on this topic in popular magazines and scientific journals (Berman and Dunbar, 1983).

Ecology

The introduction of dogs into new geographical areas frequently had ecological consequences. Dogs probably played a significant role in the extinction of native wildlife when they were introduced onto islands that were previously free of vertebrate predators (Kruuk and Snell, 1981; Barnett and Rudd, 1983). In mainland sites dog populations may have a deleterious effect on the local fauna (Whitehouse, 1977; Triggs *et al.*, 1984; Esteve, 1985). As competitors, predators, and transmitters of diseases, dogs have severely impacted populations of wolves (Boitani, 1983; Francisci *et al.*, 1985), Cape hunting dogs (*Lycaon pictus*) (Kat *et al.*, 1995; Burrows *et al.*, 1995; Laurenson *et al.*, 1997), lions (*Panthera leo*) (Harder *et al.*, 1995), white-tailed deer (*Odocoileus virginianus*) (Sweeney *et al.*, 1971), red kangaroos (*Megaleia rufa*), and emus (*Dromaius novaehollandiae*) (Caughley *et al.*, 1980). In addition, dogs may harm livestock and thus may represent a significant source of economic loss (Coman, 1972; Esteve, 1985; Coman and Robinson, 1989).

Despite biological arguments to the contrary (Wayne, 1993), *C. familiaris* is most frequently considered a species distinct from the wolf (*C. lupus*), its ancestor and the archetypal wild canid. Such a designation belies the fact that members of the genus regularly interbreed in areas where the various species are sympatric. Furthermore, hybrid offspring frequently result from such matings and this has led to some concern that a number of "pure" wild species are the victims of biological pollution, i.e. the species gene pool is being swamped with genes of other species, in this case *C. familiaris*, due to hybridization. Dingoes are currently hybridizing freely with domestic (non-dingo) dogs, raising concerns that dingoes will become extinct (Derr, 1997). Corbett, in noting that barriers between domestic dogs (feral and urban free-ranging) and dingoes are being rapidly removed, concluded that extinction of pure dingoes seems inevitable (Corbett, 1995a). In fact, in Malaysia, Indonesia, Laos, the Philippines, and India, the approximate proportion of pure dingoes remaining is less than 50% (range: 1-42%); only Australia and Thailand have dingo populations in which pure dingoes comprise more than 80% of the population (Corbett, 1995a). In Italy, hybridization with domestic dogs may be so extensive that the character of grey wolves (*C. lupus*), which enter small towns to feed because their natural prey has been depleted, may be altered (Wayne, 1993). Even the highly endangered Simien jackal (*Canis simensis*) is threatened with hybridization by feral domestic dogs (Wayne, 1993). This topic has been discussed further by a number of authors (Boitani, 1983; Ginsberg and Macdonald 1990; Macdonald and Carr, 1995).

Although dogs are the most widespread and abundant of all carnivores, our knowledge of the role of the dog in human cultures and its impact on the environment is still limited (Wandeler *et al.*, 1993). Early studies of pet populations and dog ecology were conducted with the goal of characterizing population abundance and spatial distribution. These and later studies provided data on the potential health hazards of various zoonoses, the problem of dog bites and animal aggression, and the need for population regulation. Furthermore, they raised awareness of the benefits and disadvantages of the human-animal bond, as well as concern for the welfare of dogs and cats (Nasser *et al.*, 1984 cited in Hill, 1985). Knowledge of the structure and dynamics of a population are important prerequisites for the development of effective control measures. For instance, to understand the epizootiology of canine rabies and other dog zoonoses, their ecology and population biology must be considered. Likewise, cost-benefit analyses of control strategies (such as mass vaccination) cannot be made without reliable information on the abundance of dogs and their accessibility. In the 1980s, it was recognized that in many countries few, if any, data on dog populations and ecology were available and that what did exist was insufficient to evaluate national disease control programs (Bakkali, 1985; Ben Osman and Haddad, 1988). In 1986, WHO recommended that comprehensive studies of dog populations and their ecology be conducted to provide background information for effective planning and implementation of canine rabies control programs, as well as to evaluate control measures already applied (WHO, 1984). Since then, several groups of researchers have conducted field studies to better understand the structure and dynamics of dog populations in countries with endemic dog rabies.

Terminology

In discussing aspects of the population biology of domestic dogs, including their population size, reproduction, and survival, it must be borne in mind that several distinct types of populations may be included. The first, and most common, is the free-ranging dog population encompassing both owned and ownerless dogs. These dogs are not under immediate human supervision and have unrestricted access to public property (Beck, 1973). Thus, the population will include owned animals that are cared for as well as abandoned dogs or "strays" that may receive some shelter or food from humans but which are not owned. At the extreme end of this population gradient are the feral dogs, defined as those that have become de-socialized from humans, or never became socialized, and consequently behave as untamed or wild, non-domestic animals (Daniels and Bekoff, 1989c). For reasons that will be obvious below, feral dogs will be considered separately from owned and ownerless free-ranging dogs. A third type of population is represented by the dingo. Although most feral dogs that have been studied to date represent populations that have been feral for, at most, a few generations, dingoes are an exception in that they have been feral for several thousand years, and will be addressed accordingly.

Classifying dogs into one of three types of populations, however, does not obviate confusion. Even a cursory perusal of the published literature will illustrate the variety of terms used to describe domestic dog populations. For instance, ownerless dogs may be referred to as stray, feral, abandoned, or pariah dogs, depending on the circumstances leading to their current state and/or the convention used to name dogs in a particular locale. Owned or ownerless dogs can be free-ranging or free-roaming, synonyms referring to the lack of human control over their movements. They may be family dogs (typically owned) or neighborhood dogs (usually ownerless though resources are often provided by human residents of the area). While these terms may seem like semantic distinctions only, there are real ecological differences associated with the different classes. The distinction between dogs which have a reference household (owned dogs, family dogs, and some neighborhood dogs) and those without one (ownerless dogs, feral dogs) is useful from methodological and managerial points of view. Clearly, the definitions used need to be both specific and practical, for notions of dog ownership and the responsibilities of the human populace in whose presence these dogs reside are quite variable from one area to another. Further discussion of these terms is provided below as the breadth of dog social organization is described.

Methodology

Population analysis, in general, is concerned with the numerical attributes of a population such as the number of animals, the sex ratio, turnover rates (a function of nationality, emigration, immigration, and mortality), and the characteristics of the animals and the environment that determine those values (Caughley, 1977). Once specific surveys are conducted to obtain accurate population data, appropriate statistical analyses should provide estimates of the unknown population parameters. Ease of estimation, the extent to which the parameters collectively describe the significant properties of a population, the ability to extrapolate beyond the data from which the parameters were calculated will all contribute to the completeness of the picture that is drawn.

Although dogs are ideal subjects for population biology studies, largely because they can be seen and counted, they have received little attention. This is unfortunate because knowledge of the abundance of owned and ownerless dogs is a prerequisite for the planning of animal control and vaccination campaigns as well as for epidemiological and ecological studies of this species in general. Thus, the first task must be to estimate the size of the local dog population.

Abundance can be measured in three ways: (1) as the number of animals in a population; (2) as the number of animals per unit area (absolute density); and (3) as the density of the dog population relative to that of the human population (relative density). In some cases it is not particularly useful to have an estimate of dog population size, especially when no distinct boundaries exist or when the boundaries are unknown. A more useful measure is the absolute density of the dog population, which allows comparisons between different areas and habitats. The number of human inhabitants per dog is also a useful measure because of the strong relationship between the human and canine populations, especially given the reliance health workers must place in the help of area residents to implement control/vaccination programs. However, it often is not easy, or even possible, to get reliable data on the human population. In such cases the dog population size assessment must be combined with a survey of the human population as well, whether it involves questionnaires, aerial mapping, or door-to-door surveys (Beran and Frith, 1988a).

In many situations, information on more than just the size of the population is needed. For instance, after a dog vaccination campaign is completed it will be important to know how many dogs remain unvaccinated, whether specific groups of dogs were excluded from vaccination, how often vaccination campaigns should be repeated to assure a minimum coverage within the population, etc. Unfortunately, no standardized field techniques are available that have been shown to reliably measure various dog population parameters in different habitats. Methods previously developed for the analysis of wildlife species in natural habitats can and should be adapted for future work. They should not only take into consideration the peculiarities of the target dog population but also the environment and the specific study conditions. In order to promote the development and evaluation of such techniques WHO published guidelines for the study of dog populations and a list of available techniques (WHO, 1984; WHO and WSPA, 1990). Since then, several pilot studies based on these guidelines have been conducted in different parts of the world.

From experience gained in a dog ecology study in Guayaquil, Ecuador, Beran and Frith derived guidelines for establishing the size and characteristics of a dog population and using the resulting data and interpretations to conduct and evaluate rabies elimination programs (Beran and Frith, 1988a). They defined a multi-step process which included preliminary qualitative research, planning and implementing the survey, analysis of ecological data, and applying the ecological data to a vaccination campaign. On the basis of other pilot studies initiated by WHO, Matter *et al.* proposed a possible standard protocol for the analysis of dog populations which has been shown to produce valuable data during a number of small-scale field studies in developing countries (Matter, 1998b; Matter *et al.*, 2000). Their protocol includes five principal steps: (1) marking a variable proportion of owned dogs during a vaccination campaign or a household survey; (2) collecting specific information on population parameters such as survival, fecundity, sex ratio, mortality, age structure, etc., of owned dogs by the use of a questionnaire survey. This survey also provides data on the human population, on dog-keeping practices, on the role of dogs in local human society, etc.; (3) estimating the abundance of owned dogs by a capture-mark-recapture approach at the household level; (4) estimating abundance of ownerless dogs by a capture-mark-recapture approach in the field; and (5) collecting additional information on dogs without a reference household by direct observation in the field (reproduction, survival, habitat use, food sources, restriction, social behavior and organization, etc.).

Of prime importance, as noted above, is whether or not dogs in the population are owned. The effect of ownership will be reflected in the animal's age, health, and its ability to access resources. Although it may be difficult, or even impossible, to assign every individual dog to a specific class in the field, on a population level the ratio of owned to ownerless dogs can be calculated if the number of owned dogs is established and the total population is reasonably well-estimated by comprehensive investigation. In these situations marking of dogs has been proven useful. In general, it is possible to mark a high proportion of owned dogs by dyes (using paint sticks for example) or collars during a vaccination campaign or a survey of households. Collaring an owned dog is not problematic since they can be handled by their owners. However, if ownerless and free-ranging dogs are to be marked, time-consuming efforts to capture animals must be implemented. The marking system used should be inexpensive and marks must be able to persist until the end of the study period and be visible from variable distances. Collars made of nylon (long lasting) or polypropylene (short duration) are available in different colors and have been successfully used in small-scale field studies in different countries (Matter *et al.*, 1998b; Matter, 1989; Kappeler, 1991; WHO, 1994; Childs *et al.*, 1998; Matter *et al.*, 2000). Polypropylene collars are inexpensive and can easily be adjusted to the individual dog's size. They are fixed with double-sided adhesive tape and/or with staples. Depending on the environment, these collars may last for several days or a few weeks. In some cases it may be useful to combine two marker systems (collars and paint sticks, for example) in order to estimate marker loss. If this is not possible it should be borne in mind - especially for long-term studies - that the loss of collars is not a linear function of time but that the rate of loss increases with time due to accumulated damage to the collars. In some studies, dog marking by collars was considered an indicator of accessibility of dogs to parenteral vaccination; dogs which cannot be captured and handled for marking are probably also inaccessible for parenteral vaccination (Matter, 1987; Matter *et al.*, 1998b).

A unique marker system is sufficient for most purposes though it is sometimes necessary to establish recapture histories of individual dogs in order to get more in-depth information. In many cases, dogs are so variable in size, shape, and color that they can be distinguished individually without any need of further marking. Beck was the first to take advantage of this by photographing any dog encountered in surveys through the study area (Beck, 1973). This provides the same type of data as any other capture-recapture method, but without the need to handle the dogs for marking (Heussner *et al.*, 1978; Meslin and Matter, 1994). The first photograph of a dog is equivalent to its capture; any photograph of the same dog taken in subsequent surveys is treated as a recapture. Native dogs in some geographic areas are physically more uniform in appearance and distinguishing individuals on photographic pictures is difficult or impossible (Matter, 1989). In these situations more sophisticated systems, such as color-codes, ear tags, microchips, etc., are needed.

Estimating the size of free-ranging populations is a common problem encountered by wildlife biologists. Several methods and techniques have been proposed and/or used for estimating absolute and relative densities of dog populations such as direct visual counts (WHO, 1984; Schmidt *et al.*, 1993; Matter *et al.*, 1995), rate of (physical) capture (WHO, 1984; Schmidt *et al.*, 1993), different indices such as dog feces or reports of dog bites (Anvik *et al.*, 1974; WHO, 1984;), distance sampling (Childs *et al.*, 1998; Buckland *et al.*, 1993), and marking and re-observation (Anvik *et al.*, 1974; Kappeler, 1991). Of the last, a variety of techniques exist. The earliest capture-recapture approaches to the problem of estimating animal abundance were developed by Petersen (Petersen, 1896) and Dahl (Dahl, 1919). Reviews of the different techniques have been published (Seber, 1982; Pollock *et al.*, 1990). A growing set of software has been developed and some programs are available for free via the Internet. WHO recommends the use of capture-recapture techniques for assessing dog population size and accessibility of dogs (WHO, 1984). Bailey's direct and indirect sampling, the Jolly-Seber method, Beck's method for evaluation of photo-recaptures, and other techniques have been used to estimate dog population size in rural and urban environments. For instance, in cities, where trapping is not feasible, photographic mark-recapture was used by Beck in his study of dogs in Baltimore, Maryland, USA (Beck, 1973). In that study, 232 dogs per km^2 was the estimated free-ranging dog population. Daniels used the same method to estimate a population of 154 free-ranging dogs per km^2 in Newark, (Daniels, 1983b), and subsequently found a mean density of 735 dog per km^2 at two sites in Ciudad Juarez, Chihuahua, Mexico (Daniels and Bekoff, 1989a). The method has been used successfully in less urbanized areas as well. Two communities on the Navajo Reservation were found to have an average free-ranging dog population of 330 animals per km^2 (Daniels and Bekoff, 1989a).

Although equal catchability of marked and unmarked dogs is crucial for simple mark-recapture methods such as the one proposed by Peterson-Bailey, this assumption may not be realistic. Consideration of specific characteristics of the population, such as the dogs' activity patterns and ownership status, may dictate the best time of day to conduct surveys and, therefore, maximize the likelihood of seeing recaptures. If differences in catchability are not taken into account the population size and the proportion of ownerless dogs tend to be overestimated. To produce reliable population estimates under these conditions, it has been proposed that the probability of observing confined and free-roaming dogs, i.e. their visibility, be assessed and that these estimates by used to specify the recapture probability in a Bayesian model (Matter *et al.*, 1998a, b; Matter *et al.*, 2000). Although the Bayesian model assumes a closed population, no marker loss, and equal recapture probabilities within particular population segments, as other models do, it is flexible in being able to account for different capture probabilities between these segments and generating confidence intervals. The proposed model has so far been used to assess dog population size in areas of Tunisia, Turkey, and Sri Lanka. Data for this approach are obtained using both household surveys and transects through the study area to survey marked and unmarked dogs.

Household surveys frequently involve the use of questionnaires and appropriate sampling procedures to obtain a huge amount of representative data on the owned segment of the dog population and on aspects of the human-dog relationship. In some instances household surveys have also been used to collect data on dogs which have no reference household and to estimate their abundance (Marx and Furcolow, 1969; Boitani and Fabbri, 1982; Beran and Frith, 1988b; Prosperi *et al.*, 1992).

During questionnaire surveys, households are usually visited by one or more interviewers. Considerable time may be spent on every individual interview to obtain detailed information on the household and its dogs. WHO recommends the use of questionnaires consisting of two parts: one for gathering information on the household, the human-dog relationship and on the changes in the number of dogs owned during a well-defined period preceding the interview, and the other for collecting data on each dog owned by the family (WHO, 1984). Questions in the first part provide information on the size and composition of the family, the total number of owned dogs, the reasons for keeping dogs, dog-keeping practices (e.g. supervision, feeding habits, shelter and care, etc.), the general attitude towards dogs, dog bite injuries, etc. The second part of the questionnaire provides information on the age and sex of the dogs, reproductive and rearing success (e.g. age at first whelping, fertility, litter size, puppy survival, etc.), movement constraints, and diseases of owned dogs. Although questionnaires should be as brief as possible, they should be designed to collect all the data required. Therefore, they should be unambiguous and available in an international language as well as in the local language. The forms should be pre-tested by surveyors in the field and interviewers should be from the community under study. Chief among the many reasons for recruiting community members for the survey are their knowledge of local customs and linguistic subtleties, and their access to residents; the quality of the data ultimately depends on the capability of the survey team (Beran and Frith, 1988a). Depending on the particular study area, household surveys may include a total census (especially in villages), non-random selection of a portion of households, or random selection of households or blocks of households with or without previous stratification. The sample size should be adapted to the objectives of the study, the level of certainty, and the level of variation within the population.

The relative ease with which data may be collected by a questionnaire survey says nothing of the veracity of those data. Information provided by household members are very likely to be biased. Furthermore, dog owners can only provide substantial answers to questions if the requested information is available; the fact that an interviewee provides an answer does not insure that he/she is correct. It has been observed that basic questions about age and vaccination status of the dogs were often answered inaccurately, and a second visit to the same household sometimes produced completely different answers to the same questions (Rautenbach *et al.*, 1991; Vos and Turan, 1998). It is therefore useful to combine questionnaire surveys with other more objective methods of assessing parameters, if available. Direct observations in the field frequently will be necessary to obtain data on reproduction and survival rates, habitat use, behavior, etc. This can be done by focal animal and *ad libitum* sampling in which data are obtained during predefined periods or by chance, as the opportunity arises, respectively. If the study site and time permit, radio-telemetry, which requires placing a transmitter on the dog, can provide important data that would otherwise be unavailable, such as home-range size and temporal use patterns. This technique has been used for the study of free-ranging ownerless dogs in Australia and in Tunisia (McIlroy *et al.*, 1986; Coman and Robinson, 1989; Matter, 1989). Finally, postmortem examinations provide information on age (size, weight, tooth-wear pattern, baculum size), health status, diet (stomach content), and reproduction status (Habermehl, 1975; Tarasov, 1984; WHO, 1984).

Dogs in the Americas, Asia, and Australia

Population structure and dynamics

Free-ranging dog populations tend to be higher in developing countries than in developed countries (Daniels, 1983b; Daniels and Bekoff, 1989a), in urban areas compared to rural (Beck, 1973; Fox *et al.*, 1975; Daniels and Bekoff, 1989a), and in locales with relatively high per capita garbage-producing districts (Beran, 1985). Because of differences in dog ecology that are likely from one site to another (Boitani and Ciucci, 1995), there is clearly a need to evaluate each site independently at the time a study or control program commences.

Sources of dogs depend on the population under consideration. Dingoes, having become feral several thousand years ago, maintain their population through reproduction. As with wolves and other non-domestic canids, dingoes have retained, or reacquired, the pattern of a single breeding cycle per year, with most matings occurring in April and May (Catling *et al.*, 1992). In contrast, other domestic dogs, including most feral dogs, have two cycles per year (Harrop, 1960). Because feral dog populations are generally believed to be incapable of sustaining their numbers without continued recruitment, sources of dogs often can be traced back to nearby towns. As such, the free-ranging dog population serves as a source of potential feral dogs (Daniels and Bekoff, 1989a; Boitani *et al.*, 1995), although reproduction by feral dogs may contribute to the population (Daniels and Bekoff, 1989a, b). In a study of feral dogs in Alabama, USA, it was concluded that reproduction in the wild and recruitment from "tame and free-ranging" dogs were occurring (Scott and Causey, 1973). On Isabela island in the Galapagos archipelago it was noted that domestic dogs living in nearby communities were the source of feral dogs (Barnett and Rudd, 1983). Likewise, changes in local settlements may result in the growth of feral dog populations. Gipson suggested that during construction of the Trans-Alaska Oil Pipeline in the mid-1970s additional food available at dumps near work camps and garbage discarded at construction sites led to a marked increase in dog numbers (Gipson, 1983).

One characteristic of free-ranging dog populations that has been documented at several sites is the high turnover rate. That is, a significant proportion of the population dies and is replaced by new members annually. Consequently, the age structure of the population is skewed for young individuals. 38% of dogs in Mexico City were between the ages of 3 months and 1 year (Rangel *et al.*, 1981). A mortality rate of 50% was found in dogs in Baltimore, Maryland, USA (Beck, 1973). Estimates for dogs breeding without human aid in raising the litter, suggest that pup mortality would be greater than 50% (Anonymous, 1971). In the Philippines, the average life expectancy of dogs was 2.8 years (Beran, 1985), while in Baltimore the average adult age was about 2.5 years (Beck, 1974).

Given that virtually nothing is usually done to restrict free-ranging dogs' breeding (Beran, 1985), mortality, both naturally occurring and human-induced, is primarily responsible for the age structure. Nutritional, parasite, and disease problems, both pre- and post-natally, reduce the chances of any offspring surviving up to weaning age (Fox *et al.*, 1975). Few dogs living in Isabela (Galapagos Islands) island lived longer than 5 years (Barnett and Rudd, 1983). In a study of pariah dogs in West Bengal, India, survival rates of pups in eight litters was just 33%: most mortality occurred during the first forays pups made upon leaving the den (Oppenheimer and Oppenheimer, 1975).

Mortality rates for feral dog populations are more difficult to determine because of the difficulty of conducting long-term field studies. In a study of dogs on the Navajo Reservation, it was found that just 34% of 18 pups survived past 4 months of age (Daniels and Bekoff, 1989a). 33% of pups from two feral litters in rural Alabama survived to the age of independence, at about 4 months of age (Scott and Causey, 1973). Fewer still, approximately 22%, survived to 1 year of age. In a 5-year study of feral dogs on a wildlife refuge in Illinois, USA, only 19% of 16 pups born into two litters survived to the age of 4 months, when they were then integrated into the pack (Nesbitt, 1975). It has been noted in Italy that feral dog populations as in many places were not reproductively self-sustaining, that they suffered from high rates of juvenile mortality, and that they depended indirectly upon humans for food, for dogs that might join the population, and for space (Boitani and Ciucci, 1995). Furthermore, the role that social organization (see below) has in influencing the mortality picture may be considerable. The low survival rate at 4 months of age (7.5%) is a clear indication that most mortality occurs during the period of early independence by the pups, and may be attributed to four factors (Boitani *et al.*, 1995). First, the lack of alloparental care, or helping behavior, by other group members leaves the pups unattended at the den for extended periods. In turn, this increases the risk of predation. Second, as pups leave the den and begin to explore their environment at about 6-8 weeks of age, without adult supervision, the risk of predation further increases. Third, their mother is likely to lose interest in the offspring as she enters a new estrous cycle. Fourth, the irregular breeding cycles occurring twice yearly may result in the birth of litters during periods of inclement weather. Of course, the significance of each of these factors may vary from site-to-site and from year-to-year.

During a long-term study of dingoes, it was found that packs raise an average of 1.1 litters per year, but sources of mortality were not identified (Thomson, 1992a). Pups were first seen outside dens at 20-22 days of age, and between 9 and 24 weeks of age progressively accompanied adults on longer journeys. By 16 weeks of age pups were less dependent on intensive parental care for their survival (Thomson, 1992b). Adult mortality factors in one study area included intra-specific strife; three radio-collared dingoes were killed by packs in an adjoining site (Thomson, 1992a).

Sex ratios in free-ranging dog populations generally have been skewed, ranging from 1.6:1 to 5:1 in favor of males (Beck, 1973; Daniels, 1983b; Boitani and Racana, 1984; WHO, 1988; Daniels and Bekoff, 1989a). Conversely, a female-biased ratio of one male to 1.9 females for pups has been reported, though the adult sex ratio was even (Oppenheimer and Oppenheimer, 1975). The tendency to find significantly more males in most free-ranging dog populations probably reflects their source as pets or "partially" -owned animals. Human residents more frequently choose male dogs as guardians of the owner's property, though taking no steps to prevent dogs from ranging away from the home site. Furthermore, selection of a male relieves the putative owner of the consequences of unwanted matings with neighboring dogs. In Newark, it was found that there was a bias toward euthanasia of female dogs by dog catchers since their capture could effectively cause large groups of dogs that were interested in the female during estrus to disband (Daniels, 1983a). These factors may act in concert to skew the adult sex ratio for males.

Feral dog populations exhibit a range of sex ratios that can either be male or female-biased. An even ratio for dogs in two of the three packs has been reported by Scott and Causey (1973), while the third pack consisted of just two females. Male-biased sex ratios have been reported (Boitani et al., 1995; Macdonald and Carr, 1995). In contrast, the sex ratio of the Navajo Reservation population favored females by about 3.5:1 (Daniels and Bekoff, 1989a). This was likely the result of frequent abandonment of female pups at area dumps from which the feral dog population could draw members (Daniels and Bekoff, 1989a).

For dingoes, sex ratio at birth is approximately even (Corbett, 1995a). However, adult sex ratios have been strongly biased for males, perhaps due to higher natural mortality of female pups associated with their smaller body size (Harden and Robertshaw, 1987). The lack of long-term data on sex ratios at birth makes conclusions about the origins of skewed adult ratios somewhat speculative, whether it is a feral or dingo population being considered.

Dispersal strategies have not been well-documented in free-ranging or feral dog populations, again largely due to the need for long-term studies that span several generations. Data for dingoes indicate that mean dispersal distance beyond known pack territories was 20.1 km (n = 19, range = 1-184 km), with males tending to disperse farther than females (Thomson, 1992b).

Good population data for free-ranging and feral dog populations are not easily obtained and therefore there is a high degree of variability in nearly every population parameter measured, including local environmental conditions and the role that humans play. However, trends are apparent. In general, pup mortality is quite high regardless of the population under investigation. Both free-ranging and feral dogs, exclusive of dingoes, appear to rely on continued immigration of previously owned dogs to counter population losses. And proximity to human settlements, and sources of food and shelter that are found there, strongly influence dog abundance.

Social organization

The distribution of group sizes in a population, that is whether individuals live alone or in groups, the sizes of those groups, as well as the form of leadership and the genetic relatedness of individuals in the groups, describe the social organization for that population. With respect to free-ranging and feral dogs, it is necessary first to define the term "pack". For the purposes of this chapter, a pack is defined as a group of animals that travels, rests, forages, and hunts together (Daniels and Bekoff, 1989a). Although canid packs usually are groups of related individuals (Bekoff *et al.*, 1984; Mech, 1986), the criterion of relatedness was not applied to dog groups discussed here because in many cases, relatedness could not be determined.

Surveys of three study sites in Newark, revealed that approximately 80% of all dogs observed were solitary (Daniels, 1983b). By comparison, 51% of dogs in Baltimore, were solitary, as well (Beck, 1973). In both studies, the distribution of group sizes was significantly different from that expected if dogs were aggregating with others randomly and, in fact, suggested that dogs were specifically avoiding others. Furthermore, those groups that did form were composed of dogs that were familiar with one another (Daniels, 1983a, b), regardless of whether they were owned or ownerless, based on prior social encounters. Groups are usually transitory aggregates of both owned and stray dogs (Rubin and Beck, 1982). When aggressive behavior was exhibited, it was directed against unfamiliar dogs significantly more often than at familiar dogs (Daniels, 1983b).

Familiarity has been shown to be a critical predictor of mating success in urban free-ranging dog groups as well. Estrous groups, defined as those that form around a female in breeding condition, differ from non-estrous groups in seven ways: time of day groups form, mean group size, mean duration, home range size, activities conducted, whether or not a leader is present, and hierarchy structure (Daniels, 1983a). When males were identified as either familiar or unfamiliar to the female in heat, it was discovered that unfamiliar males generally remained on the periphery of the group, that they traveled with the group for shorter periods of time, that they suffered a disproportionate number of attacks compared to familiar males, and that they never successfully mated (Daniels, 1983a). While the consequences of such mate selection may not be clear, the purported shift from monogamy (or limited polygamy) to promiscuity resulting from artificial selection may be somewhat overstated with respect to free-ranging dogs and should not automatically imply indiscriminate mating.

Free-ranging dogs living in two communities on the Navajo Reservation tended to remain solitary (Daniels, 1983a). Mean group sizes in each community were 1.29 dogs and 1.32 dogs, which were not significantly different. Thus, the questions we should ask are why "man's best friend", an animal we equate with sociality and pack-living, is frequently not social when free-ranging, and what dictates its choice to group or not group with specific individuals.

An inverse relationship has been reported between mean group size and dog population density at the Ciudad Juarez, Chihuahua, Mexico sites, suggesting that dog density may influence the observed social system (Daniels and Bekoff, 1989a). Although the effects of population density on social behavior in a number of species are well-documented (Eisenberg *et al.*, 1972; Wilson, 1975), density alone is not the most significant proximate influence on social organization. Rather, the distribution of local shelter and food resources, and how those resources change over time, more precisely dictate social organization in these dog populations (Daniels and Bekoff, 1989a, b). Urban and rural (e.g. those on the Navajo Reservation) dogs, for example, exhibited territorial behavior that was restricted to the home site. Food was provided by owners or caregivers at these sites as well, so home sites represented relatively small, easily defended pockets of abundant resources. In addition, there may not be much of an advantage to being social. Scarce resources beyond those provided by human residents at both urban and rural sites would be exploited more efficiently by individuals than by larger groups (Beck, 1973; Berman and Dunbar, 1983). Further, individual differences in behavior among dogs largely accounted for the presence of those few groups that did form in urban areas (Daniels, 1983a, b). In essence, most grouping was done by a relatively few individuals, and these tended to be dogs that shared a home site with conspecifics. Individuals that lived alone generally remained solitary, even if the opportunity to join a group presented itself. It has been concluded that social organization in some urban and rural sites was based largely on dog-ownership practices (Daniels and Bekoff, 1989a).

Human predatory behavior in the form of animal control practices also may make grouping a disadvantage. More than 50% of all complaints to "dog catchers" during the Newark study concerned groups of two or more dogs, yet these groups comprised less than 25% of the population at any time (Daniels, 1983b). Data clearly indicate that social organization within free-ranging dog populations is dynamic, with individuals leaving and joining groups as resources and social parameters allow. However, it would be inaccurate to conclude that groups were not, in one way at least, stable as well. Although it was concluded that few groups in a study appeared stable (Beck, 1973), subsequent studies revealed that dissociation and coalescence of groups is usually limited to a small number of individuals that have formed social bonds with other group members (Daniels, 1983a, b). For example, it was routinely observed that free-ranging dog groups in Newark form and break apart on a regular basis, typically with the same individuals each day (Daniels, 1983b).

Social organization in feral dog populations usually is characterized by larger mean group sizes, longer periods in which dogs remain together, and more frequent positive social interactions. Thus the term "pack" (see above) can aptly be applied. Using radio-telemetry, data on 94 feral dogs in 14 packs was collected and found that pack sizes ranged from two to six animals (Causey and Cude, 1980). Feral dog packs near Delta Junction, Alaska, USA ranged in size from as many as 11 dogs (when pups were integrated into the pack) to as few as three (when a number of dogs were killed by human residents) (Gipson, 1983). Of feral, urban and rural free-ranging dogs in one study it was found that feral dogs were the most social; of 12 dogs living near the dump outside Navajo, New Mexico, USA, nine (75%) lived in packs year-round and two (17%) were seasonal pack members (Daniels and Bekoff, 1989a). Feral dogs studied in the Galapagos Islands often were in packs of up to eight animals; mean pack size at Caleta Web was 2.6 dogs (Kruuk and Snell, 1981).

While social groups tend to be larger in feral groups, density of dogs per unit area is invariably lower. It has been estimated that the feral dog population in Alabama, USA was one dog per 78 ha (Causey and Cude, 1980). Eight feral dogs were found in three packs in Alabama, representing a density of one dog per 135 ha (Scott and Causey, 1973). Twelve feral dogs, excluding pups, were found in the vicinity of a dump located outside the community of Navajo, New Mexico (Daniels and Bekoff, 1989a). In general, numbers of feral dogs have been low in the few studies conducted to date. Despite their increased sociality, there is no reason to expect that feral dogs' pack sizes will remain static year-round (Mech, 1977). Reproductive activity of pack members contributes seasonally to increases in pack size, just as mortality reduces it. Daily changes may occur as well; feral dogs from larger packs on the Galapagos Islands were commonly seen to break off into smaller groups for a time, only to later rejoin the same or another pack (Barnett and Rudd, 1983).

By virtue of its tenure outside human society, the dingo might be considered the most accomplished feral dog. Dingo society centers around packs that comprise discrete, long-term entities that interact in a normally friendly manner, though members are not always together (Thomson, 1992d; Corbett, 1995a). As in wolves, dingo packs consist of a mated pair and their young of various years, though Thomson noted that mean monthly pack size varied from three to 12 individuals (Thomson, 1992d). However, 25% of all observations were of solitary dingoes.

An important factor contributing to successful reproduction of dingoes is the availability of helpers, i.e. non-reproductive pack members that aid in rearing the young (Corbett and Newsome, 1975). Alloparental care in the form of guarding the den site or provisioning the pups can significantly enhance the likelihood of pup survival (Thomson, 1992a, b). Helping behavior in feral dogs appears to be less obvious. For instance, denning and rearing pups apart from the group was reported in feral dogs in Illinois (Nesbitt, 1975), and on the Navajo Reservation (Daniels, 1988; Daniels and Bekoff, 1989b). Under such circumstances, group splitting during the denning period may be an adaptive strategy for pack-living canids as a way to reduce the burden of alloparental care on the pack (Daniels and Bekoff, 1989b). In the absence of selective pressure for pack splitting, and even without the display of obvious helping behavior by other group members, denning within the group's territory increases protection from intruders and potential predators (Boitani and Ciucci, 1995). It has been observed that the father of pups being reared apart from the group was "guarding" the general area, constituting a form of helping behavior (Nesbitt, 1975).

The social organization of dingoes can vary from region to region, and this flexibility is expected given the variety of habitats, prey species, climate, and levels of human exploitation encountered across Australia (Newsome *et al.*, 1983; Corbett and Newsome, 1987; Thomson, 1992c, d; Corbett, 1995a). For dingoes, pack-splitting is a common event. Solitary dingoes that belonged to socially integrated packs, but whose members met every few days or coalesced during the breeding season have been observed to mate (Corbett, 1995a). However, the highest proportion of solitary dingoes has been observed during the nursing season, suggesting that there may be competing urges among pack members to help rear the young, yet reduce the demands being placed on them to provision the bitch and her pups (Thomson, 1992d). Scent marking and howling, two forms of communication that serve to announce the presence of pack members to others, were most pronounced at these times (Corbett, 1995a).

Notable among the factors that influence pack size is the availability of prey. A total of 25 (9.2%) of 272 chases of kangaroos were successful (Thomson, 1992c). In general, dingoes in groups were more successful than those that were solitary. It is interesting that hunting packs were never observed with more than six dingoes, suggesting that an upper size limit on such packs existed (Thomson, 1992d). With a decline in the abundance of kangaroos at one site, some packs disintegrated and the dingoes became more solitary, then increasing their foraging on smaller species (Thomson, 1992c). Similar observations have been made (Mech, 1986); wolf packs frequently split in summer months when rodent prey is abundant and the need for cooperatively hunting large prey is reduced. Prevailing environmental conditions play a role in determining if packs subsequently re-form or not; if a pack splits in the face of severe food shortages there may also be territory shifts, changes in activity patterns, and increases in emigration.

Reasons for pack-splitting in feral dogs, aside from that occurring seasonally by reproductive females, can be surmised based on the distribution of food resources as well. In virtually all studies of (non-dingo) feral dogs a strong dependence on garbage (and to a lesser extent, small animals) has been documented. As discussed below, cooperative hunting of large prey is not a characteristic behavior of most feral dogs; the consensus is that free-ranging and feral dogs may harass such wildlife but rarely succeed in capturing prey. This shortcoming results in a need to forage for more accessible food items, hence the proximity to human settlements and dumps where dogs can scavenge for edible garbage. Given this resource base, there is little need to forage as a group generally, and greater efficiency may be achieved by individuals leaving the pack periodically to search for food on their own. Re-formation of packs may be dictated by competing interests, such as the need to avoid being attacked by a superior predator like a coyote or wolf. It has been suggested that one factor in the success of a feral dog pack in Alaska was its ability to avoid interactions with wolves, and it is likely this would be enhanced by maintaining pack ties (Gipson, 1983).

Although feral dogs may exhibit greater sociality than non-feral free-ranging dogs, they generally lack the higher social organization characteristic of wolf or dingo packs, with more ambiguous dominant-subordinate relationships and weaker social bonds among all group members (Boitani and Ciucci, 1995). This, in turn, may pose an upper limit to the number of feral dogs that can effectively cooperate as functional unit, as well as influence factors such as mortality and recruitment rates. However, it is important to note that this conclusion may apply primarily to feral dogs living in the wild for just one or two generations. Thus, continued isolation from non-feral populations, as in the case of dingoes, may not only lower the phenotypic variability in appearance among feral dog populations but also the behavioral differences we currently observe between other feral dog populations and dingoes.

Spatial and temporal resource use

How dogs acquire and use resources are critical aspects of their ecology. For instance, the way dogs distribute themselves in space relative to available resources may help clarify environmental variables that are important for successful colonization of an area by dogs (Daniels and Bekoff, 1989b). In this section the published data on space use patterns, i.e. home range sizes and the presence or absence of territoriality, and how dogs use that space both in the short-term (daily) and long-term (seasonally) are reviewed.

The home range is that area, usually around a primary shelter site (the home site), through which an animal travels in search of food and other resources (Burt, 1943). In general, urban dogs have relatively small home ranges that may be amoeboid in shape owing to the presence of buildings and other features of the urban landscape. These home ranges may also be three-dimensional, at least to a limited extent, because dogs have access to basements or upper floors of buildings (Daniels, 1983b). Reported home ranges varied in size from as little as 0.1 ha for an individual in Newark (Daniels, 1983b), to 61 ha for a pack of three dogs in St Louis, Missouri (Beck, 1973; Fox *et al.*, 1975; Berman and Dunbar, 1983; Daniels, 1983b), and tend to be smaller in winter than in summer. For example, Daniels recorded home ranges for individual dogs in Newark, varying in size from 0.2 to 11.1 ha in summer, and from 0.1 to 5.7 ha in winter, suggesting that the reduction in range use during winter reflected less overall activity during periods of cold weather (Daniels, 1983b). Further analysis indicated there was no relationship between home range size and either a dog's sex or body size, although owned dogs had smaller home ranges than ownerless dogs (Daniels, 1983b). The latter relationship most likely reflects the greater availability of resources owned animals have, relieving them of the need to travel extensively in search of food. Conversely, a study of dogs in Queens (New York City), New York, USA found home ranges averaged 4 ha for 13 dogs observed, and body size influenced the distance dogs traveled from home (Rubin and Beck, 1982); smaller dogs ranged significantly less than larger dogs, although reasons for this difference were not given.

Home range data for free-ranging suburban dogs are lacking, though Daniels reported home ranges for 15 dogs living in the rural Navajo Reservation community of Window Rock, Arizona, USA (Daniels, 1987b). Mean home range size for males during non-estrous periods was 0.12 km^2 while for females the mean home range size was 0.14 km^2. On average, home ranges doubled during estrous periods; the mean home range for males increased to 0.21 km^2, and that for females rose to 0.28 km^2. Even though rural dogs generally have larger home ranges than those living in urban areas, Daniels noted that space use patterns were similar to those reported for urban dogs, with activities largely restricted to home sites and grouping characterized by sociality among familiar animals (Daniels, 1987b).

Space use by feral dogs is similar to that for most other wild canids in that they utilize definite and traditional home ranges which, to varying degrees, are defended against intruders (territories) (Scott and Causey, 1973; Causey and Cude, 1980; Gipson, 1983; Daniels and Bekoff, 1989b; Boitani *et al.*, 1995). A home range of 28.5 km^2 was noted for a pack of four dogs on a wildlife refuge in Illinois (Nesbitt,

1975), and a pack of seven dogs in Alaska, USA ranged over an area of approximately 70 km² (Gipson, 1983). Data on three Alabama packs illustrate how variable home ranges can be: areas varied from 444 ha to 1050 ha for each pack (Scott and Causey, 1973). A minimum home range of 18.7 km² for a pack of dogs in Alabama has been reported (Causey and Cude, 1980).

Because home range size is intimately tied to habitat features such as food availability, and frequently to pack size as well, home range sizes can be as variable as the number of groups considered. While this realization precludes predicting home range size from one site to another, some trends have been shown consistently among populations. Chief among these is the reduction in home range immediately prior to and post-parturition, when pack activity is more limited to the area around the den site. A shift in the home range core area in response to the presence of pups has been observed, though area measurements were not provided (Scott and Causey, 1973). On the Navajo Reservation, one pack of feral dogs, mean home range size increased more than tenfold once pups were able to survive without immediate parental care, at about 4 months of age (Daniels and Bekoff, 1989b). A second pack of dogs showed no seasonal shift in home range associated with the birth and independence of pups. The authors speculated that the members of the smaller pack may have had less of a need to search for food beyond the bounds of their fairly small home range.

In urban areas, territoriality, as exhibited by the defense and/or maintenance of an area exclusive of conspecifics, typically is limited to the home site (Daniels, 1983b). Thus opportunities for social interactions are frequent (whether or not they are taken) given the degree of overlap in home ranges that is characteristic of such populations. Territorial behavior involved barking and the display of aggressive postures directed at potential intruders that wandered close to the home site, though such overt aggression was rarely observed. The lack of sociality that marked the Newark population was facilitated by mutual avoidance (Daniels, 1983b). Territorial behavior has been observed by a female whose pups were denning beneath a porch in Baltimore (Beck, 1973). Territorial behavior has also been directed at a pack of three dogs on one occasion when the pack traveled beyond its usual home range borders (Fox *et al.*, 1975). These authors also noted that this was in sharp contrast to dogs living in the pack's home range, which tolerated the animals' presence.

As with urban dogs, territorial behavior exhibited by dogs in the rural community of Window Rock, Arizona, was limited to the home site. Likewise, territory "defense" in the form of barking was displayed rarely to dogs with which they were familiar; neighbors frequently entered each other's territories with impunity (Daniels, 1987b). Territorial behavior often precedes incidents of dog bites and may be especially prevalent in urban areas where dogs' home sites are small and density of conspecifics is relatively high (Beck, 1973; Daniels, 1986). While territoriality technically refers to behavior directed at conspecifics, dogs typically generalize this behavior to humans that approach or invade the territory.

Both feral and abandoned free-ranging dogs on the Navajo Reservation exhibited territorial behavior, mainly by females during periods of pup dependence when dogs' activities were restricted to the immediate vicinity of the den (Daniels and Bekoff, 1989b). Territorial behavior involved threats by pack members directed at non pack members, but no escalation of aggression was observed.

Feral dogs on the Navajo Reservation also exhibited a form of territoriality that appeared to provide them with access to resources in the local dump. Priority of access to food at the dump on the outskirts of Navajo, New Mexico, was influenced by aggressive interactions among dogs at the dump (Daniels and Bekoff, 1989b). Specifically, members of the Canyon or Corral packs would bark as they entered the dump, essentially announcing their arrival to any dogs already present. In nine of the 11 cases in which dogs already were present and foraging, they increased their vigilance and then moved out of sight before the newcomers arrived. In another episode, the newcomers (Canyon pack) chased an early forager out of the dump. These observations contrast with that of dogs observed at dumps which were highly tolerant of each other, and may reflect the relative quantity of resources at each site (Gipson, 1983).

Studies thus far indicate that free-ranging and feral dogs exhibit a daily activity pattern that is crepuscular, with increased activity in early morning and late evening hours, at least in the summer season. At those times, human interference was likely to be minimal and potential prey would be active. Beck observed that most dogs during summer were active between 0500 and 0800 hours, and again from 1900 to 2200 hours, resting during the hottest part of the day (Beck, 1973, 1975). Fox *et al.* observed a similar pattern in St Louis, Missouri, USA (Fox *et al.*, 1975), as did Daniels both in Ciudad Juarez, Chihuahua, Mexico and on the Navajo Reservation, where temperatures in summer could be quite high (Daniels, 1987b). This bimodal pattern usually is less pronounced in cooler weather, when some dogs are always active on the streets (Beck, 1973). Daniels observed that winter activity did not begin until late morning and surmised that dogs remained sheltered until temperatures began to rise and were more comfortable (Daniels, 1983b). In Berkeley, California, dog numbers peaked at 0700 and on 1700 hours which may reflect an increased likelihood of encountering conspecifics outside the home site (Berman and Dunbar, 1983). Even with activity peaks at well-defined times of day, dogs may be active throughout the night (Adams and Johnson, 1993). Galapagos Island dogs were largely nocturnal and therefore difficult to observe (Kruuk and Snell, 1981). Feral dogs on the Navajo Reservation frequently foraged at night time, when chances of encountering local residents were much reduced.

Dingoes use space in much the same way as other feral dog populations. Thomson noted that the center of activity of dingo packs generally shifted from season to season, though somewhat unpredictably, and that most of these shifts probably were related to changes in the availability of food resources (Thomson, 1992d). However, he also noted that rearing pups was the most important seasonal factor affecting movement patterns of dingoes and as such, influenced ranging patterns. Dingo packs tend to be most active at sunrise and sunset, moderately active during the night, and least active during the heat of the day (Harden, 1985).

Studies of dingo populations have found that packs are territorial, with minimal overlap between territories of neighboring packs (Thomson, 1992d). Members use howling and scent-marking to maintain the separation between packs, and lone dingoes are known to deliberately avoid encounters with territory residents. In addition, dingoes use scent posts to indicate currently shared hunting grounds and possibly to synchronize reproduction between pairs (Corbett, 1995a). The size of a dingo pack's territory varies with prey resources and terrain but is not correlated with pack size (Thomson, 1992d; Corbett, 1995a).

Predation and food resources

Free-ranging ownerless dogs most frequently obtain their food by scavenging for edible scraps amid the refuse disposed of by human residents (Oppenheimer and Oppenheimer, 1975; Beran, 1985). As with most commensals, the clear benefit to maintaining an association with humans lies in the availability of food and shelter. Feral dogs, since they are not socialized to humans, face a somewhat harder task. In order to take advantage of the potential resources found within the proximity of human settlements, a rather rigid set of environmental conditions must be met. First, edible garbage must be disposed of where dogs have access. This means in an open dump that typically is located beyond community borders. Second, there must be adequate shelter in the surrounding area that permits dogs to remain close, yet unobtrusive. As such, feral dogs usually are not found in urban areas, although exceptions do occur when habitat requirements are met and dogs can isolate themselves from urban dwellers. Third, interactions with humans must be infrequent or feral dogs face the risk that steps will be taken to reduce their numbers.

Predatory behavior by feral dogs is assumed to be more common than is warranted on the basis of data that have been collected. Although a nationwide survey in 1964 revealed nearly every state reported feral dog populations, convincing evidence of their predatory skill is difficult to obtain (Scott and Causey, 1973). Despite reports that go back at least as far as 1938 (Gentry, 1983), free-ranging and feral dogs rarely kill white-tailed deer successfully. In Colorado and Virginia, USA, deer have been reported to being killed by feral dogs (Denney, 1974; Gavitt *et al.*, 1974). Likewise, 12 deaths occurred among 39 deer that were chased in northern Idaho, USA, although the number of such incidents actually observed by the authors was not reported (Lowry and MacArthur, 1978). A statewide California survey of problems that dogs cause to wildlife showed that predation due to feral dogs was minor. The majority of cases involved unrestrained owned dogs and were the result of both overpopulation of pet dogs and owner irresponsibility (Howard and Marsh, 1984). Likewise, it was concluded that dogs were negligible causes of direct mortality on deer in Missouri (Progulske and Baskett, 1958). Feral dogs in other studies did not appear to prey either on white-tailed deer or cattle (Scott and Causey, 1973). In fact, the foods eaten included small mammals, garbage, and vegetable material. In Alabama, coastal plain habitats feral dogs were observed to be inefficient predators of adult white-tailed deer (Causey and Cude, 1980), and that feral dogs were hardly more than a nuisance to adult deer (Gipson and Sealander, 1977). 65 chases of white-tailed deer by one to nine hounds was recorded without any deer being caught (Sweeney *et al.*, 1971). In a study of feral dogs in Illinois, they were never observed to pursue, capture or kill deer (Nesbitt, 1975). The situation for livestock in the USA is similar. Three reports of dogs chasing cattle in Alaska were reported, but no kills documented (Gipson, 1983). The author was unable to tell if the cattle had been harassed by feral or free-ranging (non-feral) dogs. This is not to say that predation does not occur. Feral dogs apparently do prey on small animals such as rodents, rabbits, and crippled waterfowl that may be locally abundant, although good data on the frequency of such behavior are lacking (Nesbitt, 1975; Daniels, 1987b). One reason for the lessened impact on local wildlife may have to do with the degree of cooperation necessary to capture prey. Feral dog groups, where leadership may be more ambiguous and social bonds among individuals are more flexible, predatory tendencies, if any, may be less effective, mostly uncoordinated, and with severe limitations (e.g. lower kill rate, smaller prey size, higher energetic cost, and longer time to functional response) (Boitani and Ciucci, 1995).

Feral dog populations outside of the USA may have more of an impact on local fauna than those studied thus far in the USA. In Venezuela's llanos feral and semi-feral dogs were reported to prey on capybaras (*Hydrochoerus hidrochaeris*) (Macdonald, 1981). Feral dogs seriously threaten populations of endemic fauna, such as giant tortoises (*Geochelone elephantopus*) and breeding colonies of flightless cormorants (*Nannopterum harrisi*) and blue-footed boobies (*Sula nebouxi*) (Barnett and Rudd, 1983), on the islands of Santa Cruz and Isabela in the Galapagos. Introduction of domestic dogs to the Galapagos followed soon after colonization of the archipelago, and feral dogs have lived continuously on both Floreana and San Cristobal islands since at least 1832 (Barnett and Rudd, 1983). By the time of Stanford Hopkins' expedition to the Galapagos in 1898, large-scale destruction of tortoise eggs by feral dogs was already apparent, and by 1913 increasing numbers of feral dogs were viewed as a "terrible plague" on cattle populations in the highlands (Barnett and Rudd, 1983). Given that cattle are the main staple of the dogs' diet in this study, it appears that the population of feral dogs is regulating numbers of introduced herbivores (Barnett and Rudd, 1983).

Marine iguanas (*Amblyrhynchus cristatus*) in the Galapagos Islands are routinely preyed upon by feral dogs (Kruuk and Snell, 1981; Barnett and Rudd, 1983). Wild dogs were first reported along the coast of Sierra Negra by a group studying marine iguanas in 1934, and recent estimates indicated a population of about 500 dogs. Most of the iguanas killed are large males which tend to be more approachable by the dogs (Kruuk and Snell, 1981). Iguana remains occurred in 58% of 185 feral dog feces found on the islands of Santa Cruz and Isabela; in 51% of the feces, iguanas were either the sole or most important item. In other parts of the islands, marine iguanas comprised 90% or more of items found in dog scats. Estimates are that dogs take approximately 27% of the marine iguana population per year, which is more than the iguana population at this site can sustain over time (Kruuk and Snell, 1981).

The issue of feral dogs' effects on native wildlife populations is fundamentally an issue of human actions that may or may not have been intentional at the start, but whose long-term outcomes generally were unforeseen. The distribution of dogs throughout the Pacific region is the result of descendants of the early domesticated dogs of Southeast Asia, the pariah dogs, accompanying humans from island to island (Titcomb and Pukui, 1969). Dingoes, most closely associated with Australia, were transported to that continent by seafaring Asians about 2000 BC (Schwartz, 1997). By the mid-1700s, when European exploration of the region began in earnest, an occasional dog, but mainly its hybrid relatives, ran wild and destroyed birds, preyed on introduced pigs that had become feral, and attacked corralled livestock (Thomson, 1922). On other islands feral dogs and pigs were scavengers able to take advantage of local resources, for instance, eating corpses on battlefields in New Zealand, the Hawaiian Islands, and in the Society Islands (Ellis, 1853, 4, p. 160; Henry, 1928, p. 313; White, 1887-1991, 4, p. 9 - cited by Luomala, 1960).

Some of the most successful animal introductions into new areas have involved species with the ability to become feral (Munton, 1984). Nowhere has the impact of introduced animals been more obvious than in New Zealand. The country had no native mammals, but early settlers felt it was desirable to introduce them under the assumption that there were empty niches (*sensu* (Elton, 1958)) that should be filled (Munton, 1984). One result has been a marked decline in the number of Kiwi (*Apteryx* sp.) on the New Zealand mainland (McLennan and Potter, 1993), and feral dogs are clearly responsible in some cases (Taborsky, 1988).

One reason for the severity of impacts feral dogs can have on local populations is that historically, native species have not faced the competitive and/or predatory threat that introduced dogs pose. For example, prior to the arrival of Polynesian colonizers in the 4th century AD, Hawaiian biota evolved for at least 40 million years in virtual isolation (Beverley and Wilson, 1985; Stone and Loope, 1987). Consequently, defensive behaviors that might have allowed the native fauna to withstand predation pressure from introduced animals had not evolved. In the case of feral dogs, although they are encountered infrequently today, they may have had a severe impact on small, localized populations of the Hawaiian Goose (*Nesochen sandvicensis*) with which they were sympatric in the past (Stone and Loope, 1987). Still, reductions in local wildlife populations will not necessarily result everywhere feral dogs occur. Bino (1996) noted that feral dogs in New Guinea were primarily scavengers on kills of other predators such as the New Guinea harpy eagle (*Harpyopsis novaeguine*). Dingoes living in the Tanami Desert of Australia occasionally feed on the rare rufous hare-wallaby (*Lagorchestes hirsutus*) but the most severe impacts have been inflicted by feral cats (*Felis catus*) and red foxes (*Vulpes vulpes*) (Lundie-Jenkin *et al.*, 1993).

As the largest extant mammalian carnivore in the Australian region, the dingo is a critically important part of the ecosystem. Insofar as this species has been feral for at least 200 generations, its impact on endemic wildlife is primarily of historic interest. Most notable among these is the disappearance of the Thylacine (*Thylacinus cynocephalus*), or "Tasmanian wolf", a dog-like marsupial predator that was once distributed throughout Australia, but which apparently could not compete with the dingo upon its arrival 3500 years BP (Archer, 1974; Corbett, 1995a). Thylacine populations were severely reduced just 500 years after the dingo's arrival, although remnant Thylacine populations managed to hold on for some time in Tasmania. The species became extinct in the 1930s and an epizootic, possibly of Toxoplasmosis, may have contributed to their demise (Nowak and Paradiso, 1983; Corbett, 1995a). Likewise, the Tasmanian native hen (*Gallinula mortierii*) is today restricted in the wild to Tasmania, possibly the result of predation from dingoes that caused extinction on the mainland (Baird, 1991).

The dingo today may still have a significant impact on prey populations, though extinction of those species is less likely. It has been suggested that dingoes may have a regulatory effect on rodents (Newsome and Corbett, 1975), and that the prime impact of dingo predation on a population of wallabies (*Wallabia bicolor*) was on recruitment (Robertshaw and Harden, 1985). Such effects are reduced by the tendency of dingoes to eat a diverse range of prey, from insects to buffalo. In particular areas they may specialize on the commonest available wildlife prey and change group size and hunting strategy accordingly to maximize hunting success (Corbett, 1995b). If common prey (e.g. of rabbits) becomes scarce, for example, dingoes may increasingly kill large prey (e.g. of red kangaroos) (Corbett, 1995b). Likewise, Corbett concluded that although dingoes have harassed livestock, especially sheep and cattle, most attacks occurred when native prey was scarce (e.g. during droughts or as result of human disturbance) (Corbett, 1995a). Conversely, some dingoes have a strong preference for swamp wallaby, the occurrence of which in the diet was disproportionate to its observed numbers (Robertshaw and Harden, 1985). Furthermore, switching was not observed even when numbers of swamp wallaby were reduced and alternative macropod prey were present.

Dingoes, as with feral dogs elsewhere (Daniels, 1987a), also may exhibit cannibalism under specific circumstances (Thomson, 1992c). Clearly, the environmental factors influencing foraging and prey selection are variable from site to site, and from year to year.

Dogs in Africa

Dog populations are a public health concern in Africa due to the ecological and demographic conditions prevailing in most human settlements and large urban areas. Although people in some urban areas keep dogs as pets (Akakpo, 1985), the practice in Africa is less common than it is in Europe or North America. Pet dogs in Africa are generally well cared for by their owners, comprise only a small proportion of the entire dog population, and likely play a marginal role in the transmission of diseases (Dar and Alkarmi, 1997). Therefore, recent studies of dogs in African countries have focused mainly on the role dogs have in disease transmission and their impact on public health. Closely related parameters such as abundance and the dogs' function in the various African societies have also been studied. Behavioral ecology data (activity patterns, habitat use, feeding habits, social organization) and information on the abundance and distribution of resources (food, water, shelter), as well as their predictability (temporal abundance), and the carrying capacity of the environment, are scarce. Despite an increasing number of dog population studies conducted in both northern and southern Africa over the last two decades, our knowledge of dog populations for much of the continent remains rather limited.

As a consequence of the plurality of culture and religion, dog populations in Africa are probably more heterogeneous than elsewhere in the world. The following review of dog studies conducted in Egypt, Morocco, Nigeria, Senegal, South Africa, Tunisia, Zambia, and Zimbabwe may corroborate this view. Data on dog populations in some countries may be more difficult to obtain than in others, partly because the information is often scattered and some studies are never published. Readers are encouraged to consult the original literature when possible, to learn more about the design and conditions of the different studies.

Population structure and dynamics

Canine abundance varies considerably among countries, as well as geographic regions within countries, and reflects the type of habitat (urban, rural), the social strata of the human population, human settlement patterns, and the epidemiological situation. For instance, the dog:human ratio reported in Africa most commonly lies between 1:12 and 1:3. Such variability dictates that the "global ratio" of 1:6 therefore be used only as an indicator for managerial purposes when no better data are available (Perry, 1993). The ratio of owned dogs to human residents is usually higher in the rural areas of a country, but there is also considerable variation within cities (Wandeler, 1985). By using a simple capture-recapture technique, an average of 6.8 inhabitants per dog in rural areas of Tunisia varying between one dog per 4.5 and 8.9 inhabitants has been estimated (Artois and Ben Osman, 1986). Another author using several methods such as full census, questionnaire surveys, and capture-recapture techniques, reported three to six and nine to 45 inhabitants per dog in rural and in urban areas of Tunisia, respectively (Matter, 1989). In the cities of Tunis and Sfax, for instance, 80-85% of households had no dogs whereas in rural areas of northern and central Tunisia more than 75% of households had dogs. In urban and suburban zones, dog population density varied between 600 and 1200 dogs per km^2. The total canine population in Tunisia was estimated at approximately one million, with a higher human to dog ratio in the northern half of the country than in the south (Chadli *et al.*, 1982).

Reasons for such variation are not always clear. Although dogs are considered impure in the Muslim religion, for example, it does not automatically mean that they are absent from Muslim areas. In North Africa the relationship between humans and dogs is actually close and has a long tradition (Frank, 1965; Aulagnier, 1990; Ibrahim and Gusbi, 1997; Ouhelli *et al.*, 1997). Islam obviously does not discourage people from keeping dogs in these countries (Bernard *et al.,* 1967; Ben Osman, 1985; Artois and Ben Osman, 1986; Artois *et al.,* 1986; Matter, 1989), while it does in other parts of the Islamic world (Beran, 1982). In a study conducted in the area of Rabat (Morocco), 96.3% of people thought the dog was a crucial and/or useful animal, while only a small proportion thought that dogs were harmful, would bite, and/or could transmit diseases. Nevertheless, some people in the latter category still had dogs in their households (Ouhelli *et al.*, 1997). In the Pikine district of Senegal, religion was not a limiting factor to dog ownership, though ethnic influences were observed (Akakpo *et al.*, 1990). In northern Kaduna State (Nigeria) less than one dog per 1000 inhabitants in the Muslim northern region were found, while in southern parts of the same state the dog to human ratio lay between 1:27 and 1:3 (Ezeokoli *et al.*, 1984). The observation that rural households have more dogs than households in urban areas is actually not without exception. 38% (range: 32.4-44.0%) of the households in an urban area of Nigeria kept dogs, compared to just 20% in rural areas (range: 2.3-58.0%). The dog-human ratio was 1:21 (range: 1:17-1:26) and 1:45 (1:33-1:62) in the urban and rural area, respectively, resulting in absolute dog densities of 131 and 15 animals per km^2 (Oboegbulem and Nwakonobi, 1989). In the Machakos District of Kenya, a household survey covering 2.5% of the district's human population revealed 1.4 dogs per household (range: 0.8-2.2), indicating a dog to human ratio of 1:9.6 (range: 1:5.5-1:16.0) and a mean of 10.4 (range: 3.5-83.4) dogs per km^2 (Kitala *et al.*,

1993). In Zimbabwe, an average of 0.9 dogs per household, a dog to human ratio of 1:6.5, and an average of 3.5 dogs per km^2 was reported (Brooks, 1990). In urban areas, the dog to human ratio was estimated to be 1:16 and 68 dogs per km^2 compared with 1:4.5 and six dogs per km^2 in a more rural community. In a survey including four high-density suburbs of Harare (Zimbabwe), an average of 0.2 dogs per household was reported (Hill, 1985). In a low income, densely populated suburb of Lusaka (Mutendere, Zambia), only 11% of the households kept dogs, with a dog-human ratio of 1:45 and 0.12 dogs per household (De Balogh *et al.*, 1993). For comparison, these authors repeated the same household study in a semi-rural area of Palabana, where dogs were kept by 42% of households (dog-human ratio: 1:6.7 and 1.0 dog per household) (De Balogh *et al.*, 1993). In Soweto, a densely populated urban area in Gauteng Province of South Africa, a survey of households revealed a dog:human ratio of 1:12.4 or 0.4 dogs per household. It has been reported that dog:human ratios varied between 1:2.9 and 1:15.6 in Natal and Kwa-Zulu (South Africa), with large variation among the different ethnic groups (Perry, 1993).

Data on the sex and age distribution of dog populations in Africa are almost exclusively based on questionnaire surveys and vaccination records. With few exceptions, a net surplus of male dogs has been reported in most dog populations. Such data collected in Tunisia (Artois and Ben Osman, 1986; Matter, 1989; BenYoussef *et al.*, 1998) and Morocco (Azlaf and Is Sidi Yahia, unpublished; Ben Kaddour *et al.*, 1990), for example, revealed that males comprised 65-78% and 68-80%, respectively, of the owned dog population. Furthermore, in Tunisia male-biased sex ratios were noted through all age classes from juvenile to adult dogs. In Kenya (Machakos District) the male to female ratio was 1:0.7 (Kitala *et al.*, 1993). Likewise, in a suburban area of Lusaka (Zambia) 54% of owned dogs were male compared to 43% of male dogs in a semi-rural area (De Balogh *et al.*, 1993). In Zimbabwe, males outnumbered female dogs, 56-44% (Brooks, 1990).

Reasons for this sex ratio bias, as noted in dog populations elsewhere, appear to be anthropogenic in nature. It has been suggested that a higher mortality rate of females in the first weeks after birth, due to selective killing and/or abandonment of female pups, accounted for the unbalanced sex ratio in favor of male dogs later in life. This hypothesis was supported by the fact that the sex ratio at birth in rural areas was not significantly different from unity (Matter, 1989). In comparison, ownerless free-ranging dogs frequently exhibit a more equitable sex ratio (Bernard *et al.*, 1967; Matter, 1989), probably because active selection against females is less intense and/or females are abandoned more often than males.

While dog owners may report the sex of their animals reliably to survey takers (at least in the case of adult animals), this is far less true for their ages; information on a dog's age provided by a household member is likely to be heavily biased (recall bias, digit preferences, information bias, etc.). For this reason, the proportion of animals under one year of age is often a better indicator of the age structure of a population than indications of the mean age.

Dog populations in Africa are characterized by a high proportion of juvenile and young adult dogs, and an accelerated turnover rate, defined as the proportion of animals leaving a population through mortality or emigration and being replaced by newborn or immigrating individuals. For example, in Tunisia the mean age of owned dogs in different populations varied between 1.9 and 3.8 years (Aulagnier, 1990; BenYoussef *et al.*, 1998; Matter *et al.*, 1998a). In Morocco 12-36% of owned dogs were under 1 year of age (Azlaf and Is Sidi Yahia, unpublished; Ben Kaddour *et al.*, 1990) while in Nigeria, 57% of dogs in urban areas, and 46% of dogs in rural areas, were less than one year old (Oboegbulem and Nwakonobi, 1989); the mean age of dogs in both sites was approximately 2 years. In Kenya (Kitala *et al.*, 1993), Zambia (De Balogh *et al.*, 1993), and Zimbabwe (Brooks, 1990), the proportion of the population under 3 months of age varied from 9-34%. Although this information is important for population management and disease control programs, annual turnover rates in dog populations are difficult to assess because reliable data on reproduction, mortality, immigration and emigration often are not available. Estimates of the turnover rate based on the proportion of dogs under 1 year of age suggest that it is usually high in free-ranging dog populations. In a rural site in northern Tunisia, 30.3% of dogs registered at the beginning of the study died or emigrated within the period of observation; 88% of these animals were replaced by newborn or immigrating dogs. Of dogs living at the end of the observation period, only 72.3% had been part of the population at the beginning. Similar results were obtained in other rural, suburban, and urban areas of Tunisia where 23%, 30%, and 40%, respectively, of the owned dog population was replaced within 6 months (Wandeler *et al.*, 1993). In rural areas of Morocco 18.5% of owned dogs died after 1 year (Ben Kaddour *et al.*, 1990). In the Masai Mara region, a growth rate of 45% per year in a dog population with an annual mortality rate of 40% was found (Coleman, 1997).

The proportion of females to males, the proportion of reproductive-age females, and puppy survival rates all contribute to a dog population's ability to reach its reproductive potential. A significant drawback to using such data is that collection is typically done through the use of questionnaires which, as noted earlier, can be fraught with inaccuracies. Matter (1989) tried to overcome this problem by interviewing dog owners monthly during a 1-year period in a village of 144 households in northern Tunisia. Of female dogs older than 6 months of age, 66% had had at least one litter and 13% had whelped two litters. Since sexual maturity is reached between 6 and 12 months of age (Kaiser, 1971; Jöchle and Andersen, 1977), such populations are characterized by early and frequent breeding. In fact, 1-2 year-old females were the most prolific group in the Tunisia study (Matter, 1989), with each female giving birth to an average of two female pups. In general, fecundity gradually declines with increasing age. Several studies suggest that dogs occupy an intermediate position between birth-pulse and birth-flow fecundity, with no distinct reproduction period as in other *Canidae* but exhibiting an increase in births during the spring and autumn (Engle, 1946; Jöchle and Andersen, 1977; Shille and Stabenfeldt, 1980; Rowlands, 1991).

The relatively high fecundity is balanced by an equally high mortality rate in young dogs. Much of the mortality is induced by humans, either by direct action or indirectly through neglect. Of 352 puppies born during the Tunisia study (Matter, 1989), 61.2% were killed by a household member, 13.9% died of other causes, 7.9% were given away, 5.7% were lost, and only 11.3% remained in the household of origin. Of 4300 pups born in households in Morocco during 1 year, 10% were still in the household, 21% were given to neighbors, 33% died or were killed, and about 30%

were abandoned (Azlaf and Is Sidi Yahia, unpublished). In other areas of Morocco, 50-55% of dogs died or were killed, 16-19% were given away, 17-21% were abandoned and 10-13% were kept in the household (Fayda, 1988; Ben Kaddour *et al.*, 1990). Kitala *et al.* reported that in Kenya 85% of adult bitches had whelped at least once with an average number of litters per bitch of 2.1 and a mean litter size of 5.2. Twenty-two per cent of puppies were lost during the pre-weaning period through natural mortality, while 58% were killed and disposed of by owners. Similar to other sites, only 16% of puppies were still alive at the time of weaning (Kitala *et al.*, 1993). Studies in both Lusaka (Zambia) (De Balogh *et al.*, 1993) and Zimbabwe (Brooks, 1990) reported that 52% of pups from recent litters had died, while just 8% and 18% of pups, respectively, remained in the household.

It is clear that despite geographic variation in population structure from one site to another, dog populations in Africa, as elsewhere, have a characteristic pattern of females reproducing early and frequently which is facilitated by ownership practices. In fact, there are four main sources of dogs for household members willing to acquire one: (1) keeping puppies from bitches already living in the household; (2) receiving dogs from relatives, neighbors and friends living in the same community; (3) adopting abandoned dogs; and (4) purchasing dogs from a dog handler. In urban areas of Tunisia, 70-90% of owned dogs were received or bought (80% as puppies) from another household (Matter, 1989). In rural areas, 30-50% of dogs were born in the same household, with female dogs being given away or received more often than males. In a Moroccan study, 40% of dogs living in households were adopted from the street, 29% were born in the household, and 32% were received from neighbors (Ben Kaddour *et al.*, 1990). In another study 54.5% were born in the household, 27.5% were received from neighbors and 18% were adopted strays (Azlaf and Is Sidi Yahia, unpublished).

Dog keeping practices

A comprehensive review of nearly 600 publications treating cultural aspects of dog keeping in Africa has been published (Frank, 1965), and the reader is referred there for a more thorough treatment of the subject. Below is a brief overview of the variety of roles dogs have played, and continue to play, in African societies.

Three major uses of dogs in Africa have been described: (1) specific functions (guard dogs, hunting dogs, etc.); (2) economic utility; and (3) religious (Akakpo, 1985). Maintenance of large numbers of dogs is actually widespread among pastoral communities in Africa, where their main roles include guarding people from predators and intruders, and scavenging on refuse, a form of waste disposal (Macpherson and Wachira, 1997). In several West African countries dogs are raised for consumption by humans and in some areas they play an important role in religious ceremonies (Akakpo, 1985). Sakiti (cited by Akakpo) reported that in Benin, dog meat was used as bait for the capture of crabs (Akakpo, 1985). In Africa, except in some Muslim areas, dog saliva has the reputation of being an antiseptic or having curative properties, and in parts of southern Africa, dogs may be prescribed for certain ritual and ceremonial sacrifices (Oboegbulem and Nwakonobi, 1989).

In North Africa, the dog population has been classified into three groups depending upon the relationship to humans and their associated livestock (Ibrahim and Gusbi, 1997). These included stray dogs, herding or sheepdogs, and farm or house dogs. In rural areas of Morocco more than 70% of dogs were used for guarding while less than 2% were used for hunting (Azlaf and Is Sidi Yahia, unpublished; Ben Kaddour *et al.*, 1990). Ouhelli *et al.* cite a study in which 71-93% of dogs were used for guarding house or herd and 1.8-16.2% were used for hunting. In Tunisia, more than 80% of dogs were kept for guarding purposes and personal security. Dogs also were used for herding cattle, sheep, and goats and, in some areas, special breeds of dogs were raised for hunting (Matter, 1989). In Zimbabwe, 70% of dog owners indicated guard duties were their dogs' main function, although herding, companionship, and hunting were each described by approximately 10% of the respondents as the main reason for keeping dogs (Brooks, 1990). More than 90% of dogs in four suburban areas of Harare were kept for security (Hill, 1985). Dogs in Zimbabwe are not only expected to guard homes but also to protect the owner's crops from marauding baboons, and to keep predators such as hyenas and jackals away from livestock. In urban areas of Nigeria, dogs were kept for guarding in 45% of cases, while in rural areas most dogs were used for both hunting (36%) and guarding (31%) (Oboegbulem and Nwakonobi, 1989). The authors concluded that the growing sense of insecurity, occasioned by a rising incidence of violent crime in the cities, may induce more and more households to own guard dogs.

In general, African dog owners take a predominantly utilitarian approach to keeping dogs and relatively few households have animals that serve only as pets. In urban areas of Morocco, just 8-30% of dogs were kept as pets (Ouhelli *et al.*, 1997). Similarly, in urban areas of Nigeria dogs were kept as pets in just 30% of households; in rural areas the figure was a mere 4% (Oboegbulem and Nwakonobi, 1989). A household survey in Soweto, South Africa, revealed that interviewees kept dogs not only for personal security, but as companions and for keeping away feral cats (McCrindle *et al.*, 1998). For fulfilling their duties, owned dogs generally receive all or part of their daily food from residents, although this is not always the case. According to a survey conducted in different parts of Tunisia, the percentage of owned dogs which had to seek a large proportion of food outside the household (in waste disposal sites, near abattoirs, etc.) varied between 1.2 and 25.6%. In a rural area of Tunisia food provided to owned dogs consisted of bread (35%), chaff-water mash (27%), offal (26%), cereals (7%), milk (4%), and offal meat (1%). Hunting dogs often receive privileged treatment in the form of supplemental food (Akakpo, 1985). Food given to dogs in Morocco was equally diverse; a survey of 400 households showed that most owned dogs were fed bread and surplus food scraps. Animal viscera and meat also constituted a substantial part of their diet (2.4-33.2%) (Ouhelli *et al.*, 1997). Owned dogs in Nigeria may be irregularly fed by owners and therefore must lead a partly self-sufficient existence (Oboegbulem and Nwakonobi, 1989). About 95% of owned dogs in Machakos District of Kenya fed on household leftovers and waste (Kitala *et al.*, 1993). In Zimbabwe very few dogs were fed by their owners every day. Among households with dogs, 23% said that dogs other than their own occasionally scavenged garbage at their household. Stray dogs in these communities may scavenge at homes, hospitals, and boarding schools (Brooks, 1990). Owned dogs in a household survey in Harare (Zimbabwe) were fed mostly on maize meal and household scraps; only about one tenth of the dog owners bought commercial dog food (Hill, 1985). In many countries owned dogs have easy access to contaminated offal, which is either fed by their owners or available around slaughterhouses and butcher shops. Under such circumstances the opportunity to become infected with *Echinococcus granulosus*, and subsequently expose people to cystic echinococcosis (Ouhelli *et al.*, 1997), is ideal.

A sub-optimal health status is characteristic for most dog populations in Africa. This does not only affect the mortality rate but may also be an important issue in regard to the control of disease by vaccination (Haddad *et al.*, 1987). The health status of a dog population in rural southern Africa revealed that a significant segment of the population was in a chronic state of starvation and malnutrition; at the time of examination more than 50% of the population had one or more serious clinical conditions such as canine ehrlichiosis (17.2%), transmissible venereal tumors (6.8%), canine distemper (5%), *Cordylobia* infestation (5.5%), trauma (4.1%), and severe malnutrition (4.1%) (Rautenbach *et al.*, 1991). Significant differences in the prevalence of diseases among hospitalized dogs in South Africa have been found (Eckersley *et al.*, 1992). Dogs from developing communities were mainly young cross-bred dogs which suffered from infectious and parasitic diseases and trauma. Although the mortality rate was high, more than 80% of dogs suffered from diseases that could have been prevented. Dogs from developed communities were mainly adult or old pure-bred dogs that suffered primarily from organ diseases that resulted in a low mortality rate.

Free-ranging dogs

In many developing countries, a large proportion of the dog population is only temporarily, if at all, restricted in their activities or movements. As an example, a survey conducted in 42 countries on six continents indicated that in eight sub-Saharan countries more than 50% of dogs, on average, were strays (Macpherson and Wachira, 1997). By comparison, data from Europe indicated that less than 1% of dogs were strays. Generally, free-roaming dogs are tolerated and may even passively be protected, though the community does not hold itself responsible for these dogs.

In many rural communities, there is little demarcation of property lines and residents maintain a strong sense of communal responsibility. In such a setting, most owned dogs are recognizable or traceable to specific owners, although the dogs can range over a relatively large area. For instance, a dog from one household may be permitted to wander the neighborhood and be offered food at other households. Thus, while 55% to 90% of all owned dogs in urban areas of Tunisia were under permanent supervision of their owners, about half of all animals in rural areas were rarely, if ever, restricted. Furthermore, of those dogs confined during daytime, 20-25% were permitted to roam freely at night. In 1 year, monthly daytime visits of 385 dogs revealed that approximately 15% of dogs were always confined and 35% were never confined (Matter, 1989). As in other studies, male dogs were found to roam significantly more often, and over greater distances, than bitches. In most cases (57.7%) dogs were observed less than 500m from their household, although some were seen up to 8 km from their homes (Wandeler *et al.*, 1993). In a review of several studies, it was found that in most regions of Morocco dogs were frequently free to stray (75-90% being occasionally astray) and that strays represented the largest category of dogs (Ouhelli *et al.*, 1997). In Nigeria, 77.6% of owned dogs were always free-roaming in an urban area, and 96% of dogs in rural areas had no movement restriction (Oboegbulem and Nwakonobi, 1989). In the Machakos District, dogs were restricted in just 19.4% of the households and 69% of dogs spent all of their time free outdoors (Kitala *et al.*, 1993). In a suburban area of Zambia, 54% of the dogs were never restrained and only 27% were restrained on occasion (De Balogh *et al.*, 1993).

The proportion of true strays, i.e. those dogs which have no reference household, is generally low. Such dogs are concentrated mainly near the huge waste disposal sites of big cities (Artois and Ben Osman, 1986) where food can be obtained readily. In Tunisia, Matter found that true strays constituted between 5% and 15% of the total dog population (Matter, 1989). In fact, the proportion of ownerless dogs exceeded 10% only in areas where an accumulation of resources was observed. A low proportion of ownerless dogs was also found in two study areas of Zambia (less than 20%) (De Balogh *et al.*, 1993). Ownerless dogs are derived from the population of owned dogs through abandonment, typically because they are sick, there is fear of transmission of diseases to household members, especially children, or they are old and no longer able to fulfill their duties to the owner's satisfaction. Environmental conditions such as the absence of resources like food and shelter may also promote movement away from the previous owner.

Puppies born to ownerless females and surviving to the adulthood are rare (Ben Osman, 1985; Matter, 1989). Of 17 ownerless bitches observed in a rural area of Tunisia over a 2-year period, 59 pups were born in 13 litters. Of these, 34% were adopted shortly after birth by humans, primarily children. In only two of these cases did the adopted puppies survive the first 3 months (Matter, 1989). Nineteen per cent of the wild-born puppies were killed by area inhabitants, 9% died of natural causes, and 36% were lost for unknown reasons. Thus, only two of the 59 puppies survived more than 3 months after birth and were integrated into an existing group of ownerless dogs. Due to a high human-induced death rate of pups during the first weeks of life, it is clear that the overall reproductive success of ownerless bitches was insufficient to compensate for mortality (Wandeler *et al.*, 1993). Death of juvenile and adult ownerless dogs is primarily the result of being hit by cars (especially in urban areas), disease, and killing through animal control measures.

Unlike free-ranging domestic pets, ownerless dogs need to forage for their food (Berman and Dunbar, 1983). In Tunisia, ownerless dogs were observed feeding on carcasses of chicken, sheep, cattle, rabbit, donkey, wild boar, dog and cat, different small animals, as well as on human feces and fruits (Wandeler *et al.*, 1993). The principal diet of the dogs, however, consisted of offal which was available in small quantities throughout the study area and in greater abundance at a central waste disposal site. Activity patterns and habitat use of 34 ownerless dogs showed two peaks of activity: between 0500 and 0900 hours and again from 1900 to 2200 hours. Periods of least activity were between 0200 and 0500 hours as well as between 0900 and 1200 hours. Activity periods did not differ between male and female dogs, however, the overall duration of activity for male dogs and younger dogs was higher than that for females and older dogs. Differences between the sexes were due primarily to reduced activity of females during pregnancy and immediately after parturition, as well as the increased activity of male dogs in estrous groups.

The home range sizes of 21 ownerless dogs in Tunisia, calculated on the basis of more than 4300 observations, averaged 2 km^2 by the Minimum Area Method and ranged from 0.1 to 8.5 km^2 (Wandeler *et al.*, 1993). Male dogs had larger home ranges than females, and core areas within the home ranges were twice as large for males than for females. In contrast, home range size estimates for groups of stray dogs in rural environments were one or two orders of magnitude larger than those reported in urban areas (Font, 1987). Generally, owned dogs have smaller home ranges than ownerless animals, and those in rural areas have bigger home ranges than dogs in urban areas.

Free-roaming dogs aggregate in groups that are not random (WHO, 1984; Font, 1987). Pack formation may be more frequent in rural than in urban areas, perhaps because of the distribution of food resources (Font, 1987). Urban stray dogs that feed chiefly on refuse and occasional handouts from local area residents live in an area where food is patchily distributed. This distribution of food resources promotes foraging on an individual basis or in a very small group. In addition, pack formation in an urban environment may even be maladaptive, since large groups of dogs are rarely tolerated by people and are often subjected to dog control measures (Font, 1987). An analysis of the structure of dog packs in relation to the dogs' ownership status found that 80% of all non-reproductive packs were exclusively composed of ownerless dogs (Matter, 1993). In just 10% of cases were ownerless dogs observed together with owned dogs. The size of non-reproductive packs varied between two and nine dogs, with groups of two (60.4% of observations) and three dogs (21.5%) most common.

The structure of packs formed around females in estrus was completely different (Matter, 1993). Generally, the presence of an estrous female leads to increased aggression among males as they congregate around the female (Daniels, 1983a). In 30% of cases in this study, the groups of dogs that formed around a female in heat consisted of both ownerless and owned dogs. The frequency of contact between ownerless dogs and free-roaming owned dogs, whether it be during mating periods or in casual interactions each day, is of special importance in the transmission of rabies and other pathogens affecting dogs and man (Wandeler *et al.*, 1993).

Conclusions: human interactions and dog population control

The ecology of dogs - whether they be well cared - for pets, free-ranging dogs living in the midst of humans, or feral-cannot be understood fully except in the context of the dog's relationship with humans. Domestication is an evolutionary process marked by both phenotypic and genotypic changes in a species that result in increased adaptation to life with the domesticator (human) population (Daniels and Bekoff, 1990). Domestication enhanced certain behavioral and morphological traits in the ancestral wolf population resulting in: (1) the retention of juvenile characters into adulthood (i.e. neoteny); (2) dogs well-suited to life in human society (e.g. lower aggressiveness, more dependence on humans, early sexual maturation, easier submission); and (3) greater plasticity in behavioral development (Frank, 1980; Frank and Frank, 1982; Price, 1984).

With the creation of a new animal, for that is what resulted from the regimen of artificial selection, comes an obligation to care for that animal (Daniels and Bekoff, 1990). Data from studies of free-ranging and feral dogs worldwide indicate that problems with such populations are linked directly to the local culture. As Brisbin noted, the pariah niche, marked by habitats with adequate food in the form of garbage, does not exist deep within wilderness areas and is found only in areas adjacent to towns or cities or where human civilization has invaded former wilderness habitats (Brisbin, 1977). Development of water resources has allowed dingoes to move beyond the range of natural water resources (Corbett, 1995a). Thus, in an ecological sense we are dealing with populations of dogs that are limited to areas dictated by humans and a lifestyle that is likewise controlled, at least indirectly, by the local human populace. The reality of this relationship is that dog populations are cosmopolitan, their numbers are frequently too high, and their presence often does not bode well for sympatric wildlife populations. Given their intimate contact with other animals and man, dogs have the potential to play a significant role as reservoirs and vectors of diseases to humans and livestock (Akakpo, 1985; Chapters 3-9). For instance, a strong correlation between the incidence of human hydatidosis in different regions of Turkana, Kenya and the time spent by dogs inside human habitations has been reported (Watson-Jones and Macpherson, 1988). Other factors such as whether they were allowed to lick young children or scavenge from eating bowls and dried animal skins also correlated with disease incidence (Watson-Jones and Macpherson, 1988). In Morocco, women were more often infected with cystic hydatidosis than men, a fact attributed to the tendency for women to take on most dog-keeping chores (Ouhelli et al., 1997). While humans may have the ability to rectify the situation, the will to do so may be lacking. For example, free-ranging dogs were accepted as part of the community and their removal or destruction was socially unaccepted, although no one wanted to accept the responsibility of having dogs vaccinated against rabies (Beran, 1985). The accessibility of the domestic dog population to rabies vaccination in and around the Masai Mara National Reserve (Kenya) and the development of long-term control strategies has been investigated (Coleman, 1997). In this area, rabies is not only a threat to human beings and livestock but it has also been implicated in the local extinction of Cape hunting dogs (L. pictus) (Kat et al., 1995) as a result of spillover from the domestic dog population. Attempts to vaccinate dogs in conjunction with livestock immunization programs, in which animals are brought to a vaccination center, is the traditional approach in Kenya but has had limited success. In one study, even though 70% of dogs were located within 2 km of the vaccination points, the overall vaccination coverage achieved was only about 15% and the farthest any one dog was brought for vaccination was 1.5 km.

Education that fosters responsible dog-ownership is a high priority. Awareness of the health risks associated with dogs and community participation on all activities directed at the control, surveillance, and vaccination of the dog population are prerequisites for successful management. This situation is more of a problem in the tropics than in temperate regions; stray dogs have been brought under control in many parts of Europe and the USA but free-ranging dogs still plague many tropical countries (Fischman, 1985). One reason for this is that an adequate food base for free-ranging dogs is dependent on a primitive form of garbage and waste disposal that is often found in small towns and villages of the tropics (Brisbin, 1977). In these situations, habitat modification may be effective in reducing the size of dog populations. Lowering the carrying capacity of a given habitat would require reducing the availability and quality of resources such as food, water, and shelter. Habitat modification requires considerable government investment and a long-term effort that lasts several years or more (Kappeler, 1989). Population control programs based primarily on the physical elimination of dogs are cost-inefficient and often create animosity in the populace against any dog control efforts. They also may disrupt the dogs' social organization which, in turn, may have undesirable consequences with respect to the control of diseases (Kappeler, 1989). No elimination campaign known thus far has met the goal of significantly reducing the dog population over a prolonged period of time. Because the high reproductive potential of dogs allows them to compensate quickly for population losses due to elimination campaigns, removal of 50-80% of the total dog population would be required annually to attain a lasting reduction of the population (Wandeler and Capt, 1985 and Kappeler, 1989). For example, efforts to reduce the numbers of dingoes and feral dogs in Australia have involved the distribution of poisoned baits. The practice of consistently replacing baits that were removed by target animals achieved a mean reduction of 76.1% of the wild dog population, encompassing both feral dogs and dingoes (Fleming, 1996). Populations returned to the pre-control levels within 1 year (Fleming *et al.*, 1996). Poisoning is problematic not only because death may not be immediate but there is the risk of poisoned baits being taken by non-target animals as well (Singer, 1997). A 91% reduction in the abundance of red foxes, which were not target animals, was recorded in areas where baits had been distributed (Fleming, 1996).

Our obligation to care for the animals we created does not rule out taking steps to limit their numbers. If it is assumed that concern for free-ranging and feral dog populations precludes actions that induce suffering in those animals, fertility control is a logical and ethically sound approach to the problem, particularly if attending to the welfare of individual dogs is at odds with the desire to preserve other aspects of the environment, such as species that are in danger (Singer, 1997). Ultimately, such steps must be taken if any effort to reduce the burden of large free-ranging dog populations is expected to work. Surgical vasectomy has been suggested as a means of controlling feral dog populations on the Galapagos Islands (Barnett and Rudd, 1983). Although it is a humane procedure it, too, would require that a large proportion of the population be captured, treated, and released.

While the use of reproductive inhibitors has clear ethical advantages, the feasibility of this method has not been shown for any mammalian wildlife species to date (Fischman, 1985; Tyndale-Biscoe, 1994). The most important question regarding the efficacy of immuno-contraceptive methods is whether or not the fecundity of a mammalian pest species can be curbed sufficiently to reduce the population (Tyndale-Biscoe, 1994). If so, and this may not be determined prior to implementing a control program, the next hurdles are to design an agent that induces sterility, followed by the need to deliver it to the target population. In the case of free-ranging dogs, some of which may be owned, the added burden of being able to reverse the sterilization (by making the effect a temporary one) may be an issue as well. Any effective strategy will have to consider the target population's social systems also because of their influence on which individuals breed and how interference with normal reproductive behavior will affect the social status of treated animals. Related to this is the need to insure that enough animals are treated to have a significant impact on the population. Another important consideration is that the cost of such a program may be prohibitive. Finally, the willingness of the human populace to implement such a plan may be insufficient. Thus, an ethically sound program to control free-ranging and feral dog populations is still a number of years off. Despite these drawbacks, it is clear that such work should continue. Harassment of deer by dogs in some instances increased as homes were built in forested areas where deer went undisturbed (Lowry and MacArthur, 1978). In the decades since then, development of residential communities and the concomitant fragmentation of forested areas has continued unabated throughout the world. Problems with free-ranging animals, not simply domestic dogs, have grown continually and the need to address the issue, all the while making the environment more conducive to the growth of such populations, is apparent. In the case of "man's best friend", the scientific knowledge that will facilitate control of dog populations may be in hand long before the collective will to use it.

References

Abou-Eisha, A.M. and Abdel-Aal, A.A. (1995) Prevalence of some zoonotic parasites in dog faecal deposits in Ismailia City. *Assiut Veterinary Medical Journal* 33, 119-126.

Adams, R.M. and Johnson, K.G. (1993) Sleep-wake cycles and other night-time behaviors of the domestic dog *Canis familiaris*. *Applied Animal Behavior Science* 36, 233-248.

Akakpo, A.J. (1985) Le chien dans la société Noire Africaine: un réservoir de rage. In: Kuwert, E., Mérieux, C., Koprowski, H. and Bögel, K. (eds) *Rabies in the Tropics*. Springer, Berlin, pp. 516-517.

Akakpo, A.J., Bornarel, P., Sarradin, P., Leye, S.M. and Alambedji, R. (1990) Socio-ethnology and role of the dog in the Pikine district (suburban zone of Dakar - Senegal). *Dakar Medicine* 35, 99-105.

Allen, K. (1998) The healthy pleasure of their company: roles of animals in enhancing human health and quality of life. In: The International Association of Human-Animal Interaction Organization (ed.) *Human-Animal Interactions and Zoonoses Prevention and Control in Developing Countries*. WHO/IAHAIO, Prague, pp. 1-4.

Anonymous (1971) The plight and threat of man's best friend. *Baltimore Magazine*, August 56, 19-21.

Anvik, J.O., Hague, A.E. and Rahaman, A. (1974) A method of estimating urban dog populations and its application to the assessment of canine fecal pollution and endoparasitism in Saskatchewan. *Canine Veterinary Journal* 15, 219-223.

Archer, M. (1974) New information about the Quaternary distribution of the

Thylacine (Marsupialia, Thylacinidae) in Australia. *Journal of the Proceedings of the Royal Society of Western Australia* 57, 43-50.

Artois, M. and Ben Osman, F. (1986) Le chien et la rage en Tunisie. *Anthropozoolica* 4, 33-37.

Artois, M., Ben Osman, F., Kilani, M. and Wandeler, A.I. (1986) New contribution to the knowledge of the ecology of stray dogs in Tunisia. *Comparative Immunology, Microbiology and Infectious Diseases* 9, 4-5.

Aulagnier, S. (1990) Zoogéographie et statut des carnivores sauvages du Maroc. *Vie Milieu* 40, 150-155.

Baird, R.F. (1991) The dingo as a possible factor in the disappearance of *Gallinula mortierii* from the Australian mainland. *Emu* 91, 121-122.

Bakkali, M.M. (1985) Epidémiologie et prophylaxie de la rage au Maroc. In: Kuwert, E., Mérieux, C., Koprowski, H. and Bögel, K. (eds) *Rabies in the Tropics.* Springer, Berlin, pp. 371-386.

Barnett, B.D. and Rudd, R.L. (1983) Feral dogs of the Galapagos islands: impact and control. *International Journal for the Study of Animal Problems* 4, 44-58.

Baxter, D.N. (1984a) The deleterious effects of dogs on human health: dog associated injuries. *Community Medicine* 6, 29-36.

Baxter, D.N. (1984b) The deleterious effects of dogs on human health: 3. miscellaneous problems and a control programme. *Community Medicine* 6, 198-203.

Baxter, D.N. and Leck, I. (1984) The deleterious effects of dogs on human health: 2. canine zoonoses. *Community Medicine* 6, 185-197.

Beck, A.M. (1973) *The Ecology of Stray Dogs: a Study of Free-ranging Urban Animals.* York Press, Baltimore, Maryland.

Beck, A.M. (1974) The ecology of urban dogs. In: Noyes, J.N. and Progulske, D.R. (eds) *Wildlife in an Urbanizing Environment.* University of Massachusetts Cooperative Extensive Service, Amherst, Massachusetts.

Beck, A.M. (1975) The ecology of "feral" and free-roving dogs in Baltimore. In: Fox, M.W. (ed.) *The Wild Canids: Their Systematics, Behavioral Ecology and Evolution.* Van Nostrand Reinhold, New York, pp. 380-390.

Bekoff, M., Daniels, T.J. and Gittleman, J.L. (1984) Life history patterns and the comparative social ecology of carnivores. *Annual Review of Ecology and Systematics* 15, 191-232.

Ben Kaddour, M., Fartah, K., Kamili, A., Moussaoui Rahhali, S. and Ouahri, M. (1990) *Ecologie Canine et Prophylaxie de la Rage dans la Zone Rurale de Zemamra (Safi). Rapport de Stage de Développement 4ème Année Vétérinaire.* Institut Agronomique et Vétérinaire Hassan II, Rabat, Morocco.

Ben Osman, F. (1985) Le chien errant en Tunisie. *Revue Ecologique (Terre vie)* 40, 197-201.

Ben Osman, F. and Haddad, N. (1988) Experience in field rabies control programs. *Review of Infectious Diseases* 10, S703-S706.

BenYoussef, S., Matter, H.C., Schumacher, C.L., Kharmachi, H., Jemli, J., Mrabet, L., Gharbi, M., Hammami, S., ElHicheri, K., Aubert, M.F. and Meslin, F.X. (1998) Field evaluation of a dog owner, participation-based, bait delivery system for the oral immunization of dogs against rabies in Tunisia. *American*

Journal of Tropical Medicine and Hygiene 58, 835-845.

Beran, G.W. (1982) Ecology of dogs in the central Philippines in relation to rabies control efforts. *Comparative Immunology, Microbiology and Infectious Diseases* 5, 265-270.

Beran, G.W. (1985) Ecology of dogs in developing countries in relation to rabies control programs. In: Kuwert, E., Mérieux, C., Koprowski, H. and Bögel, K. (eds) *Rabies in the Tropics*. Springer-Verlag, Berlin, pp. 691-697.

Beran, G.W. and Frith, M.F. (1988a) *Guidelines for Urban Dog Ecology Surveys*, Iowa State University.

Beran, G.W. and Frith, M.F. (1988b) Domestic animal rabies control: an overview. *Reviews of Infectious Diseases* 10, S672-S677.

Berman, M. and Dunbar, I. (1983) The social behavior of free-ranging suburban dogs. *Applied Animal Ethology* 10, 5-17.

Bernard, J., Ben Osman, F. and Juminer, B. (1967) Enquêtes sur les helminthes parasites du chien (CFL) à Tunis-Ville. *Archives de l'Institut Pasteur de Tunis* 44, 1-89.

Beverley, S.M. and Wilson, A.C. (1985) Ancient origin for Hawaii Drodophilinae inferred from protein comparisons. *Proceedings of the National Academy of Sciences of the United States of America* 82, 4753-4757.

Bino, R. (1996) Notes on behavior of New Guinea singing dogs (*Canis lupus dingo*). *Science in New Guinea* 22, 43-47.

Boitani, L. (1983) Wolf and dog competition in Italy. *Acta Zoologica Fennica* 174, 259-264.

Boitani, L. and Ciucci, P. (1995) Comparative social ecology of feral dogs and wolves. *Ethology, Ecology, and Evolution* 7, 49-72.

Boitani, L. and Fabbri, M.L. (1982) Censimento dei cani in Italia con particolare riguardo al fenomeno del randagismo. *Ricerche di Biologia della Selvaggina* 73, 1-51.

Boitani, L. and Racana, A. (1984) Indagine eco-etologica sulla popolazione di cani domestici e randagi di due comuni della Basilicata. *Silva Lucana, Bari* 3, 1-86.

Boitani, L., Francisci, F., Ciucci, P. and Andreoli, G. (1995) Population biology and ecology of feral dogs in central Italy. In: Serpell, J. (ed.) *The Domestic Dog: its Evolution, Behavior, and Interactions With People*. Cambridge University Press, Cambridge, England, pp. 217-244.

Brisbin, I.L. (1977) The pariah: its ecology and importance to the origin, development, and study of pure bred dogs. *Pure-Bred Dogs American Kennel Gazette* 94, 22-29.

Brooks, R. (1990) Survey of the dog population of Zimbabwe and its level of rabies vaccination. *Veterinary Record* 127, 592-596.

Buckland, S.T., Anderson, D.R., Burnham, K.P. and Laake, J.L. (1993) *Distance Sampling. Estimating Abundance of Biological Populations*. Chapman and Hall, London.

Bukowski, J.A. and Wartenberg, D. (1997) An alternative approach for investigating the carcinogenicity of indoor air pollution: Pets as sentinels of environmental cancer risk. *Environmental Health Perspectives* 105, 1312-1319.

Burrows, R., Hofer, H. and East, M.L. (1995) Population-dynamics, intervention and survival in African wild dogs (*Lycaon pictus*). *Proceedings of the Royal Society of London Series B Biological* 262, 235-245.

Burt, W.H. (1943) Territoriality and home range concepts as applied to mammals. *Journal of Mammalogy* 24, 346-352.

Carding, A.H. (1969) The significance and dynamics of stray dog populations with special reference to the UK and Japan. *Journal of Small Animal Practice* 10, 419-446.

Catling, P.C., Corbett, L.K. and Newsome, A.E. (1992) Reproduction in captive and wild dingoes (*Canis familiaris dingo*) in temperate and arid environments of Australia. *Wildlife Research* 19, 195-209.

Caughley, G. (1977) *Analysis of Vertebrate Populations.* John Wiley & Sons, Chichester.

Caughley, G., Grigg, G.C., Caughley, J. and Hill, G.J.E. (1980) Does dingo predation control the densities of kangaroos and emus? *Australian Wildlife Research* 7, 1-12.

Causey, M.K. and Cude, C.A. (1980) Feral dog and white-tailed deer interactions in Alabama. *Journal of Wildlife Management* 44, 481-484.

Chadli, A., Bahmanyar, M. and Chaabouni, A. (1982) Epidémiologie de la rage en Tunisie. Etude comparative des résultats des 28 dernières années. *Archives de l'Institut Pasteur de Tunis* 59, 5-21.

Childs, J.E., Robinson, L.E., Sadek, R., Madden, A., Miranda, M.E. and Miranda, N.L. (1998) Density estimates of rural dog populations and an assessment of marking methods during a rabies vaccination campaign in the Philippines. *Preventive Veterinary Medicine* 33, 207-218.

Clutton-Brock, J. (1977) Man-made dogs. *Science* 197, 1340-1342.

Coleman, P. (1997) *Short Report of the Work Presented by Paul Coleman at the Southern and Eastern African Rabies Group (SEARG)/World Health Organization (WHO) International Meeting on the Epidemiology and Control of Rabies, Nairobi, 4-6 March 1997.* WHO, Nairobi.

Collins, S. (1998) Change and continuity in human relationships with companion animals, 1500 to 1900. In: The International Association of Human-Animal Interaction Organization (ed.) *Human-Animal Interactions and Zoonoses Prevention and Control in Developing Countries.* WHO/IAHAIO, Prague, pp. 48-49.

Coman, B.J. (1972) Helminth parasites of the dingo and feral dog in Victoria with some notes on the diet of the host. *Australian Veterinary Journal* 48, 456-461.

Coman, B.J. and Robinson, J.L. (1989) Some aspects of stray dog behavior in an urban fringe area. *Australian Veterinary Journal* 66, 30-32.

Corbett, L.K. (1995a) *The Dingo in Australia and Asia.* Cornell University Press, Ithaca, New York.

Corbett, L.K. (1995b) Does dingo predation or buffalo competition regulate feral pig populations in the Australian wet-dry tropics? An experimental study. *Wildlife Research* 22, 65-74.

Corbett, L.K. and Newsome, A.E. (1975) Dingo society and its maintenance: a preliminary analysis. In: Fox, M.W. (ed.) *The Wild Canids: Their Systematics, Behavioral Ecology, and Evolution.* Van Nostrand Reinold, New York, pp. 369-

379.

Corbett, L.K. and Newsome, A.E. (1987) The feeding ecology of the dingo. III. Dietary relationships with widely fluctuating prey populations in arid Australia: an hypothesis of alternation of predation. *Oecologia* 74, 215-227.

Dahl, K. (1919) Studies of trout and trout-waters in Norway. *Salmon and Trout Magazine* 18, 16-33.

Daniels, T.J. (1983a) The social organization of free-ranging urban dogs. II. Estrous groups and the mating system. *Applied Animal Ethology* 10, 365-373.

Daniels, T.J. (1983b) The social organization of free-ranging urban dogs. I. Non-estrous social behavior. *Applied Animal Ethology* 10, 341-363.

Daniels, T.J. (1986) A study of dog bites on the Navajo Reservation. *Public Health Report* 101, 50-59.

Daniels, T.J. (1987a) Conspecific scavenging by a young domestic dog. *Journal of Mammalogy* 68, 416-418.

Daniels, T.J. (1987b) The social ecology and behavior of free-ranging dogs. PhD dissertation, University of Colorado, Boulder, Colorado.

Daniels, T.J. (1988) Down in the dumps. *Natural History* 97, 8-12.

Daniels, T.J. and Bekoff, M. (1989a) Population and social biology of free-ranging dogs, *Canis familiaris*. *Journal of Mammalogy* 70, 754-762.

Daniels, T.J. and Bekoff, M. (1989b) Spatial and temporal resource use by feral and abandoned dogs. *Ethology* 181, 300-312.

Daniels, T.J. and Bekoff, M. (1989c) Feralization: the making of wild domestic animals. *Behavioral Processes* 19, 79-94.

Daniels, T.J. and Bekoff, M. (1990) Domestication, exploitation, and rights. In: Bekoff, M. and Jamison, D. (eds) *Explanation, Evolution, and Adaptation.* Westview Press, Boulder, Colorado, pp. 345-377.

Dar, F.K. and Alkarmi, T. (1997) Cystic echinococcosis in the Gulf Littoral States. In: Andersen, F.L., Ouhelli, H. and Kachani, M. (eds) *Compendium on Cystic Echinococcosis in Africa and in Middle Eastern Countries With Special Reference to Morocco*, Brighman Young University, Provo, Utah, USA, pp. 281-291.

Davis, S.J.M. (1978) Evidence for domestication of the dog 12,000 years ago in the Natufian of Israel. *Nature* 276, 608-610.

De Balogh, K.K., Wandeler, A.I. and Meslin, F.X. (1993) A dog ecology study in an urban and a semi-rural area of Zambia. *Onderstepoort Journal of Veterinary Research* 60, 437-443.

Denney, R.N. (1974) The impact of uncontrolled dogs on wildlife and livestock. *Transactions of the Thirty-ninth North American Wildlife and Natural Resources Conference* 39, 257-291.

Derr, M. (1997) *Dog's Best Friend*. Henry Holt and Co., New York.

Eaton, R.L. (1969) Cooperative hunting by cheetahs and jackals and a theory of domestication of the dog. *Mammalia* 33, 87-92.

Eckersley, G.N., Hohn, E., Reyers, F., Turner, G.V. and Wolmarans, L. (1992) A comparison between the disease status of hospitalized dogs from developed and those from developing communities. *Journal of the South African Veterinary Association* 63, 2-6.

Eisenberg, J.F., Muckenhirn, N.A. and Rudran, R. (1972) The relation between ecology and social structure in primates. *Science* 176, 863-874.

Elton, C.S. (1958) *The Ecology of Invasions by Animals and Plants.* Methuen, London, England.

Engle, E.T. (1946) No seasonal breeding cycle in dogs. *Journal of Mammalogy* 27, 79-81.

Esteve, R. (1985) Importance des chiens errants dans les causes de mortalité des animaux sauvages et domestiques en Haute-Savoie. *Revue Ecologique (Terre vie)* 40, pp. 206.

Ezeokoli, C.D., Ogunkoya, A.B., Beran, G., Belino, E.D. and Eze, E.U. (1984) The epidemiology of rabies in Kaduna State. *Bulletin Animal Health Production, Africa* 32, 378-384.

Fayda, M. (1988) Etude socioécologique dans la population canine en zone rurale et son application à la prophylaxie de la rage. PhD thesis, Institut Agronomique et Vétérinaire Hassan II, Rabat, Morocco.

Feldmann, B.M. and Carding, T.H. (1973) Free-roaming urban pets. *Health Services Reports* 88, 956-962.

Fischman, H.R. (1985) Rabies in wildlife and tropical canines - a population problem. In: Kuwert, E., Mérieux, C., Koprowski, H. and Bögel, K. (eds) *Rabies in the Tropics.* Springer-Verlag, Berlin, pp. 662-668.

Fleming, P.J.S. (1996) Ground-placed baits for the control of wild dogs: evaluation of a replacement-baiting strategy in north-eastern NSW. *Wildlife Research* 23, 729-740.

Fleming, P.J.S., Thompson, J.A. and Nicol, H.I. (1996) Indices for measuring the efficacy of aerial baiting for wild dog control in north-eastern NSW. *Wildlife Research* 23, 665-674.

Font, E. (1987) Spacing and social organization: Urban stray dogs revisited. *Applied Animal Behavior Science* 17, 319-328.

Fox, M.W., Beck, A.M. and Blackman, E. (1975) Behavior and ecology of a small group of urban dogs (*Canis familiaris*). *Applied Animal Ethology* 1, 119-137.

Francisci, F., Giovannini, A., Fabbri, M.L., Boitani, L. and Spagnesi, M. (1985) The management of canids in Italy: its relationship with public health and conservation problem. *Revue Ecologique (Terre vie)* 40, p. 206.

Frank, B. (1965) *Die Rolle des Hundes in Afrikanischen Kulturen.* Franz Steiner Verlag GMBH Wiesbaden.

Frank, H. (1980) Evolution of canine information processing under conditions of natural and artificial selection. *Zeitschrift für Tierpsychologie* 53, 389-399.

Frank, H. and Frank, M.G. (1982) On the effects of domestication on canine social development and behavior. *Applied Animal Ethology* 8, 507-525.

Gavitt, J.D., Downing, R.L. and McGinnes, B.S. (1974) Effects of dogs on deer reproduction in Virginia. *Proceedings of the Annual Conference of the Southeastern Association of State Game & Fish Commissioners* 28, 532-539.

Gentry, C. (1983) *When Dogs Run Wild: the Sociology of Feral Dogs and Wildlife.* McFarland and Company, Jefferson, New York.

Ginsberg, J. and Macdonald, D.W. (1990) *Foxes, Wolves, Jackals, and Dogs: Action Plan for the Conservation of Canids.* Gland, Switzerland: IUCN Publications.

Gipson, P.S. (1983) Evaluation and control implications of behavior of feral dogs in interior Alaska. In: Kaukeinen, D.E. (ed.) *Vertebrate Pest Control and Managment Materials: Fourth Symposium*. American Society for Testing and Materials. Philadelphia, Pennsylvania, pp. 285-294.

Gipson, P.S. and Sealander, J.A. (1977) Ecological relationships of white-tailed deer and dogs in Arkansas. In: Phillips, R.L. and Jonkel, C. (eds) *Proceedings of the 1975 Predator Symposium*. University of Montana, Missoula, Montana, pp. 3-16.

Goldstein, E.J.C. (1992) Bite wounds and infection. *Clinical Infectious Diseases* 14, 633-640.

Grimason, A.M., Smith, H.V., Parker, J.F.W., Jackson, M.H., Smith, P.G. and Girdwood, R.W.A. (1993) Occurrence of *Giardia* sp. cysts and *Cryptosporidium* sp. oocysts in faeces from public parks in the west of Scotland. *Epidemiology and Infection* 110, 641-645.

Habermehl, K.H. (1975) *Die Altersbestimmung bei Haus- und Labortieren*. Verlag Paul Parey, Berlin.

Haddad, N., Blancou, J., Gritli, A. and Ben Osman, F. (1987) Etude de la réponse immunitaire des chiens tunisiens à la vaccination antirabique. *Maghreb Vétérinaire* 3, 61-64.

Harden, R.H. (1985) The ecology of the dingo in North-Eastern New South Wales. I. Movements and home range. *Australian Wildlife Research* 12, 25-37.

Harden, R.H. and Robertshaw, J.D. (1987) Ecology of dingo in northeastern New South Wales. V. Human predation on the dingo. *Australian Zoology* 24, 65-72.

Harder, T.C., Kenter, M., Appel, M.J.G., Roelke-Parker, M.E., Barrett, T. and Osterhaus, A.D.M.E. (1995) Phylogenetic evidence of canine distemper virus in Serengeti's lions. *Vaccine* 13, 521-523.

Harrop, A.E. (1960) The physiology of reproduction in the dog and bitch. In: Harrop, A.E. (ed.) *Reproduction in the Dog*. Balliere, Tindall and Cox., London, England, pp. 64-86.

Hartung, J. (1997) Influence of companion dog on the indoor air and surface hygiene. *Atemwegs- und Lungenkrankheiten* 23, S82-S85.

Hejny-Brandl, M. (1995) Contamination of open spaces and children's play areas in Vienna with eggs of canine endoparasites pathogenic for human beings. Original language title: Zur Kontamination öffentlicher Grünflächen und Kinderspielplätze in Wien mit Dauerstadien humanpathogener Endoparasiten vom Hund. *Wiener Tierärztliche Monatsschrift* 82, p. 397.

Heussner, J.C., Flowers, A.I., Williams, J.D. and Silvy, N.J. (1978) Estimating dog and cat populations in an urban area. *Animal Regulation Studies* 1, 203-212.

Hill, F.W.G. (1985) A survey of the animal population in four high density suburbs in Harare. *Zimbabwe Veterinary Journal* 16, 31-36.

Hommel, M., Jaffe, C.L., Travi, B. and Milon, G. (1995) Experimental models for leishmaniasis and for testing anti-leishmanial vaccines. *Annals of Tropical Medicine and Parasitology* 89, 55-73.

Horn, K., Schnieder, T. and Stoye, M. (1990) Contamination of public children's playgrounds with helminth eggs in Hannover. Original language title: Kontamination öffentlicher Kinderspielplätze Hannovers mit Helmintheneiern.

Deutsche Tierärztliche Wochenschrift 97, 122-125.

Howard, W.E. and Marsh, R.E. (1984) Ecological implications and management of feral animals in California. In: Munton, P.N. (ed.) *Feral Mammals - Problems and Potential.* IUCN, Lucerne, Switzerland, pp. 33-41.

Ibrahim, M.M. and Gusbi, A.M. (1997) Cystic echinococcosis in Northern Africa (excluding Morocco): veterinary aspects. In: Andersen, F.L., Ouhelli, H. and Kachani, M. (eds) *Compendium on Cystic Echinococcosis in Africa and in Middle Eastern Countries With Special Reference to Morocco.* Brighman Young University, Provo, Utah, USA, pp. 207-222.

Jöchle, W. and Andersen, A.C. (1977) The estrous cycle in the dog: A review. *Theriogenology* 7, 113-140.

Kaiser, G. (1971) Die Reproduktionsleistung der Haushunde in ihrer Beziehung zur Körpergrösse und zum Gewicht der Rassen. *Zeitschrift für Tierzüchtung und Züchtungsbiologie* 88, 118-168.

Kappeler, A. (1989) *Does a Technology Package Exist.* WHO, Geneva.

Kappeler, A. (1991) *Dog Population Studies Related to a Vaccination Campaign Against Rabies in Lalitpur City, Nepal.* WHO, Geneva.

Kass, P.H. and Hart, L.A. (1998) An epidemiologic study of determinants of dog and cat relinquishment to animal shelters in Sacramento County, California. In: The International Association of Human-Animal Interaction Organization, (ed.) *Human-Animal Interactions and Zoonoses Prevention and Control in Developing Countries.* WHO/IAHAIO, Prague, pp. 57.

Kat, P.W., Alexander, K.A., Smith, J.S. and Munson, L. (1995) Rabies and African wild dogs in Kenya. *Proceedings of the Royal Society of London[Biol]* 262, 229-233.

Kitala, P.M., McDermott, J.J., Kyule, M.N. and Cathuma, J.M. (1993) Features of dog ecology relevant to rabies spread in Machakos District, Kenya. *Onderstepoort Journal of Veterinary Research* 60, 445-449.

Kruuk, H. and Snell, H. (1981) Prey selection by feral dogs from a population of marine iguanas (*Amblyrhynchus cristatus*). *Journal of Applied Ecology* 18, 197-204.

Laurenson, K., Van Heerden, J., Stander, P. and Van Vuuren, M.J. (1997) Seroepidemiological survey of sympatric domestic and wild dogs (*Lycaon pictus*) in Tsumkwe district, north-eastern Namibia. *Onderstepoort Journal of Veterinary Research* 64, 313-316.

Lawrence, B. (1967) Early domestic dogs. *Zeitschrift für Säugetierkunde* 32, 44-59.

Lowry, D.A. and MacArthur, K.L. (1978) Domestic dogs as predators on deer. *Wildlife Society Bulletin* 6, 38-39.

Lundie-Jenkin, G., Corbett, L.K. and Phillips, C.M. (1993) Ecology of the rufous hare-wallaby, *Lagorchestes hirsutus* Gould (Marsupialia: Macropodidae), in the Tanami Desert, Northern Territory. III. Interactions with introduced mammal species. *Wildlife Research* 20, 495-511.

Luomala, K. (1960) The native dog in the Polynesian system of values. In: Diamond, S. (ed.) *Culture in History: Essays in Honor of Paul Radin.* Columbia University Press, New York, pp. 190-240.

Macdonald, D.W. (1981) Dwindling resources and the social behavior of Capybaras

(*Hydrochoerus hydroheaeris*). *Journal of Zoology* 194, 371-391.

Macdonald, D.W. and Carr, G.M. (1995) Variation in dog society: between resource dispersion and social flux. In: Serpell, J. (ed.) *The Domestic Dog: its Evolution, Behavior, and Interactions With People.* Cambridge University Press, Cambridge, England, pp. 199-216.

Macpherson, C.N.L. and Wachira T.W.M. (1997) Cystic echinococcus in Africa south of the Sahara. In: Andersen, F.L., Ouhelli, H. and Kachani, M. (eds) *Compendium on Cystic Echinococcosis in Africa and in Middle Eastern Countries With Special Reference to Morocco.* Brighman Young University, Provo, Utah, pp. 245-277.

Marx, M.B. and Furcolow, M.L. (1969) What is the dog population. *Archives of Environmental Health* 19, 217-219.

Matter, H.C. (1987) Etude écologique d'une population canine. *Maghreb Vétérinaire* 3, 65-68.

Matter, H.C. (1989) Populationsbiologische Untersuchungen an Hundepopulationen in Tunesien. PhD thesis, University of Berne, Switzerland.

Matter, H.C. (1993) Canine ecology and rabies vaccination. In: Fondation Marcel Mérieux and WHO (eds) *Proceedings of the Symposium on Rabies Control in Asia. Jakarta, Indonesia,* Fondation Marcel Mérieux, Lyon, April 27-30, 1993 pp. 75-94.

Matter, H.C. (1998a) The epidemiology of bite and scratch injuries by vertebrate animals in Switzerland. *European Journal of Epidemiology* 14, 483-490.

Matter, H.C. (1998b) Analysis of canine populations and bait delivery techniques for the oral immunization of dogs against rabies. In: WHO, (ed.), *WHO/MZCP Workshop on Strengthening Rabies Surveillance and Control in the MZCP Countries.* WHO/MZCP, Istanbul, pp. 1-7.

Matter, H.C., Kharmachi, H., Haddad, N., Ben Youssef, S., Sghaier, C., Ben Khelifa, R., Jemli, J., Mrabet, L., Meslin, F.X. and Wandeler, A.I. (1995) Test of three bait types for oral immunization of dogs against rabies in Tunisia. *American Journal of Tropical Medicine and Hygiene* 52, 489-495.

Matter, H.C., Fico, R. and Neuenschwander, B.E. (1998) Study of the structure and density of a dog population in Tekirdag (Turkey). *The Journal of Etlik Veterinary Microbiology* 9, 9-24.

Matter, H.C., Schumacher, C.L., Kharmachi, H., Hammami, S., Tlatli, A., Jemli, J., Mrabet, L., Meslin, F.-X., Aubert, M.F.A., Neuenschwander, B. and El Hicheri, K. (1998) Field evaluation of two bait delivery systems for the oral immunization of dogs against rabies in Tunisia. *Vaccine* 16, 657-665.

Matter, H.C., Wandeler, A.I., Neuenschwander, B.E., Harischandra, P.A.L. and Meslin, F.X. (2000) Study of the dog population and the rabies control activities in the Mirigama area of Sri Lanka. *Acta Tropica* 75, 95-108.

McCrindle, C.M.E., Cornelius, S.T., Schoeman, H.S. and Gallant, J. (1998) Changing roles of dogs in urban African society - a South African perspective. In: The International Association of Human-Animal Interaction Organization (ed.) *Human-Animal Interactions and Zoonoses Prevention and Control in Developing Countries.* WHO/IAHAIO, Prague, pp. 62.

McIlroy, J.C., Cooper, R.J., Gifford, E.J., Green, B.F. and Newgrain, K.W. (1986)

The effect on wild dogs, *Canis f. familiaris*, of 1080-poisoning campaigns in Kosciusko National Park, N.S.W. *Australian Wildlife Research* 13, 535-544.

McLennan, J.A. and Potter, M.A. (1993) Juveniles in mainland populations of kiwi. *Notornis* 40, 294-297.

Mech, L.D. (1977) Productivity, mortality, and population trends of wolves in northeastern Minnesota. *Journal of Mammalogy* 58, 559-574.

Mech, L.D. (1986) *The Wolf: the Ecology and Behavior of an Endangered Species.* Natural History Press, New York.

Meggitt, M.J. (1965) The association between Australian Aborigines and Dingoes. In: Leeds, A. and Vayda, A.P. (eds) *Man, Culture and Animals.* American Association for the Advancement of Science, Washington, DC, pp. 7-26.

Meslin, F.X. (1995) Zoonoses in the world: current and future trends. *Schweizerische Medizinische Wochenschrift* 125, 875-878.

Meslin, F.X. and Matter, H.C. (1994) *Assignment Report on Rabies Control in Yemen. 19-24 July 1993.* Alexandria: WHO. Regional Office for the Eastern Mediterranean.

Meslin, F.X., Fishbein, D.B. and Matter, H.C. (1994) Rationale and prospects for rabies elimination in developing countries. In: Rupprecht, C.E., Dietzschold, B. and Koprowski, H. (eds) *Lyssaviruses.* Springer-Verlag, Berlin, pp. 1-26.

Munton, P. (1984) Problems associated with introduced species. In: Munton, P.N. (ed.) *Feral Mammals - Problems and Potential.* IUCN, Lucerne, Switzerland, pp. 127-142.

Nesbitt, W.H. (1975) Ecology of a feral dog pack on a wildlife refuge. In: Fox, M.W. (ed.) *The Wild Canids.* Van Nostrand Reinhold., New York, pp. 391-396.

Newsome, A.E. and Corbett, L.K. (1975) Outbreaks of rodents in semi-arid and arid Australia: causes, preventions, and evolutionary considerations. In: Prakash, I. and Ghosh, P.K. (eds) *Rodents in Desert Environments.* Junk, The Hague, pp. 117-153.

Newsome, A.E., Catling, P.C. and Corbett, L.K. (1983) The feeding ecology of the dingo II. Dietary and numerical relationships with fluctuating prey populations in south-eastern Australia. *Australian Journal of Ecology* 8, 345-366.

Nowak, R.M. and Paradiso, J.L. (1983) *Walker's Mammals of the World.* Johns Hopkins University Press, Baltimore, Maryland.

Oboegbulem, S.I. and Nwakonobi, I.E. (1989) Population density and ecology of dogs in Nigeria: A pilot study. *Revue Scientifique et Technique de l'Office International des Epizooties* 8, 733-745.

OLorcain, P. (1994) Prevalence of *Toxocara canis* ova in public playgrounds in the Dublin area of Ireland. *Journal of Helminthology* 68, 237-241.

Oppenheimer, E.C. and Oppenheimer, J.R. (1975) Certain behavioral features in the pariah dog (*Canis familiaris*) in West Bengal. *Applied Animal Ethology* 2, 81-92.

Ouhelli, H., Kadiri, A., El Hasnaoui, M. and Kachani, M. (1997) Prevalence of *Echinococcus granulosus* in dogs in Morocco and potential role of dogs in transmission of cystic echinococcosis. In: Andersen, F.L., Ouhelli, H. and Kachani, M. (eds) *Compendium on Cystic Echinococcosis in Africa and in Middle Eastern Countries With Special Reference to Morocco.* Brigham Young

University, Provo, Utah, USA, pp. 145-155.

Perry, B.D. (1993) Dog ecology in eastern and southern Africa: implications for rabies control. *Onderstepoort Journal of Veterinary Research* 60, 429-436.

Petersen, C.G.J. (1896) The yearly immigration of young plaice into Limfjord from the German sea. *Report of the Danish Biological Station* 6, 1-48.

Pollock, K.H., Nichols, J.C., Brownie, C. and Hines, J.E. (1990) Statistical inference for capture-recapture experiments. *Wildlife Monographs* 107, 1-97.

Price, E.O. (1984) Behavioral aspects of animal domestication. *Quarterly Review of Biology* 59, 1-32.

Progulske, D.R. and Baskett, T.S. (1958) Mobility of Missouri deer and their harassment by dogs. *Journal of Wildlife Management* 22, 184-192.

Prosperi, S., Giovannini, A., Ostanello, F. and Rossi, T. (1992) Evaluation of the size of stray dog population and of related problems in Emilia-Romagna. *Annali dell'Istituto Superiore di Sanita* 28, 485-491.

Rangel, M.C.F., Lara, J.C. and Aluja, A.S. (1981) The canine population of Mexico City: an estimative study. *Animal Regulation Studies* 3, 281-290.

Rautenbach, G.H., Boomker, J. and De Villiers, I.L. (1991) A descriptive study of the canine population in a rural town in southern Africa. *Journal of the South African Veterinary Association* 62, 158-162.

Robertshaw, J.D. and Harden, H. (1985) The ecology of the dingo in North-Eastern New South Wales. II. Diet. *Australian Wildlife Research* 12, 39-50.

Robinson, R.D., Thompson, D.L. and Lindo, J.F. (1989) A survey of intestinal helminths of well-cared-for dogs in Jamaica West Indies and their potential public health significance. *Journal of Helminthology* 63, 32-38.

Rowlands, I.W. (1991) Some observations on the breeding of the dog. *Proceedings of the Society for the Study of Fertility* 1, 40-55.

Rubin, H.D. and Beck, A.M. (1982) Ecological behavior of free-ranging urban pet dogs. *Applied Animal Ethology* 8, 161-168.

Sacks, J.J., Sattin, R.W. and Bonzo, S.E. (1989) Dog bite-related fatalities from 1979 through 1988. *Journal of the American Medical Association* 262, 1489-1492.

Schmidt, C.G., Margolles, C.C., Curdi, L.J. and Igarza, A.A. (1993) Population densities of feral dogs in north-eastern Spain, estimated using two different methods. *Revue Scientifique et Technique de l'Office International des Epizooties* 12, pp. 189.

Schöttler, G. (1998) Studie zum Vorkommen von Wurmeiern - insbesondere von Eiern des Hundespulwurmes (Larva migrans visceralis-Syndrom) im Strandsand von Warnemünde 1997. *Gesundheitswesen* 60, 766-767.

Schwartz, M. (1997) *A History of Dogs in the Early Americas*. Yale University Press, New Haven, Connecticut.

Scott, M.D. and Causey, K. (1973) Ecology of feral dogs in Alabama. *Journal of Wildlife Management* 37, 253-265.

Scrimgeour, E.M., Smith, H.V., Prentice, M. and McGahy, I. (1996) Toxocara control: failure of dog-owners to carry out regular deworming of their pets. *International Journal of Environmental Health Research* 6, 27-30.

Seber, G.A.F. (1982) *The Estimation of Animal Abundance and Related Parameters*. Edward Arnold, London.

Serpell, J.A. (1998) Demonic pets: the concept of the witch's familiar in early modern England. In: The International Association of Human-Animal Interaction Organization (ed.) *Human-Animal Interactions and Zoonoses Prevention and Control in Developing Countries*. WHO/IAHAIO, Prague, pp. 83.

Shille, V.M. and Stabenfeldt, G.H. (1980) Current concepts in reproduction of the dog and cat. *Advances in Veterinary Science and Comparative Medicine* 24, 211-243.

Singer, P. (1997) Neither human nor natural: ethics and feral animals. *Reproduction Fertility and Development* 9, 157-162.

Stone, C.P. and Loope, L.L. (1987) Reducing negative effects of introduced animals on native biotas in Hawaii: what is being done, what needs doing, and the role of the national parks. *Environmental Conservation* 14, 245-258.

Sweeney, J.R., Marchinton, R.L. and Sweeney, J.M. (1971) Responses of radio-monitored white-tailed deer chased by hunting dogs. *Journal of Wildlife Management* 35, 707-716.

Taborsky, M. (1988) Kiwis and dog predation: observations in Waitangi State Forest. *Notornis* 35, 197-202.

Talan, D.A., Citron, D.M., Abrahamian, F.M., Moran, G.J. and Goldstein, E.J.C. (1999) Bacteriologic analysis of infected dog and cat bites. *New England Journal of Medicine* 340, 85-92.

Tarasov, S.A. (1984) Age pecularities of baculum in some mammals. *Zoologicescij Zhurual* 63, 120-125.

Thomson, G.M. (1922) *The Naturalization of Animals and Plants in New Zealand*. Cambridge, England.

Thomson, P.C. (1992a) The behavioral ecology of dingoes in North-western Australia. I. The Fortescue River study area and details of captured dingoes. *Wildlife Research* 19, 509-518.

Thomson, P.C. (1992b) The behavioral ecology of dingoes in North-western Australia. II. Activity patterns, breeding season, and pup rearing. *Wildlife Research* 19, 519-530.

Thomson, P.C. (1992c) The behavioral ecology of dingoes in North-western Australia. III. Hunting and feeding behavior, and diet. *Wildlife Research* 19, 531-541.

Thomson, P.C. (1992d) The behavioural ecology of dingoes in North-western Australia. IV. Social and spatial organization, and movements. *Wildlife Research* 19, 543-563.

Titcomb, M. and Pukui, M.K. (1969) *Dog and Man in the Ancient Pacific With Special Attention to Hawaii*. Bernice P. Bishop Museum Special Pub. 59, Honolulu, Hawaii.

Topal, J. and Csanyi, V. (1998) Evaluation of the dog-owner bond: a new application of the Ainsworth's strange situation test. In: The International Association of Human-Animal Interaction Organization (ed.) *Human-Animal Interactions and Zoonoses Prevention and Control in Developing Countries*. WHO/IAHAIO, Prague, pp. 89.

Triggs, B., Brunner, H. and Cullen, J.M. (1984) The food of fox, dog and cat in Crajingalong National Park, South-Eastern Victoria. *Australian Wildlife*

Research 11, 491-499.

Tyndale-Biscoe, C.H. (1994) Virus-vectored immunocontraception of feral mammals. *Reproduction Fertility and Development* 6, 281-287.

Vos, A. and Turan, B. (1998) Study of the dog population in Istanbul, Turkey. *The Journal of Etlik Veterinary Microbiology* 9, 25-34.

Waltner-Toews, D. (1993) Zoonotic disease concerns in animal-assisted therapy and animal visitation programs. *Canine Veterinary Journal* 34, 549-551.

Wandeler, A.I. (1985) Ecological and epidemiological data requirements for the planning of dog rabies control. In: Kuwert, E., Mérieux, C., Koprowski, H. and Bögel, K. (eds) *Rabies in the Tropics.* Springer-Verlag, Berlin, pp. 657-661.

Wandeler, A.I. and Capt, S. (1985) Ecologie du chien. In: Rosset, R. (ed.) *Pasteur et la Rage.* Informations Techniques des Services Vétérinaires, pp. 115-120.

Wandeler, A.I., Matter, H.C., Kappeler, A. and Budde, A. (1993) The ecology of dogs and canine rabies: a selective review. *Revue Scientifique et Technique de l'Office International des Epizooties* 12, 51-71.

Watson-Jones, D.L. and Macpherson, C.N.L. (1988) Hydatid disease in the Turkana district of Kenya. VI. Man:dog contact and its role in the transmission and control of hydatidosis amongst the Turkana. *Annals of Tropical Medicine and Parasitology* 82, 343-356.

Wayne, R.K. (1993) Molecular evolution of the dog family. *Trends in Genetics* 9, 218-224.

Whitehouse, S.J.O. (1977) The diet of the Dingo in Western Australia. *Australian Wildlife Research* 4, 145-150.

Wilson, E.O. (1975) *Sociobiology: the New Synthesis* Belknap/Harvard University Press, Cambridge, Massachusetts.

WHO (1984) *Guidelines for Dog Rabies Control.* WHO, Geneva.

WHO (1988) *Report of WHO Consultation on Dog Ecology Studies Related to Rabies Control. Geneva, 22-25 February 1988.* WHO, Geneva.

WHO (1994) *Report of the Fifth Consultation on Oral Immunization of Dogs Against Rabies: Organized by WHO With the Participation of the Office International des Epizooties (OIE). Geneva, 20-22 June 1994.* WHO, Geneva.

WHO (1998) *World Survey of Rabies N° 32 for the Year 1996.* WHO, Geneva.

WHO and WSPA (1990) *Guidelines for Dog Population Management.* WHO, Geneva.

Wright, J.C. (1991) Canine aggression toward people. Bite scenarios and prevention. *Veterinary Clinics of North America: Small Animal Practice* 21, 299-314.

Chapter Three

Dogs and Rabies

Alexander I. Wandeler and John Bingham

Rabies is a zoonosis. Perhaps it would be better to say: Rabies are zoonoses in a number of different mammalian hosts caused by a variety of lyssaviruses. As a disease entity with distinctive clinical and epidemiological features, it has been recognized since antiquity. However, its ranking among all human health concerns is difficult; too many imponderabilities are attached to it. It is a reportable disease in most countries, and most countries provide legislation for controlling it. Rabies control programs aim at protecting human health and preventing economic losses. The occurrence of rabies in humans can be controlled by prophylactic vaccination and postexposure treatment and reducing the risk of exposure, or conclusively, by disease elimination in the host species. The easiest way to reduce the incidence of human infection is by prophylactic immunization of those domestic animals which are the most common source of human exposure. It is a considerably more ambitious task to eliminate rabies in its principal host populations.

Although a large number of mammalian species are susceptible to infection with rabies viruses, only a few are recognized as important for the persistence of the disease in nature. In these principal host species, a prolonged enzootic existence is possible because of sets of coadapted traits of susceptibility, viral evasion of immune surveillance, long incubation, excretion in saliva, neurological disorders that promote transmission, host life history traits, social behavior, and population biology. *Chiroptera* (bats) are identified as hosts of lyssaviruses in Africa, the Americas, Australia, and Europe. Different *Carnivora*, including domestic dogs, are the principal hosts for classical rabies (serotype 1) in Asia, Africa, Europe, and in the Americas. From a human health and disease control standpoint one may distinguish between bat rabies, rabies maintained by terrestrial wildlife, and dog rabies.

The rabies virus

Rabies virus and related viruses constitute the genus *Lyssavirus* (Murphy *et al.*, 1995). Lyssaviruses are members of the family *Rhabdoviridae* (Greek *rhabdos* =

rod) and of the order *Mononegavirales*. All rhabdoviruses share a common morphology, genome structure, and replication mechanisms (Tordo *et al.*, 1998).

Rabies virus structure

The rabies virus genome is an unsegmented negative strand RNA molecule of approximately 12,000 nucleotides in length, coding for the five rabies structural proteins designated N, P (formerly M1 or NS), M (formerly M2), G, and L (Tordo, 1996). Rabies viruses are enveloped short cylindrical rods of approximately 75 nm in diameter and 100 to 300 nm in length. They are often described as bullet-shaped, rounded at one end, and more or less flat at the other. The virion envelope is composed of membrane (matrix) protein (M) and glycoprotein (G-protein) molecules, the G-protein forming spikes that cover the surface. Inside the virion is a dense helical ribonucleocapsid cylinder consisting of the viral genome RNA covered with N, P, and L-protein molecules.

Virus replication

Rabies virions bind to cell surface receptors with the assistance of specific regions of the G-protein. One of these binding sites is the nicotinic acetylcholine receptor (Baer and Lentz, 1991). Other receptors may also be important, but they are not yet well characterized. Bound virions are internalized into endosomes, from where the ribonucleoprotein (RNP) complexes are released into the cytoplasm. The genomic negative-strand rabies RNA is transcribed into positive-strand "anti-genome" for replication and messenger RNA's for protein synthesis (Tordo and Kouznetzoff, 1993). The newly made G-proteins are incorporated into the host cell membrane, while the other synthesized viral protein encapsidate the RNA progeny to form RNP. RNP accumulates in inclusion bodies, which are visible in histological preparations as Negri bodies. RNP strands are coiled into dense helices before they are incorporated into virions budding from cellular membranes fitted with G-protein spikes.

Physical properties

Rabies viruses are quite fragile. They are readily inactivated by elevated temperatures, UV light, detergents and organic solvents, and by extreme pH values. The destructive influence of physical and chemical agents is greatly modified by stabilizing effects of polypeptides and other compounds (Michalski *et al.*, 1976). This signifies in practical terms that most of the virus on the exposed surface of a dead animal is inactivated within a few hours, and that the infectivity in internal organs is lost within a few days in summer, but can persist for many weeks under cool weather conditions.

Other lyssaviruses

The genus *Lyssavirus* contains numerous distinct viruses isolated from mammals, fish, and arthropods (Rupprecht *et al.*, 1991). Some rabies-related Lyssaviruses have been grouped into four serotypes: rabies (serotype 1), Lagos bat (serotype 2), Mokola (serotype 3), and Duvenhage (serotype 4). Serotypes 2, 3, and 4 have so far been found in Africa only. The serological classification is now becoming obsolete with the accumulation of virus genome sequence data and their phylogenetic analysis. Based on such information it has been suggested to group the rabies-related viruses into six genotypes (Bourhy *et al.*, 1993). Genotype 1 accommodates the old serotype 1, the classical rabies virus strains. It occurs on all continents, except Australia and Antarctica. Genotype 2 replaces serotype 2: Lagos bat virus. Mokola viruses are genotype 3 (serotype 3). Duvenhage viruses are genotype 4 (serotype 4). Genotype 2, 3, and 4 viruses have so far been found in Africa only (King *et al.*, 1994). European bat lyssavirus type 1 (EBL1) is genotype 5. European bat lyssavirus type 2 (EBL2) is genotype 6. EBL viruses are restricted to Europe (Eurosiberia). Lyssaviruses isolated from bats in Australia, which are closely related to genotype 1, may be considered an additional genotype 7. Viruses of all genotypes cause rabies-like clinical disease in mammals.

Antigenic and genetic variation

The mutation rate of RNA virus genomes is a thousand to a millionfold higher than that of DNA genomes. This is due largely to the absence of intrinsic proofreading mechanisms in RNA replication. Average frequencies of base substitutions in rhabdoviruses are estimated to be 10^{-4} to 4×10^{-4} per base incorporated. Such a level of base change dictates that RNA viruses exist as heterogeneous populations. The expression "quasispecies" is frequently applied to such polymorphic populations. It should be noted that the predictions from a mathematical model describing populations of self-replicating RNA molecules characterized by a high rate of erroneous copying are only partially fulfilled. Despite the obvious potential for random viral mutation, overall high levels of conservation are found in wild rabies isolates. This suggests that substantial selective pressures do operate. The quasispecies concept highlights the evolutionary potential of genetic variation. A polynucleotide can guide itself along fitness gradients to fitness peaks. If "self-guided tours" in the fitness landscape were a possibility for rabies virus, one would expect that it should switch principal hosts opportunistically. This is obviously not the case; rabies genomes appear to be trapped at local fitness optima. Adaptations to new hosts or the adoption of other transmission strategies may both be difficult due to structural and functional constraints or may need too many simultaneous coadapted changes. Though intricate, future invasions of new hosts are possible at a similar frequency as occurred in the past.

Despite the obvious constraints on random variability, hosts do permit some viral polymorphism. Such heterogeneities have been described in individual hosts (Morimoto *et al.*, 1998) as well as in host populations (Nadin-Davis *et al.*, 1993). Molecular genome analysis is necessarily more apt to uncover polymorphism than phenotypic analysis with Mabs. There are essentially two reasons for this: More mutants are synonymous than non-synonymous, and a fair number of non-synonymous mutants are not detected by monoclonal antibodies (Mabs), both indicating functional constraints on the phenotypic structure.

The viral polymorphism poses some diagnostic challenges, particularly when examining individual infected hosts. Neither molecular analysis of a PCR product with REA nor consensus sequencing, nor the application of Mabs for a phenotypic examination will necessarily detect viral heterogeneity. In the best case these methods detect one of several variants present, in the worst they let a mixture of variants appear as a new version of the virus.

Virus variants occurring in dogs

In Europe and North America dogs are frequently infected with the rabies virus variants circulating in populations of wild *Carnivora*, such as red foxes, striped skunks, and raccoons. Only rarely are dogs infected with American bat rabies variants. All these cases are considered spillover from a host that permits a particular virus variant to enzootic persistence, to dogs, a species that is susceptible, but does not have the appropriate biological attributes for continuous transmission of this virus in its populations. The situation is a bit more complicated in Southern Africa, where rabies epizootics in dogs and in jackals (*Canis mesomelas* and *Canis adustus*) appear to be independent, though caused by identical virus variants (King and Turner, 1993; Bingham *et al.*, 1999a,b).

Virus variants from areas with predominant dog rabies are all very similar when analyzed with monoclonal antibodies (Wandeler, 1991a). This may indicate functional constraints in their adaptation to the species, but more likely it is reflecting a common ancestry. Smith *et al.* (1992) have analyzed the genetic relatedness of rabies virus isolates using N-gene sequence data. They concluded that the similarity of many dog rabies virus variants from around the world is most likely the result of the introduction of European dogs and their viruses in colonial periods.

Pathogenesis

Rabies has a peculiar pathogenesis that is characterized by virus dissemination within nerve fibers rather than by blood and lymph, the rapid expansion of the infection within the central nervous system (CNS) after a variable, but generally long incubation period, virus excretion with saliva toward the end of the incubation, and the almost invariably fatal outcome.

Transmission

Rabies virus is normally transmitted from dog to dog with virus-laden saliva of the diseased animal via bite wounds. Non-bite transmission (ingestion, inhalation and other mucosal exposure) has been occasionally implicated. It has been suggested that infection may result from mouth-licking and through consumption of regurgitated food, both common practices in many social canids. Such forms of transmission may have occurred in outbreaks which have decimated packs of Cape Hunting dogs (*Lycaon pictus*) (Kat *et al.*, 1996).

Susceptibility

Dogs were not very susceptible to a European fox virus in experiments conducted by Blancou (1985). The LD_{50} (dose required to kill 50% of the animals inoculated) for dogs inoculated intramuscularly was between 10^5 and 10^6 mouse intracerebral LD_{50} ($MicLD_{50}$), this is about one million times more than required for foxes. In contrast, foxes were susceptible to low doses of a canine rabies virus from North Africa, but they resisted the injection of higher doses and became immune (Blancou *et al.*, 1983). Fekadu *et al.* (1982) inoculated dogs with Ethiopian and Mexican street rabies viruses and found significant mortality with doses as low as 1.7 $MicLD_{50}$. Dogs are also susceptible to Mokola virus and to experimental Lagos bat virus infection (Percy *et al.*, 1973; Tignor *et al.*, 1973; Foggin, 1983).

No mammal studied so far is completely refractory to rabies virus infection under experimental conditions. There are marked differences in susceptibility to intramuscular injection as demonstrated by Sikes (1962), Parker and Wilsnack (1966), Blancou (1988a), Steck and Wandeler (1980) and others. The outcome of an exposure is not only subject to the host in question, but also dependent on properties of the infecting virus variant (Blancou, 1988a). The basis for species differences in susceptibility and how susceptibility is linked to specific properties of virus variants is not understood, though Baer *et al.* (1990) speculated that the abundance of nicotinic acetylcholine receptors at the entry port would explain the contrast in susceptibility.

Incubation

The time between exposure and first appearance of clinical signs of disease may range from days to years, but the majority of incubation periods observed after experimental inoculation are between three and six weeks. Incubation periods in dogs observed after natural exposure in Zimbabwe are mostly between two to five weeks (Foggin, 1988). Usually, greater viral input leads to a shortened course and vice versa (Fekadu *et al.*, 1982; Fekadu, 1991b), but these often cited relationships are not entirely clear, they are complicated by site of viral entry, immune status, origin of virus, etc.

At the entry (inoculation) site virus replication can be detected in myocytes or in other cells. It is not entirely clear if that is an obligatory step before it gains access to the nervous system or if direct entry into peripheral nerves is the rule (Charlton, 1988, 1994). The transport of rabies virus (genomic RNA, RNP, or virions?) to the CNS may occur in motor and/or sensory fibers in the axons by retrograde axoplasmic flow (Tsiang *et al.*, 1991). Combined active and passive immunization very shortly after exposure mediates the elimination of the virus before it enters the nervous system. In laboratory rodents it is possible to interrupt the transport to the CNS by amputation of the inoculated limb or by neurectomy within a short period after inoculation (Baer *et al.*, 1968).

There is usually no measurable immune response to rabies during incubation period, except when animals are inoculated with relatively high doses (including massive amounts of dead antigen?) of a virus variant adapted to a different species

(Blancou *et al.*, 1983; Hill and Beran, 1992). Several factors may contribute to this phenomenon: low antigenicity of the inoculum and rapid sequestration within peripheral cells and nerves, immunosuppressive effects of rabies virus (Wiktor *et al.*, 1977), and possibly immunodepressive properties of saliva (Tsiang and Lagrange, 1980).

The CNS infection

The virus arrives in the area of the brain or spinal cord having direct neural connections with the inoculation site. In the CNS the virus replicates in the perikarya of neurons; other cell types are only sporadically infected (Iwasaki, 1991). The transmission of virus from one neuron to another is probably mostly by budding on postsynaptic or adjacent plasma membranes followed by endocytosis on or near synaptic junctions (Charlton and Casey, 1979). There is also some virus budding into the intercellular space. Viral dissemination within the CNS is due mainly to retrograde and anterograde axonal transport. The pathology and the distribution of rabies virus antigen in the CNS are well described (Charlton, 1988; Perl and Good, 1991). Antigen distribution is quite variable. It depends on the site of inoculation and on the infecting virus variant, and may also be more visible in certain (large) cells. Lesions, as visible by standard histology, are usually relatively mild and include some perivascular cuffing, slight neuronophagia and gliosis, and moderate inflammation of meninges. The extent of inflammatory lesions appears to be proportional to the length of the morbidity period (Fekadu *et al.*, 1982). The clinical symptoms resulting from CNS infection are certainly the expression of damaged neuronal functions. Not all behavioral changes are easily explained by the areas of the CNS most obviously affected.

Peripheral organ involvement and excretion

There is extensive infection of peripheral organs in late stages of the disease. Virus replication in the CNS allows a centrifugal spread. Again the virus moves passively inside axons. Rabies virus antigen can then be detected in most organs (Charlton and Casey, 1979; Balachandran and Charlton, 1993). Often it is limited to nerve fibers and ganglia. Replication in extraneuronal tissues is evident in the exocrine cells of salivary glands, lachrymal glands, and pancreas, frequently in myocytes of muscles, occasionally in other tissues such as tonsils and cornea. The virus concentration in peripheral organs can be high, often reaching titers of more than 10^6 MicLD$_{50}$ per gram of tissue (Fekadu and Shaddock, 1984; Baer and Wandeler, 1987; Fekadu, 1988; Fekadu, 1991b). A possible role of tonsil infection and virus excretion by asymptomatic "carrier state" animals is discussed by Fekadu *et al.* (1983).

    The WHO Expert Committee on Rabies recommends that clinically normal dogs and cats having bitten a person be observed for 10 days. The recommendation is based on two observations: First that virus excretion with saliva occasionally occurs a few days before clinical symptoms are detectable, and second that antigen detection in the brain of an infected animal during incubation or in prodromal phases is not always possible. In experimentally infected dogs Vaughn *et al*. (1965) and Fekadu *et al*. (1982) observed virus excretion up to 7 days, but in one case 14 days before the onset of clinical symptoms. Some animals never excrete virus with their saliva, some may excrete intermittently. Foggin (1988) found that only 72% of rabid dogs had viable virus in the salivary glands. Histological examination revealed that some salivary glands in which no virus could be isolated had inflammatory lesions consistent with those found with rabies infection (Foggin, 1988).

Clinical symptoms

There is no single symptom that would unfailingly identify a clinically ill animal as rabid. The clinical symptoms are highly variable (Tierkel, 1975; Baer and Wandeler, 1987; Fekadu, 1991b). During the initial period of sickness there may be increased nervousness and irritability, hyperactivity, tremor, hypersensitivity, abnormal vocalization, abnormal sexual behavior, dyspnoea, sometimes accompanied by elevated body temperature. These prodromal symptoms evolve usually very rapidly, within hours or a few days, into more advanced stages. Based on the manifestation of predominant paralysis or of excitability, the clinical syndrome is classified as dumb (paralytic) or furious. Animals displaying the dumb form may lie quiet for extended periods. Other frequently observed symptoms are pupillary dilatation, protrusion of the third eyelid, and partial paralysis of the lower jaw and tongue leading to drooling of saliva. The dumb form is common in dogs. The furious form is characterized by marked irritability and restlessness; objects within reach are attacked and if small enough often devoured (allotriophagia). However, dumb phases may alternate with furious stages in a single individual. Even animals in a dumb phase may have a tendency to bite when they are provoked and they may snap into the air. In all species the clinical illness progresses toward extensive paralysis, with or without convulsions, and then stupor and death. The range in length of illness from the onset of symptoms to death is from a few hours to a week, and rarely longer than 10 days. Numerous authors provide evidence that rabies virus infection with involvement of the central nervous system is not invariably fatal (Bell, 1975; Fekadu and Baer, 1980; Fekadu, 1991a). Bell *et al*. (1972) did not find any cerebrospinal fluid antibodies in clinically healthy dogs in a survey in an enzootic area in South America and concluded that nonfatal rabies is very uncommon.

Diagnosis and surveillance

Clinical diagnosis

Often rabies is diagnosed on the basis of clinical symptoms. Rapidly worsening symptoms in a dog as described above, and the almost invariably fatal outcome are strong indications for the presence of a rabies virus infection. There is considerable variation in the clinical course within and between species. In addition, symptoms that are considered pathognomonic may never develop. It is therefore advisable to consider as suspect rabies cases all instances of rapidly progressing neurologic disorder in the absence of binding alternate diagnosis. Distemper, infectious canine hepatitis, pseudorabies and a number of other canine diseases causing neurological disorders may be considered differential diagnoses. It is suggested that clinically suspect cases of rabies be submitted for laboratory confirmation when they have contaminated (bitten) humans or when essential for epidemiological surveillance.

Laboratory diagnosis

Current laboratory tests are described in detail in WHO's *Laboratory Techniques in Rabies* (Meslin *et al.*, 1996), in the OIE Manual of Standards (OIE, 1996), and in numerous other publications (Webster and Casey, 1988; Sureau *et al.*, 1991; Trimarchi and Debbie, 1991).

The method of choice is immunofluorescence for the detection of viral antigen in brain impression smears. Impression smears of selected parts (which must include hippocampus, brainstem and medulla oblongata) of the dissected brain are made on microscopic slides. The air-dried smears are fixed in acetone and then incubated with a fluorescein-labeled anti-rabies (preferably anti-RNP) immunoglobulin preparation. The smears are then washed in buffer to remove excess conjugate and examined with a UV microscope. Cytoplasmic viral antigen accumulations, mostly in the form of RNP, appear as fluorescing polymorphic inclusion bodies in perikarya and dendrites. The method is highly specific. Nevertheless, the diagnostician has to take into account that naturally occurring pigments may fluoresce, and that conjugates bind nonspecifically to a number of structures (sometimes by mediation of Fc receptors), especially to contaminating bacteria. The maintenance of proficiency of diagnosticians must be assured.

The demonstration of inclusion bodies in neurons with histological staining methods is less reliable. It gives accurate results in only about 80% of the positive cases when compared with immunofluorescence. Highly reliable is immunohistochemistry on paraffin or frozen sections. This is the method of choice if formalin-fixed tissue is the only material available (Bourgon and Charlton, 1987; Feiden *et al.*, 1988). This method is relatively slow, costly, and requires histology equipment.

A number of other methods (ELISA, PCR, etc.) have been described. They cannot be recommended for general use at present, although most of these methods work quite reliably in specialized laboratories. It is advisable that microscopic findings are confirmed by an additional test, preferably a procedure to isolate and identify the virus in either mice or in tissue culture. Confirmatory tests are especially important when microscopic findings are negative in suspicious cases with histories of human exposure.

Material suitable for surveillance

Specimens can be brought or shipped to the diagnostic center as whole carcasses, heads, extracted whole brains or brain samples collected through the foramen magnum or the orbita with a straw or another suitable probe. The specimens should be transported frozen or refrigerated. It is advisable to transport small pieces of brain (brainstem, medulla oblongata, hippocampus) in 50% buffered glycerol if circumstances do not permit a rapid and refrigerated delivery to the laboratory. One might also consider submitting fresh material and in addition fix half of each brain in formalin for histological or immunohistological processing.

Brain specimens from animals that have acted suspiciously or that have contaminated humans are the material most desirable and suitable for surveillance. Their submission to a diagnostic laboratory should be encouraged. Dogs, wild *Carnivora*, and bats are the species most often recognized as principal hosts. Other domestic *Carnivora* (cats, etc.), domestic herbivores, and wild ruminants are quite often victims of the disease, but they only rarely support epizootics independent from the before-mentioned species. Clearly not suitable for surveillance are rodents and birds, as well as clinically normal animals and roadkill. Not that such material should never be examined in well-defined projects, but it is very likely that the disease prevalence among them is extremely low. It is also not recommended to base rabies surveillance on serology.

There is a host of reasons why serology can be misleading. Antibodies can be measured in neutralization tests (assayed in mice or in tissue culture). The most outstanding but rarely acknowledged problem in neutralization assays are virus inactivating properties that occur quite frequently in blood collected under suboptimal conditions. The problems with nonspecificity that must be overcome in hemagglutination inhibition tests and ELISA's are profound. If one accepts a positive result as real, then one is left with the question of the cause for their presence. Serum antibodies are usually not of very high titer and are not accompanied by cerebrospinal fluid (CSF) antibodies if they are the result of vaccination. Antibody titers are very high in serum and in CSF if they are the corollaries of survival of clinical disease, which is considered to be exceptional. We do not know what antibody levels to expect as results from different forms of abortive infections and non-infective natural exposures (e.g. oral). In addition, the possibility of crossreacting rhabdovirus antibodies has never been investigated properly.

Obligations of the diagnostic center

The most obvious duty of the diagnostic center is to achieve diagnosis rapidly and to report quickly to permit timely postexposure treatment and disease control decisions. A diagnostic center is more useful if it serves a large area and not only its immediate vicinity. It is a formidable task to ensure the submission of specimens from all regions that require diagnostic services and/or need surveillance. It might not be achievable without a network of motivated and well-instructed personnel in agricultural and health services in all regions concerned.

The diagnostic center should give instructions for sample conservation, packaging, completion of submission forms, and transport. The field personnel must also be advised on the purpose of sample submissions and on what categories of specimens to collect. The diagnostic center has to supply material for conservation and packaging if these are not readily available in the field. It also should provide blank submission forms. Submission forms should accompany every specimen. They should furnish the following information: species, date (of submission), location (where animal was found), owner name and address (for domestic animals), type of human exposure (none, bite, other), date of exposure, and names and addresses of exposed people. A number of supplementary information might also be collected, such as clinical symptoms, whether the animal was killed or found dead, age and sex of the animal, and observations on the source of infection.

The diagnostic center should perform a number of additional duties aside from assisting sample submission and achieving laboratory diagnosis. A serotype/genotype identification and/or rabies virus variant characterization should be performed on some, possibly all, specimens found positive in routine testing. Selected samples should be forwarded to laboratories qualified to perform this task if it cannot be achieved in the diagnostic center. Reference samples need to be set aside. They should be stored as original rabid brain samples, or as virus isolates made thereof, at minus 70°C, or better in liquid nitrogen or in lyophilized condition. The strategies of specimen selection for long-term storage is to cover epizootic events spatially and temporally and to represent all virus variants that might circulate independently.

Last but not least, it is the diagnostic center's duty to analyze the findings or to make them available for analysis, and to produce monthly, quarterly or yearly reports. None of the classical epidemiological parameters such as incidence and prevalence are very useful: the specimens submitted to the diagnostic center do not constitute a random sample. A random sample, if one would attempt to analyze one, would have to be enormously large due to the very low prevalence of detectable rabies infections in a population (the infection is not readily detectable in its incubation stage). Simple periodical maps and tables listing by species and area of origin the numbers examined and the numbers found rabid will indicate trends and movements.

Rabies surveillance and rabies-free status

The objective of rabies diagnosis of an individual suspect animal is to enable postexposure treatment decisions. Disease surveillance has additional objectives, such as:

- to establish an understanding of the epidemiology (this will allow the formulation of strategies for public health measures, which includes postexposure treatment policies);
- to promote public awareness;
- to permit disease control planning;
- to monitor the impact of disease control operations;

- to maintain rabies-free status.

According to the OIE International Code the recognition of rabies-free status of a country or area is dependent on the following preconditions:

- Rabies is a notifiable disease.
- An effective system of disease surveillance is in operation.
- All regulatory measures for the prevention and control of rabies have been implemented including effective importation procedures.
- No case of indigenously acquired rabies infection has been confirmed in humans or any animal species during the past 2 years (some exceptions may apply).
- No imported case in *Carnivora* has been confirmed outside a quarantine station for the past 6 months.

Epidemiology

Rabies viruses must be adapted to the physiological traits and the population biology of their hosts (Bacon, 1985; Wandeler, 1991a; Wandeler *et al.*, 1994). They must have a host-specific pathogenicity and pathogenesis. Adaptation of a particular virus strain to its principal host is indicated by the frequency and magnitude of its excretion on one hand and by the host's high susceptibility to it on the other hand. These properties allow for transmission from an infective to a susceptible individual in the event of a biting incident. This has been documented to some extent by *in vivo* experiments on susceptibility and by observations on virus excretion in experimentally infected animals and in field specimens submitted for diagnosis (Blancou, 1988a; Blancou *et al.*, 1991). Viruses must either take advantage of normal mechanisms of social interaction or they must promote infectious contacts by altering host physiology and behavior. Rabies virus, possibly by altering specific neural functions (Charlton, 1994), causes aggressiveness as a prevailing feature among induced behavioral changes. However, susceptibility, aggressiveness, and virus excretion are insufficient attributes for insuring a prolonged persistence of the virus in a host population. Encounters between infective and susceptible individuals leading to transmission must occur at the correct frequency. These and other significant aspects of viral host adaptations are more difficult to explore experimentally.

Dog rabies in different regions of the world

One can easily differentiate between areas where we observe enzootic dog rabies, and areas where the disease in dogs must be considered as spillover from wildlife rabies. Domestic dogs have been the principal hosts of rabies in Europe, the Middle East and Asia for thousands of years (Baer *et al.*, 1996). In contrast, dog rabies has been a more recent phenomenon in other parts of the world. In North

America it was first reported in Mexico in the first years of the 18th century (Baer et al., 1996). It was first recorded in South America in the early years of the 19th century (Steele and Fernandez, 1991). In sub-Saharan Africa rabies was noted for its absence by early European explorers in the middle 19th century and was first reported in dogs in several countries in the early 20th century (Swanepoel, 1994). Probably it was only relatively recently introduced into regions where it is now endemic. In recent decades in large parts of Asia, Africa, and Latin America, rabies virus circulates in the dog population. Between 75% and 99% of all reported cases are in dogs (Turner, 1976; WHO, 1984; Acha and Arambulo, 1985; Blancou, 1988b). Canine rabies is occasionally coined urban rabies. In many countries it is more a problem of periurban and densely populated rural areas, while the case load in cities remains relatively low.

In Europe dog rabies declined after World War I. In the USA rabies was maintained principally by dogs until after World War II. In the second half of the 20th century rabies is prevalent in wild *Carnivora* in Europe, North America north of Mexico, and in parts of southern Africa. In those areas only 0.1-5% of the rabies cases reported annually are in dogs (Tabel et al., 1974; Steck and Wandeler, 1980). Three factors may account for the low prevalence of rabies in dogs: most dogs are restricted in their movements; they are kept indoors or in enclosures and leashed when outside; dog vaccination is strongly recommended or even compulsory. It may also be that virus strains adapted to wild species are not very well suited for propagation within dog populations. There is no recent evidence that wildlife rabies provoked epizootics in stray dog populations in the US or in Europe.

Canine rabies

The epidemiology of rabies is generally not very well understood. Incidence, prevalence, and recovery rates are difficult to record. Unfortunately this holds also for dog rabies in spite of the easy access to dog populations. From information given by Glosser et al. (1970), Beran et al. (1972), Belcher et al. (1976), Mitmoonpitak et al. (1998), and Fekadu (1982), one gets the impression that dog rabies is highly enzootic with only moderate fluctuations in prevalence. This picture is only partially correct, since epizootic patterns have also been described, e.g. by Waltner-Toews et al. (1990) and Eng et al. (1993). Eng et al. (1993) speculate that the outbreak in Hermosillo, Mexico, may have been linked to an increase in population density and a drop in vaccination coverage.

Rabies in dogs generally does not follow a marked seasonal trend in prevalence as it does in many wildlife maintenance hosts (Blancou et al., 1991; Bingham et al., 1999a), although Swanepoel (1994) does record a pronounced seasonal trend for dog rabies in the Natal Province of South Africa. Seasonality in wildlife hosts has been hypothesized to occur as a result of their highly seasonal breeding patterns and strong seasonal territorial instincts, both characteristics which are less well developed in dogs. Domestic dogs tend to breed throughout the year and may frequently breed twice in 1 year.

Epidemics of rabies in dogs are usually not clearly confined behind advancing geographical fronts as has been reported for a number of wild carnivores (Bingham *et al.*, 1999). This may be due to the poor surveillance of dog rabies in countries which do not have developed infrastructures. A spatially less-structured epidemiology may be typical of the disease in this species. Dog rabies epidemics are probably spread to a large degree by human activities, for example in cars and buses as dogs incubating the disease will be moved by their owners to new homes. In addition, dogs will often accompany their owners on foot over long distances, well out of their normal home ranges and rabid dogs will move long distances on their own (Butler, 1998).

Rabies in many dog populations appears to rank high as a cause of adult dog deaths. Although official statistics will often not indicate high prevalence rates of rabies the disease is frequently found when actively searched for. For example, Beran *et. al.* (1972) found that 23.6% of deaths in adult dogs in the Philippines were due to rabies.

Ecology and population biology of dog rabies

How rabies is maintained in dog populations is not very well understood. The rate at which infected hosts transmit rabies to healthy animals depends on the density of the host population and on aspects of the social system of the host which enhance contact between infected and non-infected individuals. Dogs are kept and tolerated at very high numbers in most human societies. Dog population densities may reach several thousand per km^2 (Wandeler *et al.*, 1988, 1993; Chapter 2). This is considerably more than any wild carnivore population ever achieves. It is assumed that high-density dog populations permit the occurrence of enzootic canine rabies. However, rabies persists also in dog populations of densities below 10 individuals per km^2 (Foggin, 1988).

The effective reproductive rate of the disease must average unity in order to permit enzootic persistence. Most canid species, including dogs, are highly adaptable with respect to their social systems (Macdonald and Carr, 1995) and this allows for considerable variation in the social parameters which determine transmission rates.

Rabid dogs will frequently display aggression and actively seek other dogs and other animals to bite. Rabid dogs may also bite following stimuli which would not normally elicit an aggressive response. There is evidence that disoriented rabid foxes (*Vulpes vulpes*) wander into their neighbors' range and are there attacked by the territory owner, this conflict leading to the transmission of the infection (Artois and Aubert, 1985; Wandeler, 1991a). It is quite likely that similar behavioral mechanisms operate in dogs, provoking a healthy dog to get in conflict with a diseased one. Butler (1998), in a study carried out in rural Zimbabwe, found that 15 of 24 rabid dogs wandered from their homes, some wandering considerable distances. These dogs approached homesteads and other dogs and provoked conflicts in the process. Six of 16 dogs for which Butler (1998) obtained detailed records were seen to bite 11 other dogs (all unvaccinated) resulting in transmission to seven of the dogs.

Rabies control

Dog population management

Rabies has a high incidence in dogs in areas where dog populations reach high densities and where the animals are poorly supervised. Attempts to reduce dog numbers and to educate owners toward responsible ownership should therefore be attempted. For this purpose the WHO/WSPA *Guidelines for Dog Population Management* (WHO/Zoon/90.165) should be consulted (Chapter 11; Larghi *et al.*, 1988). Recommended control measures include movement restrictions, reproduction control, habitat control, and removal of straying dogs. The control of movements is intended to limit social contact and access to resources (both leading to disease transmission and uncontrolled reproduction). Reproduction control may be achieved through mating restrictions, surgical sterilization, and drugs (injectable, oral). Habitat control is meant to reduce the availability of resources (litter, waste, shelter). The concept of responsible dog ownership (WHO/WSPA, 1990) as applied in industrialized western nations needs to be adapted to different contexts, taking into account economic, social and cultural constraints. The removal of straying dogs usually has only insignificant effects on population densities and is therefore not a productive method of population control, but it may serve law enforcement and is an aid to education in responsible ownership.

Prophylactic vaccination of dogs, veterinary vaccines for parenteral use

Most of the rabies vaccines used today for the immunization of dogs and other domestic animals contain inactivated rabies virus and dead antigen. Modern inactivated tissue culture vaccines combine safety with high immunogenicity (Chappuis and Tixier, 1982; Bunn, 1988, 1991; Precausta and Soulebot, 1991) and are efficacious in the field (Chomel *et al.*, 1987, 1988; Aubert, 1993; Carlos *et al.*, 1997). Cell lines and primary cell cultures are used as substrates for a number of virus strains. Several manufacturers include a variety of different antigens (distemper, adenovirus, leptospirosis, parainfluenza, parvovirus) in combined vaccines. No indications of competitive inhibition have been noted, but every new product should be investigated for its overall immunogenic potency. Inactivated nerve tissue vaccines may be prepared from brains from lambs or suckling mice inoculated newborn i.c. with fixed viruses. They may be adjuvanted. These vaccines do not always have an efficacy comparable to the efficacy of inactivated tissue culture vaccines. The use of modified live (attenuated) vaccines is no longer recommended for dog immunization, except for special situations (e.g. national campaigns under economic constraints). Live attenuated virus vaccines, such as LEP (low egg passage), HEP (high egg passage), and ERA (Evelyn Rokitniki Abelseth) have been significant components of rabies control in the past. Recombinant vaccines and other products of genetic engineering will probably become available soon (Chappuis, 1997).

Rabies vaccines for dogs should satisfy efficacy and safety requirements as they are described by WHO (1992), OIE (1996), and by national regulatory agencies. It is recommended that vaccines are completely innocuous, even for very young animals, and that they confer immunity for one, preferably 2 years after one injection in all dogs above an age of 3 months.

There are no treatment schedules or vaccines licensed for post-exposure treatment of dogs. The eighth report of the WHO Expert Committee on Rabies states that post-exposure vaccination of a previously unvaccinated animal is of uncertain effectiveness and should be discouraged (WHO, 1992).

Dog vaccination in areas with wildlife rabies

In industrialized nations with predominant wildlife rabies, dog vaccination is recommended or compulsory. Owners have to register (or license) dogs. Registration can be made dependent on the production of a certificate that the animal has been vaccinated against rabies when over 3 months old and has been revaccinated at periods of not more than 2 (1) years. Vaccinations should be done by parenteral inoculation of a product recognized by the national authorities, usually an inactivated vaccine conferring 2 years of immunity after one injection.

Rabies control in areas with canine rabies

Successful attempts at the control of rabies have generally occurred where both vaccination and dog control (destruction, confinement, breeding restrictions) have been practiced simultaneously (Tierkel *et al.*, 1950; Fredrickson *et al.*, 1953; Wells, 1954). Rabies control in areas with canine rabies is usually not a simple application of regulations on dog ownership. Their enforcement is impeded by a number of ecological and cultural constraints. But well planned and executed campaigns may reduce rabies incidence in dogs drastically and may even eliminate the disease in areas where it is not maintained by wildlife. Taking the cost and benefits of a campaign into consideration, we suggest that disease eradication should be the goal rather than a temporary reduction of the incidence rate. Comprehensive national, rather than temporary, local plans are imperative. These plans have to identify a goal, and they have to consider national structures and resources. Effective cooperation among all involved ministries and national and local agencies is necessary. WHO provides useful guidelines for program management (WHO, 1984; WHO/FAO, 1990). These documents give detailed guidance on the planning and management of control programs, on legislation, and on techniques in local program execution.

For planning a comprehensive control program it is necessary to consider a number of dog population parameters (size, turnover, accessibility). A vaccination coverage of about 75% of the total population should be attempted. This goal should be achieved in a particular area within a relatively short time period (a few weeks). Pilot projects may help in assessing: (1) dog accessibility; (2) ways of cooperating with local residents; and (3) avenues to provide information and education. Plans for large-scale operations, vaccination strategies and logistic aspects can then be adjusted according to findings in the pilot phase. An effective maintenance program must be part of the plan. Operational research for monitoring campaign efficiency is strongly recommended.

A number of different approaches can be taken. Firstly, dog owners may take their pets to private or state veterinarians for vaccination. This is the most important way in which population immunity is achieved in the more affluent parts of the world, whereas it only accounts for a small proportion of vaccinations in less wealthy countries where there are few veterinarians within communities or where the cost of a veterinary consultation is too expensive for many people. Secondly the state veterinary services may conduct campaigns of which the most common is the central point campaign where owners are required to bring their pets to a designated place at a particular time. Such campaigns require a considerable amount of prior advertising, using loud-hailers, posters and informal local news networks. Because of this and also because dog owners often have other priorities, or they may not be able to take all their dogs to the central point, this method usually does not reach more than 10% to 40% of dogs (Beran, 1982; Brooks, 1990), but can be much better if properly implemented (De Balogh *et al.*, 1993; Wandeler *et al.*, 1993). A third method of population immunization is the house-to-house vaccination campaign, where the state vaccination teams visit each household and vaccinate every dog which they are able to catch. The latter method, although very demanding of resources, is usually successful in achieving the 70% coverage (Korns and Zeissig, 1948; Beran, 1991; Coleman and Dye, 1996) thought to be necessary to eradicate dog rabies. In many African and Asian countries it is not used extensively because due to resource constraints.

Oral vaccination of dogs against rabies

The high number of human casualties caused by dog transmitted rabies clearly indicates that dog rabies control either is not applied or is failing. There may be many reasons for not reaching a sufficient herd immunity in dog populations by parenteral vaccination: inadequate logistics, insufficient community participation, large numbers of ownerless dogs, etc. It is often thought that a majority of these problems could be solved with an oral vaccine for dogs. Oral vaccination of wildlife has been applied for rabies control since 1978 (Steck *et al.*, 1982; Wandeler, 1991b). A number of live attenuated and genetically engineered vaccines have been tested for safety and efficacy in a variety of species, including dogs (Chappuis *et al.*, 1994; Fekadu *et al.*, 1996). It is essential that oral rabies vaccines for dogs meet higher safety standards than those presently applied to wildlife immunization. At present there are no vaccines licensed for oral immunization of dogs. Such vaccines are under development.

Compared to parenteral inoculation, a vaccine that can be administered orally will reduce distress in the vaccinator, the animal owner, and the animal to be vaccinated. This permits to immunize dogs that otherwise cannot be handled and facilitates community participation if properly advertised. Nevertheless, to achieve a vaccination coverage sufficient for the elimination of dog rabies remains a formidable task (Frontini *et al.*, 1992; Matter, 1997; Ben Youssef *et al.*, 1998). In view of the advantages WHO supports the concept and convened a number of consultations to outline efficacy, safety, and logistic aspects. The WHO consultations recommend that only "door to door" and "hand out" techniques with recuperation of baits and bait fragments if not taken are considered for initial field trials. First field trials using live attenuated vaccines and a vaccinia rabies glycoprotein recombinant are currently under assessment (Bishop *et al.*, 1999). For a more detailed review of oral immunization of dogs against rabies see chapter 12.

Maintenance of rabies-free status

The WHO Expert Committee on Rabies recommends that countries free from rabies should prohibit the importation of certain species of mammals and/or permit their entry only under the authority of a license granted previously. Earlier WHO Expert Committee reports state that "on entry, such animals should be subjected to a prolonged period of quarantine, preferably 4 months or more, on premises approved by the Government veterinary service" (WHO Expert Committee 7th Report, 1984). Only in their 8th report (1992) the Committee is discussing a system of animal identification, vaccination and serology, as an alternative where strict quarantine measures are impractical. The Committee recommends taking into account a number of considerations when contemplating import regulations:

- incubation periods are variable, from a few weeks to more than 6 months; very long incubation periods are rare;
- the immune response to vaccine in immature animals is inadequately defined; certain is that circulating neutralizing antibodies persist for shorter time periods than in adult individuals;
- immune responses vary not only with age, vaccine type, immunization procedure, condition of animal (e.g. parasite load), etc.;
- animals vaccinated during incubation may develop antibody, but disease may not be prevented;
- false positive results occur in current serological tests;
- misidentification of animals, certificates, serum samples, occur;
- the impact of rabies-related viruses and variants of low pathogenicity for dogs is unknown.

Some additional important aspects were addressed during a PAHO/WHO "Expert Consultation on the Technical Bases for the Recognition of Rabies-free Areas and Animal Rabies Quarantine Requirements", held in Santo Domingo, Dominican Republic, in 1994 (PAHO/WHO, 1994). Aside from addressing the question of effective surveillance, it was pointed out that rabies-free countries must have an adequate border control to prevent illegal entry. It was also recommended that all rabies-free countries cooperate with PAHO/WHO for developing contingency plans in case of introduction of rabies infection.

A.I. Wandeler and J. Bingham

The prevention of human rabies

Important components of the prevention of human rabies are the avoidance of potentially infectious contacts, and the proper prophylaxis after exposure. Both should be advocated by public health education. Such education should include information on the epidemiology, clinical signs in animals, zoonosis control, wound treatment after exposure, and should indicate that proper immunotherapy should begin as quickly as possible. Prophylactic immunization is recommended only for people with an elevated exposure risk, such as veterinarians, laboratory personnel.

Post-exposure treatment (PET) should follow national guidelines, which are usually based on WHO recommendations. It should be noted that the PET recommendations of the eighth report of the WHO Expert Committee on Rabies (WHO, 1992) are superseded by the WHO document WHO/EMC/ZOO.96.6 (WHO, 1997), which can be consulted on the WHO web site under Communicable diseases/zoonoses/rabies. Immediate and thorough cleansing of bite wounds is an important first step. The circumstances and nature of the suspected exposure should be considered in all decisions for further treatment. Immunoprophylaxis should be given when a bite by a suspicious animal or a contamination of mucosa or broken skin with potentially infectious material has occurred. Combined active immunization with vaccine and passive immunization with rabies immune globulin is considered the best post-exposure prophylaxis.

Rabies in dogs is a significant threat to human health. Worldwide an estimated 30,000 to 60,000 people die of rabies every year. The number of people receiving postexposure treatment - mostly after dog bites - was judged to be about 3.5 million per year (Bögel and Motschwiller, 1986; Bögel and Meslin, 1990), while a 1997 WHO document puts this figure to 7 to 8 million PET applications each year. Almost all human rabies deaths and the vast majority of treatments after bite exposures occur in developing countries (Acha and Arambulo, 1985), in areas where dog rabies is prevalent (Baer and Wandeler, 1987). This may in part be due to a high rate of exposure to biting dogs (Eng *et al.*, 1993). The highest figures come from South and Southeast Asia, where the annual exposure to dog bites is between 0.1 and 1% of the population. Not all biting dogs are infected with rabies, and not all bites by rabid dogs lead to clinical rabies in the bite victim. Still, up to four human rabies deaths per 100,000 inhabitants are recorded in some areas (Wandeler *et al.*, 1988, 1993).

The widespread occurrence of human rabies is not only due to the frequency of exposures, but also to the failure of applying proper treatment after bites from rabid animals. The appropriate treatment may not be available (spatially, temporally, socially, economically), or the appropriate treatment is not in compliance with traditional (religious) beliefs. It is also possible that the necessity of the appropriate treatment is not recognized because other treatments are considered equivalent or superior, or because the disease entity is not recognized. An inquiry into rabies deaths in Sri Lanka revealed that a good proportion of dog-bite victims resort to traditional dog-bite specialists, some with, some without also seeking post-exposure immunoprophylaxis. The success rate of the traditional healer may appear to the casual observer as respectable in view of the low frequency of rabies transmission by mostly healthy biting dogs (Wandeler *et al.*, 1993).

Questions, research needs, operational research

While we believe understanding rabies epidemiology in red foxes (*Vulpes vulpes*) and some other wildlife species fairly well (Steck and Wandeler, 1980; Wandeler *et al.*, 1994), we feel to be quite ignorant when it comes to dog rabies. There are also significant differences between wild carnivore and domestic dog populations. Dog populations reach much higher densities than all wild *Carnivora*, reproduction in dogs is less seasonal, and social organization (the "social use of space") and dynamics are quite different. It is rather awkward that more thorough studies on dog rabies epidemiology are so rare (Butler, 1998). It is sometimes questionable if canine rabies is really independent from a wildlife reservoir. Structural constraints and a shortage of resources may often preclude a suitable epidemiological surveillance and data analysis. On the other hand, the easy access to dog populations should allow collection of valuable data. A systematic collection of detailed case histories could identify possible sources of infection, incubation periods, vaccination records, and contacts with other animals and humans.

A number of dog populations in different parts of the world and in different ecological and cultural settings have been studied in recent years (see chapter 2). Dog population biology is reasonably well explored. Although, one has to remember that tolerance, supervision, availability (accessibility) of resources, and other aspects of the "habitat carrying capacity" are human cultural traits that vary dramatically from area to area. Attributes of culture not only determine dog population characteristics, but also their accessibility for control operations. Questionnaire surveys produce information on dog to human ratios, dog keeping practices, reproduction, morbidity and mortality, etc. Such data relate only to the owned segment of a dog population, taking into account that the ownership status of a dog may change according to criteria applied. If there is a suspicion that a substantial proportion of dogs escape recording, one should resort to an experimental approach as used by wildlife biologists. Modified mark-recapture techniques can be implemented without too many difficulties during mass vaccination campaigns. Such "operational research" conducted in conjunction with pilot projects may provide a large amount of useful data. Pilot projects in general may help in assessing: (1) dog accessibility; (2) ways of cooperating with local residents; and (3) avenues to provide information and education. Plans for large-scale operations, vaccination strategies and logistic aspects can then be adjusted according to findings in the pilot phase. We also suggest that in future programs, some operational research be conducted in order to monitor campaign efficiency.

Human-dog relations are significant factors in dog rabies epidemiology and control. Studies on this topic in non-industrialized nations (Luomala, 1960; Frank, 1965; Meggitt, 1965; Latocha, 1982; Savishinsky, 1994; and others) are usually ignored, while the affinity of people to their pets in industrialized societies has received considerable attention by human-animal-bond champions (see Chapter 1). Dog ownership can have very different meanings in different cultures and is not always easy to define in Western legalistic terms. The tolerance granted to dogs must find explanation in processes of socialization and psychology. Cultural conventions determine the level of supervision of their social interactions and access to resources (food, water, shelter, mates), which is partially a function of the density and structure of human settlements. Education toward responsible dog ownership and disease prevention must conform with cultural conditions.

The ultimate purpose of rabies control is the protection of humans from both infection and economic loss. It is obvious that the elimination of dog rabies, but also the prevention of human rabies has not made the progress one once expected (Bögel *et al.*, 1982). In view of the high efficacy of modern postexposure treatment, nearly all human rabies cases must be considered as failures of the medical system; the correct treatment was not applied, or not applied in time. We will have to pay more attention to the ethnomedical aspects of human rabies. More inquiries into health systems and the ethnology and sociology of preventing and curing dog-transmitted diseases are clearly indicated.

References

Acha, P.N. and Arambulo III, P.V. (1985) Rabies in the tropics - history and current status. In: Kuwert, E., Mérieux, C., Koprowski, H. and Bögel, K. (eds) *Rabies in the Tropics*. Springer-Verlag, Berlin, pp. 343-359.

Artois, M. and Aubert, M.F.A. (1985) Behavior of rabid foxes. *Revue d'Ecologie (Terre et Vie)* 40, 171-176.

Aubert, M.F.A. (1993) Can vaccination validated by the titration of rabies antibodies in serum of cats and dogs be an alternative to quarantine measures? *Abstracts on Hygiene and Communicable Diseases* 68, R1-R22.

Bacon, P.J. (1985) A systems analysis of wildlife rabies epizootics. In: Bacon, P.J. (ed.) *Population Dynamics of Rabies in Wildlife*. Academic Press, London, pp. 109-130.

Baer, G.M. and Lentz, T.L. (1991) Rabies pathogenesis to the central nervous system. In: Baer, G.M. (ed.) *The Natural History of Rabies,* 2nd edn. CRC Press, Boca Raton, Florida, pp. 105-120.

Baer, G.M. and Wandeler, A.I. (1987) Rabies virus. In: Appel, M.J. (ed.) *Virus Infections of Carnivores*. Elsevier Science Publishers, Amsterdam, pp. 167-182.

Baer, G.M., Shantha, T.R. and Bourne, G.H. (1968) The pathogenesis of street rabies in rats. *Bulletin of the World Health Organisation* 38, 119-125.

Baer, G.M., Shaddock, J.H., Quirion, R., Dam, T.V. and Lentz, T.L. (1990) Rabies susceptibility and acetylcholine receptor. *Lancet* 335, 664-665.

Baer, G.M., Neville, J. and Turner, G.S. (1996) *Rabbits and Rabies: a Pictorial History of Rabies Through the Ages*. Laboratorios Baer, Mexico, D.F.

Balachandran, A. and Charlton, K.M. (1993) Experimental rabies infection of non-nervous tissues in skunks (*Mephitis mephitis*) and foxes (*Vulpes vulpes*). *Veterinary Pathology* 31, 93-102.

Belcher, D.W., Wurapa, F.K. and Atuora, D.O.C. (1976) Endemic rabies in Ghana. Epidemiology and control measures. *American Journal of Tropical Medicine and Hygiene* 25, 724-729.

Bell, J.F. (1975) Latency and abortive rabies. In: Baer, G.M. (ed.) *The Natural History of Rabies*. Academic Press, New York, pp. 331-354.

Bell, J.F., Sancho, M.I., Diaz, A.M. and Moore, G.J. (1972) Nonfatal rabies in an enzootic area: results of a survey and evaluation of techniques. *American Journal of Epidemiology* 95, 190-198.

Ben Youssef, S., Matter, H.C., Schumacher, C.L., Kharmachi, H., Jemli, J., Mrabet, L., Gharbi, M., Hammami, S., El Hicheri, K., Aubert, M.F.A. and Meslin, F.X. (1998) Field evaluation of dog owner, participation-based, bait delivery system for the oral immunization of dogs against rabies in Tunisia. *American Journal of Tropical Medicine and Hygiene* 58, 835-845.

Beran, G.W. (1982) Ecology of dogs in the central Philippines in relation to rabies control efforts. *Comparative Immunology, Microbiology and Infectious Diseases* 5, 265-270.

Beran, G.W. (1991) Urban rabies. In: Baer, G.M. (ed.) *The Natural History of Rabies,* 2nd edn. CRC Press, Boca Raton, Florida, pp. 427-443.

Beran, G.W., Nocete, A.P., Elvina, O., Gregorio, S.B., Moreno, R.R., Nakao, J.C., Burchett, G.A., Canizares, H.L. and Macasaet, F.F. (1972) Epidemiology and control studies on rabies in the Philippines. *Southeast Asian Journal of Tropical Medicine and Public Health* 3, 433-445.

Bingham, J., Foggin, C.M., Wandeler, A.I. and Hill, F.W.G. (1999a) The epidemiology of rabies in Zimbabwe. 1. Rabies in dogs (*Canis familiaris*). *Onderstepoort Journal of Veterinary Research* 66, 1-10.

Bingham, J., Foggin, C.M., Wandeler, A.I. and Hill, F.W.G. (1999b) The epidemiology of rabies in Zimbabwe. 2. Rabies in jackals (*Canis adustus* and *Canis mesomelas*). *Onderstepoort Journal of Veterinary Research* 66, 11-23.

Bishop, G.C., Berthon, A.F., Schumacher, C., Bingham, J., Byebwa, B. and Aubert, A. (1999) The first field trials in dogs using Rabidog SAG2 oral vaccine baits. In: *The 10th Annual Rabies in the America Meeting.* San Diego, California, USA, 14-19 November 1999, pp. 78.

Blancou, J. (1985) La rage animale, de Pasteur à nos jours - Evolution de son épidémiolgie et de sa prophylaxie. *Bulletin de l'Academie Vétérinaire de France* 58, 455-461.

Blancou, J. (1988a) Ecology and epidemiology of fox rabies. *Reviews of Infectious Diseases* 10, Supplement 4, S606-S609.

Blancou, J. (1988b) Epizootiology of rabies: Eurasia and Africa. In: Campbell, J.B. and Charlton, K.M. (eds) *Rabies*. Kluwer Academic Publishers, Boston, pp. 243-265.

Blancou, J., Aubert, M.F.A. and Soulebot, J.P. (1983) Différences dans le pouvoir pathogène de souches de virus rabique adaptées au renard ou au chien. *Annales de Virologie* 134 E, 523-531.

Blancou, J., Aubert, M.F.A. and Artois, M. (1991) Fox rabies. In: Baer, G.M. (ed.) *The Natural History of Rabies*, 2nd edn. CRC Press, Boca Raton, Florida, pp. 257-290.

Bögel, K. and Meslin, F. (1990) Economics of human and canine rabies elimination: guidelines for programme orientation. *Bulletin of the World Health Organisation* 68, 281-291.

Bögel, K. and Motschwiller, E. (1986) Incidence of rabies and post-exposure treatment in developing countries. *Bulletin of the World Health Organisation* 64, 883-887.

Bögel, K., Andral, L., Beran, G., Schneider, L.G. and Wandeler, A. (1982) Dog rabies elimination. *International Journal of Zoonoses* 9, 97-112.

Bourgon, A.R. and Charlton, K.M. (1987) The demonstration of rabies antigen in paraffin-embedded tissues using the peroxidase-antiperoxidase method: A comparative study. *Canadian Journal of Veterinary Research* 51, 117-120.

Bourhy, H., Kissi, B. and Tordo, N. (1993) Molecular diversity of the lyssavirus genus. *Virology* 194, 70-81.

Brooks, R. (1990) Survey of the dog population of Zimbabwe and its level of rabies vaccination. *Veterinary Record* 127, 592-596.

Bunn, T.O. (1988) Vaccines and vaccination of domestic animals. In: Campbell, J.B. and Charlton, K.M. (eds) *Rabies*. Kluwer Academic Publishers, Boston, pp. 323-333.

Bunn, T.O. (1991) Canine and feline vaccines, past and present. In: Baer, G.M. (ed.) *The Natural History of Rabies*, 2nd edn. CRC Press, Boca Raton, Florida, pp. 415-425.

Butler, J.R.A. (1998) The ecology of domestic dogs, *Canis familiaris*, in the communal lands of Zimbabwe. Doctor of Philosophy thesis, University of Zimbabwe, Harare.

Carlos, E.T., Mangahas, L.C., Batungbacal, M.R., Carlos, R.S., Dubourget, P., Lomabard, M., Miranda, E.G., de la Cruz, E.C. and Hufano, J.N. (1997) Comparison of rabies vaccines in the field. In: Dodet, B. and Meslin, F.X. (eds) *Rabies Control in Asia*. Elsevier, Amsterdam, pp. 71-78.

Chappuis, G.E. (1997) Development of rabies vaccines. In: Dodet, B. and Meslin, F.X. (eds) *Rabies Control in Asia*. Elsevier, Amsterdam, pp. 61-69.

Chappuis, G.E. and Tixier, G. (1982) Étude de la corrélation existant entre le test NIH et les anticorps séroneutralisants obtenus après vaccination chez le chien. *Comparative Immunology, Microbiology and Infectious Diseases* 5, 151-157.

Chappuis, G., Languet, B., Duret, C. and Desmettre, P. (1994) Dog rabies vaccination: The use of recombinant poxviruses by oral and parenteral route. *Proceedings of the Symposium on Rabies Control in Asia*, Jakarta, Indonesia 27-30 April 1993. Fondation Mérieux, Lyon.

Charlton, K.M. (1988) The pathogenesis of rabies. In: Campbell, J.B. and Charlton, K.M. (eds) *Rabies*. Kluwer Academic Publishers, Boston, pp.101-150.

Charlton, K.M. (1994) The pathogenesis of rabies and other lyssaviral infections: recent studies. In: Rupprecht, C.E., Dietzschold, B. and Koprowski, H. (eds), *Lyssaviruses*. Springer-Verlag, Berlin pp. 95-119.

Charlton, K.M. and Casey, G.A. (1979) Experimental rabies in skunks: Immunofluorescent, light and electron microscopic studies. *Laboratory Investigation* 41, 36-44.

Chomel, B., Chappuis, G.B., Cardenas, E., De Beublain, T.D., Maufrais, M.C. and Giambruno, E. (1987) Serological results of a dog vaccination campaign against rabies in Peru. *Revue Scientifique et Technique de l'Office Internationale des Epizooties* 6, 97-113.

Chomel, B., Chappuis, G.B., Cardenas, E., De Beublain, T.D., Maufrais, M.C. and Giambruno, E. (1988) Mass vaccination campaign against rabies: are dogs correctly protected? The Peruvian experience. *Reviews of Infectious Diseases* 10, Supplement 4, S697-S702.

Coleman, P.G. and Dye, C. (1996) Immunization coverage required to prevent outbreaks of dog rabies. *Vaccine* 14, 185-186.

De Balogh, K.K.I.M., Wandeler, A.I. and Meslin, F.X. (1993) A dog ecology study in an urban and a semi-rural area of Zambia. *Onderstepoort Journal of Veterinary Resesearch* 60, 437-443.

Eng, T.R., Fishbein, H.E., Talamante, H.E., Hall, D.B., Chavez, G.F., Dobbins, J.G., Muro, F.J., Bustos, J.L., De Los Angeles Ricardt, M., Munguia, A., Carrasco, J., Robles, A.R. and Baer, G.M. (1993) Urban epizootic of rabies in Mexico: epidemiology and impact of animal bite injuries. *Bulletin of the World Health Organisation* 71, 615-624.

Feiden, W., Kaiser, E., Gerhard, L., Dahme, E., Gylstorff, B., Wandeler, A. and Ehrensberger, F. (1988) Immunohistochemical staining of rabies virus antigen with monoclonal and polyclonal antibodies in paraffin tissue sections. *Journal of Veterinary Medicine* B 35, 247-255.

Fekadu, M. (1982) Rabies in Ethiopia. *American Journal of Epidemiology* 115, 266-273.

Fekadu, M. (1988) Pathogenesis of rabies virus infection in dogs. *Reviews of Infectious Diseases* 10, Supplement 4, S678-S683.

Fekadu, M. (1991a) Latency and aborted rabies. In: Baer, G.M. (ed.) *The Natural History of Rabies*, 2nd edn. CRC Press, Boca Raton, Florida, pp. 191-198.

Fekadu, M. (1991b) Canine rabies. In: Baer, G.M. (ed.) *The Natural History of Rabies,* 2nd edn. CRC Press, Boca Raton, Florida, pp. 367-387.

Fekadu, M. and Baer, G.M. (1980) Recovery from clinical rabies of 2 dogs inoculated with a rabies virus strain from Ethiopia. *American Journal of Veterinary Research* 41, 1632-1634.

Fekadu, M. and Shaddock, J.H. (1984) Peripheral distribution of virus in dogs inoculated with two rabies virus strains. *American Journal of Veterinary Research* 45, 724-729.

Fekadu, M., Chandler, F.W. and Horizon, A.K. (1982) Pathogenesis of rabies in dogs inoculated with an Ethiopian rabies virus strain. Immuno-fluorescence histologic and ultrastructural studies of central nervous system. *Archives of Virology* 71, 109-126.

Fekadu, M., Shaddock, J.H., Chandler, F.W. and Baer, G.M. (1983) Rabies virus in the tonsils of a carrier dog. *Archives of Virology* 78, 37-47.

Fekadu, M., Nesby, S.L., Shaddock, J.H., Schumacher, C.L., Linhart, S.B. and Sanderlin, D.W. (1996) Immunogenicity, efficacy and safety of an oral rabies vaccine (SAG-2) in dogs. *Vaccine* 14, 465-468.

Foggin, C.M. (1983) Mokola virus infection in cats and a dog in Zimbabwe. *Veterinary Record* 113, 115.

Foggin, C.M. (1988) Rabies and rabies-related viruses in Zimbabwe: Historical, virological and ecological aspects. Doctor of Philosophy thesis, University of Zimbabwe, Harare.

Frank, B. (1965) *Die Rolle des Hundes in Afrikanischen Kulturen.* Franz Steiner Verlag, Wiesbaden.

Fredrickson, L.E., Willett, J.C., Smith, J.E. and Price, E.R. (1953) Mass immunization of dogs against rabies. Its influence on a rabies epizootic in St. Louis. *American Journal of Public Health* 43, 399-404.

Frontini, M.G., Fishbein, D.B., Ramos, J.G., Collins, E.F., Torres, J.M.B., Huerta, G.Q., Rodriguez, J.D.G., Belotto, A.J., Dobbins, J.G., Linhart, S.B. and Baer, G.M. (1992) A Field Evaluation in Mexico of Four Baits for Oral Rabies Vaccination of Dogs. *American Journal of Tropical Medicine and Hygiene* 47, 310-316.

Glosser, J.W., Hutchinson, L.R., Rich, A.B., Huffaker, R.H. and Parker, R.L. (1970) Rabies in El Paso, Texas, before and after institution of a new rabies control program. *Journal of the American Veterinary Medical Association* 157, 820-825.

Hill, R.E. and Beran, G.W. (1992) Experimental inoculation of raccoons (*Procyon lotor*) with rabies virus of skunk origin. *Journal of Wildlife Diseases* 28, 51-56.

Iwasaki, Y. (1991) Spread of virus within the central nervous system. In: Baer, G.M. (ed.) *The Natural History of Rabies,* 2nd edn. CRC Press, Boca Raton, Florida, pp. 121-132.

Kat, P.W., Alexander, K.A., Smith, J.S., Richardson, J.D. and Munson, L. (1996) Rabies among African wild dogs (*Lycaon pictus*) in the Masai Mara, Kenya. *Journal of Veterinary Diagnostic Investigation* 8, 420-426.

King, A.A. and Turner, G.S. (1993) Rabies: a review. *Journal of Comparative Pathology* 108, 1-39.

King, A.A., Meredith, C.D. and Thomson, G.R. (1994) The biology of southern African lyssavirus variants. In: Rupprecht, C.E., Dietzschold, B. and Koprowski, H. (eds) *Lyssaviruses. Current Topics in Microbiology and Immunology,* 187. Springer-Verlag, Berlin, pp. 267-295.

Korns, R.F. and Zeissig, A. (1948) Dog, fox, and cattle rabies in New York State. *American Journal of Public Health* 38, 50-65.

Larghi, O.P., Arrosi, J.C., Nakajata, A.J. and Villa-Nova, A. (1988) Control of urban rabies. In: Campbell, J.B. and Charlton, K.M. (eds) *Rabies.* Kluwer, Boston, pp. 407-422.

Latocha, H. (1982) *Die Rolle des Hundes bei Südamerikanischen Indianern.* Renner, Hohenschäftlarn, Germany.

Luomala, K. (1960) The native dog in the Polynesian system of values. In: Diamond, S. (ed.) *Culture in History.* Columbia University Press, New York, pp. 190-240.

Macdonald, D.W. and Carr, G.M. (1995) Variation in dog society: between resource dispersion and social flux. In: Serpell, J. (ed.) *The Domestic Dog: its Evolution, Behavior and Interactions With People.* Cambridge University Press, Cambridge, pp. 199-216.

Matter, H.C. (1997) Oral immunization of dogs: analysis of dog populations and bait delivery systems. In: Dodet, B. and Meslin, F.X. (eds) *Rabies Control in Asia.* Elsevier, Amsterdam, pp. 47-59.

Meggitt, M.J. (1965) The association between Australian aborigines and dingoes. In: Leeds, A. and Vayda, A.P. (eds) *Man, Culture, and Animals.* AAAS, Washington, DC, pp. 7-26.

Meslin, F.X., Kaplan, M.M. and Koprowski, H. (eds) (1996) *Laboratory Techniques in Rabies,* 4th edn. WHO, Geneva.

Michalski, F., Parks, N.F., Sokol, F. and Clark, H.F. (1976) Thermal inactivation of rabies and other rhabdoviruses: stabilization by the chelating agent ethylenediaminetetraacetic acid at physiological temperatures. *Infection and Immunity* 14, 135-143.

Mitmoonpitak, C., Tepsumethanon, V. and Wilde, H. (1998) Rabies in Thailand. *Epidemiology and Infection* 120, 165-169.

Morimoto, K., Hooper, D.C., Carbaugh, H., Fu, Z.F., Koprowski, H. and Dietzschold, B. (1998) Rabies virus quasispecies: implications for pathogenesis. *Proceedings of the National Academy of Sciences of the United States of America* 95, 3152-3156.

Murphy, F.A., Fauquet, C.M., Bishop, D.H.L., Ghabrial, S.A., Jarvis, A.W., Martelli, G.P., Mayo, M.A. and Summers, M.D. (1995) *Virus Taxonomy.* Springer-Verlag, Vienna.

Nadin-Davis, S.A., Casey, G.A. and Wandeler, A. (1993) Identification of regional variants of the rabies virus within the Canadian province of Ontario. *Journal of General Virology* 74, 829-837.

Office International Des Epizooties (1996) *Manual of Standards for Diagnostic Tests and Vaccines.* OIE, Paris.

PAHO/WHO (1994) 'Expert Consultation on the Technical Bases for the Recognition of Rabies-free Areas and Animal Rabies Quarantine Requirements', held in Santo Domingo, Dominican Republic, in 1994.

Parker, R.L. and Wilsnack, R.E. (1966) Pathogenesis of skunk rabies virus: quantitation in skunks and foxes. *American Journal of Veterinary Research* 27, 33-38.

Percy, D.H., Bhatt, P.N., Tignor, G.H. and Shope, R.R. (1973) Experimental infection of dogs and monkeys with two rabies serogroup viruses, Lagos bat and Mokola (ib An 27377). *Veterinary Pathology* 10, 534-549.

Perl, D.P. and Good, P.F. (1991) The pathology of rabies in the central nervous system. In: Baer, G.M. (ed.) *The Natural History of Rabies,* 2nd edn. CRC Press, Boca Raton, Florida, pp. 163-190.

Precausta, P. and Soulebot, P.J. (1991) Vaccines for Domestic Animals. In: Baer, G.M. (ed.) *The Natural History of Rabies,* 2nd edn. CRC Press, Boca Raton, Florida, pp. 445-459.

Rupprecht, C.E., Dietzschold, B., Wunner, W.H. and Koprowski, H. (1991) Antigenic relationships of lyssaviruses. In: Baer, G.M. (ed.) *The Natural History of Rabies,* 2nd edn. CRC Press, Boca Raton, Florida, pp. 69-100.

Savishinsky, J.S. (1994) *The Trail of the Hare - Environment and Stress in a Sub-arctic Community,* 2nd edn. Gordon and Breach Science Publishers, Yverdon, Switzerland.

Sikes, R.K. (1962) Pathogenesis of rabies in wildlife. I. Comparative effect of varying doses of rabies virus inoculated into foxes and skunks. *American Journal of Veterinary Research* 23, 1041-1047.

Smith, J.S., Orciari, L.A., Yager, P.A., Seidel, H.D. and Warner, C.K. (1992) Epidemiologic and historical relationships among 87 rabies virus isolates as determined by limited sequence analysis. *Journal of Infectious Diseases* 166, 296-307.

Steck, F. and Wandeler, A. (1980) The epidemiology of fox rabies in Europe. *Epidemiological Reviews* 2, 71-96.

Steck, F., Wandeler, A., Bichsel, P., Capt, S., Häfliger, U. and Schneider, L. (1982) Oral immunization of foxes against rabies. Laboratory and field studies. *Comparative Immunology, Microbiology and Infectious Diseases* 5, 165-171.

Steele, J.H. and Fernandez, P.J. (1991) History of rabies and global aspects. In: Baer, G.M. (ed.) *The Natural History of Rabies,* 2nd edn. CRC Press, Boca Raton, Florida, pp. 1-24.

Sureau, P., Ravisse, P. and Rollin, P.E. (1991) Rabies diagnosis by animal inoculation, identification of Negri bodies, or ELISA. In: Baer, G.M. (ed.) *The Natural History of Rabies,* 2nd edn. CRC Press, Boca Raton, Florida, pp. 203-217.

Swanepoel, R. (1994) Rabies. In: Coetzer, J.A.W., Thomson, G.R. and Tustin, R.C. (eds) *Infectious Diseases of Livestock With Special Reference to Southern Africa,* vol. 1. Oxford University Press, Oxford, pp. 493-552.

Tabel, H., Corner, A.H., Webster, W.A. and Casey, G.A. (1974) History and epizootiology of rabies in Canada. *Canadian Veterinary Journal* 15, 271-281.

Tierkel, E.S. (1975) Canine rabies. In: Baer, G.M. (ed.) *The Natural History of Rabies.* Academic Press, New York, pp.123-137.

Tierkel, E.S., Groves, L., Tuggle, H. and Wadley, S. (1950) Effective control of an outbreak of rabies in Memphis and Shelby County, Tennessee. *American Journal of Public Health* 40, 1084-1088.

Tignor, G.N., Shope, R.E., Gershon, R.K. and Waksman, B.H. (1973) Immunopathologic aspects of infection with Lagos bat virus of the rabies serogroup. *Journal of Immunology* 112, 260-265.

Tordo, N. (1996) Characteristics and molecular biology of the rabies virus. In: Meslin, F.X., Kaplan, M.M., Koprowski (eds) *Laboratory Techniques in Rabies,* WHO, Geneva, pp. 28-51.

Tordo, N. and Kouznetzoff, A. (1993) The rabies virus genome: an overview. *Onderstepoort Journal of Veterinary Research* 60, 263-269.

Tordo, N., Charlton, K. and Wandeler, A. (1998) Rhabdoviruses: Rabies. In: Collier, L., Balows, A. and Sussman, M. (eds) *Topley and Wilson's*

Microbiology and Microbial Infections, 9th edn., vol.1. Arnold, London, pp. 665-692.

Trimarchi, C.V. and Debbie, J.G. (1991) The fluorescent antibody in rabies. In: Baer, G.M. (ed.) *The Natural History of Rabies,* 2nd edn. CRC Press, Boca Raton, Florida, pp. 219-233.

Tsiang, H. and Lagrange, P.H. (1980) *In vivo* detection of specific cell-mediated immunity in street rabies virus infection in mice. *Journal of General Virology* 47, 183-191.

Tsiang, H., Ceccaldi, P.E. and Lycke, E. (1991) Rabies virus infection and transport in human sensory dorsal root ganglia neurons. *Journal General of Virology* 72, 1191-1194.

Turner, G.S. (1976) A review of the world epidemiology of rabies. *Transactions of the Royal Society of Tropical Medicine and Hygiene* 70, 175-178.

Vaughn, J.B., Gerhardt, P. and Newell, K.W. (1965) Excretion of street rabies virus in the saliva of dogs. *Journal of the American Medical Association* 193, 363-368.

Waltner-Toews, D., Maryono, A., Akoso, B.T., Wisynu, S. and Unruh, D.H.A. (1990) An epidemic of canine rabies in Central Java, Indonesia. *Preventive Veterinary Medicine* 8, 295-303.

Wandeler, A.I. (1991a) Carnivore rabies: ecological and evolutionary aspects. *Hystrix*, n.s. 3, 121-135.

Wandeler, A.I. (1991b) Oral immunization of wildlife. In: Baer, G.M. (ed.) *The Natural History of Rabies,* 2nd edn. CRC Press, Boca Raton, Florida, pp. 485-503.

Wandeler, A.I., Budde, A., Capt, S., Kappeler, A. and Matter, H. (1988) Dog ecology and dog rabies control. *Reviews of Infectious Diseases* 10, Supplement 4, S684-S688.

Wandeler, A.I., Matter, H.C., Kappeler, A. and Budde, A. (1993) The ecology of dogs and canine rabies: a selective review. *Revue Scientifique et Technique de l'Office International des Epizooties* 12, 51-71.

Wandeler, A.I., Nadin-Davis, S.A., Tinline, R.R. and Rupprecht, C.E. (1994) Rabies epidemiology: some ecological and evolutionary perspectives. In: Rupprecht, C.E., Dietzschold, B. and Koprowski, H. (eds) *Lyssaviruses. Current Topics in Microbiology and Immunology* 187. Springer-Verlag, Berlin, pp. 297-324.

Webster, W.A. and Casey, G.A. (1988) Diagnosis of rabies infection. In: Campbell, J.B. and Charlton, K.M. (eds) *Rabies*. Kluwer Academic Publishers, Boston, pp. 201-222.

Wells, C.W. (1954) The control of rabies in Malaya through compulsory mass vaccination of dogs. *Bulletin of the World Health Organisation* 10, 731-742.

Wiktor, T.J., Doherty, P.C. and Koprowski, H. (1977) Suppression of cell-mediated immunity by street rabies virus. *Journal of Experimental Medicine* 145, 1617-1622.

WHO/WSPA (1990) *Guidelines for Dog Population Management* (WHO/Zoon/90.165). WHO, Geneva.

WHO Expert Committee on Rabies (1984) *Seventh report. WHO Technical Report Series* 709. WHO, Geneva.

WHO Expert Committee on Rabies (1992) *Eighth report. WHO Technical Report Series* 824. WHO, Geneva.

WHO (1984) *Guidelines for Dog Rabies Control* (VPH/83.43). WHO, Geneva.

WHO (1997) *WHO Recommendations on Rabies Post-exposure Treatment and the Correct Technique of Intradermal Immunization Against Rabies* (WHO/EMC/ZOO.96.6). WHO, Geneva.

WHO/FAO (1990) *Guiding Principles for Planning, Organization and Management of Veterinary Public Health Programmes* (ISS/WHO/FAO-CC/IZSTe/90.11). Rome, WHO/FAO Collaborating Centre for Research and Training in Veterinary Public Health.

Chapter Four

Dogs and Bacterial Zoonoses

Bruno B. Chomel and Jonathan J. Arzt

The pleasures of dog ownership are certainly evident by the popularity of pet dogs in the human population. Such a relationship with dogs started with their domestication in the Mesolithic times. This brought many advantages, but also placed human beings at a greater risk for exposure to dog parasites and pathogens. For example, it has been hypothesized that measles, which today is a specific viral human disease, could have been derived from a close related virus of dogs, the distemper virus, which is specific to dogs at present. The discovery of parvovirus infection in dogs in the late 1970s has raised concern on the role of dogs in the transmission of that agent to humans as well as the potential role of dogs in the transmission of rotavirus and coronavirus. Several parasitic, mycotic and infectious agents can infect both human beings and dogs, and are therefore called zoonoses. There are more than 150 zoonoses, but only a few are associated with dogs. However, some of them are widespread and others can be severe to fatal. Prevalence of zoonoses transmitted from dogs to humans is rather difficult to estimate and will depend on numerous factors: number of infected animals, mode of transmission of the agent, behavioral characteristics of the owners, and existing measures of prevention. Usually, children are at greater risk than adults, because of their closer physical contact with household dogs and their own behavior, including pica and exploration of the environment, through putting objects in their mouth. The present chapter will focus on the bacterial zoonoses associated with dogs. A review of current concepts of bacterial dog-associated human diseases is useful to provide objective information to the dog owner and pet care and management.

Bite-associated bacterial zoonoses

Animal bites represent about 1% of all emergency department visits. Between 70% and 90% of these visits are caused by dog bites (Tan, 1997). Children are more likely to be bitten than adults, and males are twice as likely to be bitten by dogs as females. It is estimated that only 3% to 5% of dog bites will become infected. Most infections associated with dog bites are polymicrobial, with *Staphylococcus* spp., *Streptococcus* spp., and *Corynebacterium* spp. as the most frequently isolated aerobic organisms (Griego *et al.*, 1995). Additionally, anaerobic bacteria, including *Bacteroides* and *Prevotella* species, are present in 38% to 76% of dog bite wounds (Brook, 1987; Alexander *et al.*, 1997). *Porphyromonas* species have been isolated from 28% (31 of 110) of specimens from infected dog and cat bite wounds of humans (Citron *et al.*, 1996). Human cases of infection after dog bites also include septicemia caused by commensal bacteria of the oral flora of dogs, such as *Weeksella zoohelcum, Neisseria weaveri* (Canton *et al.*, 1987). However, bite-related zoonotic bacteria mainly include *Pasteurella* species and *Capnocytophaga canimorsus*.

Pasteurellosis

Pasteurellosis is commonly associated with dog bites and even more frequently with cat bites. *Pasteurella* are commensal bacteria of the oral cavity of dogs and cats. Carriage rates of *Pasteurella* in dogs range from 22% to 81%, but Ganière *et al.* (1993) indicated that pathogenic strains were found in 28% of the dogs tested (versus 77% of the cats). *Pasteurella canis* is the most common isolate from dog bites and *Pasteurella multocida* subspecies *multocida* and *P. septica* were the most common isolates from cat bites (Talan *et al.*, 1999). Several new bacterial species have been isolated from dog and cat bites, including *Reimerella anipestifer, Bacteroides tectum* and *Prevotella heparinolytica*. Swelling, inflammation and intense pain at the bite site a few hours after the exposure are the typical symptoms of *Pasteurella* infection. Penicillin is the antibiotic of choice for treatment, but most patients are more frequently treated with a combination of a β-lactam antibiotic and a β-lactamase inhibitor (Talan *et al.*, 1999). Usually, dog bite treatment includes the administration of amoxicillin-clavulanate (250 mg orally three times a day). Untreated affection can lead to severe complications, including abscess formation, septic arthritis, osteomyelitis, endocarditis, pneumonia or meningitis (Griego *et al.*, 1995).

Capnocytophaga canimorsus infection

Capnocytophaga canimorsus (formerly DF-2), a thin, Gram-negative rod, is reported as part of the normal oral flora of 16% of dogs (Underman, 1987). Most (91%) of the known *C. canimorsus* bite-related human cases resulted from a dog bite (Lion *et al.*, 1996). More than 100 human cases, with a fatality rate of 30%, have been reported from North America, Europe and Australia, since the first described case of *C. canimorsus* septicemia in 1976 (Lion *et al.*, 1996). Because of low virulence, *C. canimorsus* systemic infections occur more often in immunosuppressed or immuno-impaired individuals, such as splenectomized individuals (33%), alcohol abusers (24%) or persons following an immunosuppressive treatment (5%). Most cases have also been reported in persons 50 years old or more. Therefore, when fever occurs in immunosuppressed patients after a dog bite, *C. canimorsus* infection should be considered. Talan *et al.* (1999) recovered *Capnocytophaga* species from 4.7% of the dog and cat bite wounds they cultured. Onset of clinical signs of *C. canimorsus* infection is variable ranging from one day to several weeks (Krol-van Straaten *et al.*, 1990). The condition of the initial wound at time of diagnosis may range from gangrenous to completely healed. Almost all patients present with severe sepsis and fever. Additional symptoms include shock, disseminated intravascular coagulation, meningitis, endocarditis, macular or maculo-papular rash, pneumonia, and peripheral cyanosis. *C. canimorsus* is susceptible to most antibiotics, and penicillin G is recommended as the drug of choice (Lion *et al.*, 1996). The use of amoxicillin/clavulanic acid is a good alternative.

Other bacterial zoonoses accidentally transmitted by dog bites

Other bacterial diseases can accidentally be transmitted by dog bites, such as brucellosis (*Brucella suis*), tularemia (a few cases have been associated to dog or coyote bites), *Erysipelothrix insidiosa* infection (Abedini and Lester, 1997) and leptospirosis.

Cat scratch disease

Reports of human cases of cat scratch disease (CSD) following dog contact have been made. According to Margileth (1993), 95% of his patients had a cat-contact history and 4% a dog-contact history. However, Carithers (1985) reported in his large series (1200 cases) that 99.1% of them had a history of cat contact and was not supportive for any other animal source. No bacteremic dog and a very limited number of seropositive dogs were reported from Hawaii (Demers *et al.*, 1995). A recent report from Japan of a possible case of CSD caused by a dog contact suggests that dogs could also play a role in human *B. henselae* infection (Tsukahara *et al.*, 1998). However, such conclusions need further confirmation.

Gastrointestinal zoonoses

Campylobacteriosis

Campylobacter jejuni, a Gram-negative enteric organism, is a leading cause of human enteritis. Food animals, especially poultry, are the major reservoirs of the organisms, and human infection usually occurs following consumption of contaminated, untreated surface water, unpasteurized milk or undercooked meat. Campylobacteriosis has a higher incidence in AIDS patients than in the general population, causing severe, often bloody, diarrhea and cramping, nausea and fever (Glaser *et al.*, 1994). Most *Campylobacter* infections in dog and man are caused by *C. jejuni*, though *Campylobacter coli* infection does occur. *Campylobacter upsaliensis* has also been reported to cause gastroenteritis in humans. Evidence indicates that contact with infected dogs, especially diarrheic dogs can increase risk of acquiring *C. jejuni* (Blaser *et al.*, 1978; Salfield and Pugh, 1987). Prevalence rates are ranging from 10% to 30% in healthy dogs to 50% to 75% in diarrheic dogs and puppies for *C. jejuni* and *C. coli*. In a cross-sectional study in Denmark (Hald and Madsen, 1997), 29% (21) of the 72 healthy puppies (11-17 weeks old) and 5% (2) of 42 healthy kittens tested were infected with *Campylobacter* (dogs: *C. jejuni* 76%, *C. upsaliensis* 19% and *C. coli* 5%). Puppies are more likely to acquire the infection and show clinical signs (watery diarrhea lasting 3 to 7 days). Infection can also occur after contact with healthy dogs which are intermittently shedding the organism. It is estimated that approximately 6% of enteric campylobacteriosis is transmitted from pet animals (Saeed *et al.*, 1993).

In dogs, symptomatic puppies usually show a 3- to 7-day course of diarrhea with or without anorexia, fever and vomiting (Willard *et al.*, 1987). The diarrhea may be watery, mucoid, or bloody. Infected dogs may or may not show clinical signs of disease. Risk factors associated with non-clinical shedding include high-density housing, age less than 6 months, and autumn seasonality. Fecal shedding of *C. jejuni* in the dog is age dependent and peaks in the first year of life. In humans, the clinical picture of *Campylobacter* infection is an acute onset of fever, headache, abdominal pain and severe watery to bloody diarrhea usually lasting less than a week. Rare cases of relapse, colitis, arthritis and septicemia have been reported.

Diagnosis of infection is based on culture of fecal material on specific media for *Campylobacter* isolation and identification of the isolate. Control and prevention of zoonotic infection depends on interrupting contact with contaminated materials. Infected animals should be isolated from other animals and from children. Hands should be washed after handling the pet, pet's toys, feeding utensils and premises should be disinfected (bleach, quaternary ammonium compounds). Symptomatic treatment (fluid and electrolyte therapy) is recommended for most patients, antimicrobial therapy being reserved for severely ill individuals. Most strains of *Campylobacter* are susceptible to macrolides and fluoroquinolones (Tan, 1997), and erythromycin remains the treatment of choice for *C. jejuni* infections.

Salmonellosis

Salmonella spp. are ubiquitous Gram-negative bacilli which are capable of colonizing the gastrointestinal tracts of humans, dogs and many other species of mammals, but also birds and reptiles. Salmonellosis is one of the best-known gastrointestinal zoonoses (Willard *et al.*, 1987). *Salmonella* are shed in the feces, thus the most common mode of transmission amongst animals or between animal and human is the fecal-oral route. Salmonellosis is an extremely important zoonosis with broad economic and public health ramifications. Typically, millions of cases occur worldwide every year. It has been estimated that 1% of the 40,000 annually-reported salmonellosis cases in the US are associated with companion animals (Stehr-Green and Schantz, 1987). The true incidence of salmonellosis in dogs is unknown, as it is not a reportable disease and most infections are subclinical. Furthermore, fecal samples of dogs with clinical signs of diarrhea and vomiting are not commonly submitted for culture (McDonough and Simpson, 1996).

From 1% to 30% of the fecal samples or rectal swabs taken from healthy domestic pet dogs, 16.7% of dogs boarded in kennels, and 21.5% of dogs hospitalized were found to be positive on bacteriological culture for *Salmonella* (McDonough and Simpson, 1996). Young dogs (< 6 months of age) may have higher prevalences than older dogs and dogs may shed more than one serotype in their feces (Willard *et al.*, 1987). However, transmission of *Salmonella* species from dogs to humans is rare (Tan, 1997).

Most adult dogs shedding *Salmonella* in their stool are asymptomatic. Salmonellosis causes clinical signs mainly in young puppies, pregnant animals or aging dogs. Main clinical signs, after an incubation of 3 to 5 days, include diarrhea, fever, vomiting, malaise, anorexia, dehydration, and possible vaginal discharge especially following abortion in bitches. The acute phase lasts 4 to 10 days. Mortality is usually low (< 10%). Recovering dogs may have intermittent diarrhea for up to 3 to 4 weeks and can shed *Salmonella* in the stools for up to 6 weeks (Willard *et al.*, 1987; McDonough and Simpson, 1996). In humans, gastroenteritis with fever, vomiting, abdominal pain and watery to mucoid diarrhea occurs within a few hours to 2 to 3 days after exposure to infection.

Diagnosis of the infection in dogs, based on culture of feces or rectal swab, often follows identification of human cases in the pet owner's family. Confirmed salmonellosis or undiagnosed gastroenteritis in a family member without a known focus of exposure should prompt a testing of the house pet, even if the dog appears healthy. Young children are more likely to be at risk of developing salmonellosis from either close contact with pets or failure to properly wash their hands after handling animals. Strict hygiene and antibiotherapy, when necessary, should be recommended. Treatment is usually supportive rather than antimicrobial, as antibiotics have been shown capable of extending the period of shedding and triggering systemic disease (Willard *et al.*, 1987).

Yersiniosis

Because of their close contact with humans, pets have been suspected as possible reservoirs for human infection with *Yersinia* species. Such suspicions were based on the isolation of the human-pathogenic serotypes O:3 and O:9 from dogs and cats on several occasions. Although *Yersinia enterocolitica* has been isolated from dogs, sometimes up to 30%, with serotype O:3 accounting for 17% of the *Y. enterocolitica* isolates (Fantasia *et al.*, 1993), data on clinical manifestations have been very limited and the pathogenicity of *Y. enterocolitica* in dogs is still uncertain (Hurvell, 1981; Kapperud, 1994). In an experimental infection of dogs with *Y. enterocolitica* biotype 4, serotype O:3, dogs shed the organism for up to 23 days, and it was readily transmitted between dogs, despite the absence of any clinical sign (Fenwick *et al.*, 1994). Limited reports of diarrhea or bloody, mucoid stools in dogs caused by *Y. enterocolitica* have been published (Willard *et al.*, 1987). Only a few outbreaks have been documented where the likely source of human infection may have been the family's pet dog. In the USA, one case involved a 4-month-old child and puppies born a few weeks prior to the child's illness. The same serotype O:20 was isolated from the child and 3 puppies. Similarly, a child was reported to have been possibly infected from an asymptomatic dog in France (Hurvell, 1981). For infections caused by either *Yersinia pseudotuberculosis* or *Y. enterocolitica*, the role of dogs towards human contamination seems very limited by comparison to cats (Mollaret and Affre, 1981).

   In humans, infection may be asymptomatic. In clinical cases, after an incubation of 4 to 10 days, acute gastro-enterocolitis presents with fever, mucoid diarrhea and abdominal pain, especially in children. Extra-intestinal manifestations include cutaneous lesions, arthritis and possibly septicemia. Diagnosis in humans and animals is mainly based on culture of fecal materials, and identification of the serotype should be performed when a pet origin is suspected. Serodiagnosis is helpful in humans, but of limited value in dogs. Prevention of infection is based on standard hygienic measures, such as quick removal of feces, washing of hands and fomites, use of disinfectants (Willard *et al.*, 1987). Antibiotics of choice for treatment of *Y. enterocolitica* are aminoglycosides and trimethoprim-sulfamethoxasole.

Helicobacter infections

The bacterial genus *Helicobacter* contains at least 18 species. These organisms colonize the gastrointestinal tracts of several mammalian and avian hosts (Foley *et al.*, 1999). Some helicobacters, such as *Helicobacter canis*, *Helicobacter pullorum*, *Helicobacter heilmannii*, and *Helicobacter cinaedi* may be zoonotic. The original description of *H. canis* were from the feces of healthy and diarrheic dogs, and a child with enteritis. *Helicobacter* species have been involved in human peptic ulcer and neoplasia, enteritis and inflammatory bowel disease. Household pets could serve as a reservoir for the transmission of *Helicobacter* spp. to humans (Stolte *et al.*, 1994; McDonough and Simpson, 1996). Thomson *et al.* (1994) reported the transmission from a pet dog to a 12-year-old girl of *Gastrospirillum hominis* (now *Helicobacter heilmannii*) which caused gastric disease in both that was eradicable with treatment. Chronic vomiting and subclinical gastritis are the main manifestations of dog infection with *Helicobacter* (McDonough and Simpson, 1996).

Zoonoses of the respiratory tract

Bordetella bronchiseptica infection

Bordetella bronchiseptica infections have been reported in several instances in humans (reviewed by Ford, 1995), causing mainly pneumonia and upper respiratory tract infections in immunocompromised individuals (Ford, 1995; Woodard *et al.*, 1995; Dworkin *et al.*, 1999). More than 35 cases of human infection due to *B. bronchiseptica* have been reported (Dworkin *et al.*, 1999). *B. bronchiseptica* is a Gram-negative coccobacillus commonly isolated from the respiratory tract of various mammals. Dogs may be healthy carriers of a small number of *B. bronchiseptica* in their pharynx. It was first described in 1910 as a respiratory tract pathogen in dogs (Ferry, 1910). It is one of the infectious agents involved in the highly contagious Kennel Cough syndrome. In the few human cases, pneumonia with interstitial infiltrate is the main clinical feature (Ford, 1995). Treatment with ceftazidine and ciprofloxacin cleared all respiratory symptoms in one case (Decker *et al.*, 1991). Immunocompromised persons should restrict themselves and their dogs to any dog gathering, such as dog shows, boarding kennels (Angulo *et al.*, 1994). Vaccination of the dogs may help reduce such a risk, but will not eliminate it, as these dogs can still be potential carriers of the bacterium.

Mycobacterium tuberculosis, *Mycobacterium bovis* and other mycobacterial infections

Tuberculosis (TB) caused by *Mycobacterium tuberculosis* is certainly a rare disease in dogs, most often resulting from a human source (Acha and Szifres, 1989; Anonymous, 1999). However, the infected dog can become the source of other human infections. The increase in human cases of tuberculosis worldwide, in association with the spread of the AIDS epidemic, is of major public health concern. There is potential for infection of pet dogs, especially those owned by homeless or economically impaired persons. Because canine tuberculosis often is the marker of the disease in humans, its early recognition in dogs is essential (Clercx *et al.*, 1992). Dogs get infected by infectious aerosols from the tuberculous owner or by sniffing infectious sputum. In developing countries, where bovine tuberculosis is still enzootic, dogs can be infected by *Mycobacterium bovis* by consumption of raw milk or possibly raw meat or offal from affected cattle. It may be a potential risk for dogs living on farms that have tuberculosis-infected cattle. In dogs, tuberculosis caused by *M. tuberculosis*, which was reported to account for more than 65% of dog cases in France more than 30 years ago (Clercx *et al.*, 1992), is clinically characterized by a pleuro-pneumonia. Unfortunately, clinical signs, such as fever, weight loss and coughing, are not specific. Infection by *M. bovis* induces more commonly a digestive form of tuberculosis. In dogs, tuberculous lesions resemble sarcomatous lesions, rather than the typical tubercles, as caseation is rarely seen (Clercx *et al.*, 1992). Atypical mycobacteria often gain entry via the skin and wounds, and so cause cutaneous signs, such as nodules and pyogranulomas. Human contamination from a *M. tuberculosis*-infected dog results from infective aerosols or contact with urine, saliva or cutaneous lesions. Alimentary tuberculosis is the most likely result of *M. bovis* infection in dogs, making fecal excretion a possible zoonotic risk from affected dogs. Infection of dogs with other *Mycobacterium* species is rare and their zoonotic potential is still questioned. However, in immunocompromised patients, animal infections may be a potential source of human infection. *Mycobacterium genavense*, a recently reported cause of a wasting illness in patients with AIDS, was isolated from a cervical lymph node from a dog with severe hind-limb weakness and from tracheal tissue from a parrot with acute onset of a respiratory distress syndrome (Kiehn *et al.*, 1996). Diagnosis is a complex task, as skin test is not very reliable in the dog. Any suspicion of a human case of tuberculosis in a household where pets are present, especially dogs, should lead to the clinical examination of the dog. The most consistent methods for the diagnosis of tuberculosis in dogs have been the histopathological examination of appropriate specimens and the isolation of the bacteria by culture (Aranaz *et al.*, 1996). However, histopathology is performed usually after the death of the animal and microbiological diagnosis requires several weeks. The use of PCR has brought major improvement in the diagnosis of canine TB and reduces to a few days the time for identification of the organism (Aranaz *et al.*, 1996). Infected dogs should be destroyed and not treated, as diagnosis is often late and treatment lasts for several months, with the great risk of selecting multidrug resistant strains.

Q fever

Caused by *Coxiella burnetii*, Q fever is mainly transmitted to humans and other mammals through inhalation of infectious particles. In nature, *C. burnetii* is maintained by a wildlife-tick cycle. However, infection through tick bites has been reported for various species, including humans. Highly infectious dust from tick feces deposited on animal skin and from dried placenta following parturition are major sources of *C. burnetii* infections in these animals and humans. *Dermacentor*, *Rhipicephalus* and *Amblyomma* ticks are probably responsible for the transmission of *C. burnetii* among dogs and wildlife (Hibler *et al.*, 1985). The primary reservoir hosts for *C. burnetii* are ticks, and vertical transmission (transovarial and trans-stadial) is common. Infection in domestic and wild carnivores has been reported from various areas of the world. In a survey of 1040 dogs in California, Williberg *et al.* (1980) showed a 53% antibody prevalence (agglutinin). They found that 63% of the coyotes and 26% of the bobcats tested in that state were seropositive. In Nova Scotia, it was found that a high prevalence of Phase II antibodies were present in cattle, but also in cats (24.1% of 216 cats). None of the 447 dogs tested had antibodies. Such results could be associated to the lack of tick infection in Nova Scotia (Marrie *et al.*, 1985). *C. burnetii* has been demonstrated in the blood of cats, following laboratory induced infection, for up to 1 month and in urine for 2 months.

The organism can be isolated frequently from the placenta of cattle, sheep and goats. In several instances, human infections resulted from exposure to parturient carnivores, as high concentrations of the organism are found in the products of conception. Laughlin *et al.* (1991) reported an outbreak in a family after exposure to a deer and infected pregnant dog. In late November 1989, seven members of a family from New Brunswick became ill with headache, fever, myalgia, fatigue, sweats and a mild non-productive cough. Six of the seven family members had abnormal chest X-rays and a fourfold or more rise in Phase II antibody titer to *C. burnetii* antigen with immunoflorescent antibodies (IFA). A detailed history revealed that one family member shot a deer in early November and some of the deer liver was fed to the family dog. One week later, the dog gave birth to pups, one was stillborn and two died within the first week of life. The pups were born under the bed of one of the family members. The children, who were present in the room at the time of the puppies birth, became sick 10 days later. In this outbreak, it was strongly suspected that the dog was responsible for the outbreak. It was seropositive and *C. burnetii* was isolated from the dog's uterus. Similarly, Q fever pneumonia developed in all three members of one family 8 to 12 days after exposure to an infected parturient dog, which gave birth to four puppies that all died within 24 hours after birth (Buhariwalla *et al.*, 1996). Because of the close contact between dogs and cats and their owners, pets can be considered as sentinel animals for the presence of *C. burnetii* in the household environment (Williberg *et al.*, 1980).

Diagnosis of Q fever is based on culture of *C. burnetii*, but is rarely performed for safety reasons in the laboratory (inoculation of guinea-pigs, embryonated eggs, tissue cultures). One could consider PCR on biological products available only in very specialized laboratories. Mainly, diagnosis is based on serology using IFA, ELISA, complement fixation or microagglutination. No specific study has been conducted on treatment efficacy in domestic dogs and cats, but it is likely that tetracyclines and chloramphenicol would be effective, as in humans. Preventing farm dogs from close contact with sheep, goat or cattle is difficult, but farmers having Q fever outbreaks in their flocks or herds should be aware of the risk associated with their pets. Tick prevention and control is also important, especially in dogs.

Streptococcosis

In one report, recurrent group A beta-hemolytic streptococcus (*Streptococcus pyogenes*) pharyngitis was not eradicated until the family dog was treated (Mayer and VanOre, 1983). Canine reservoir for human pharyngitis may occur, but is still controversial (Wilson *et al.*, 1995).

Zoonoses of the genito-urinary tract

Brucellosis

Organisms of the genus *Brucella* are small, non-motile, Gram-negative coccobacilli capable of causing disease in man, dog, cattle, sheep, goats, swine, and various wildlife species. Brucellosis in humans is most commonly a foodborne disease caused by *Brucella melitensis*, as seen in California (Chomel *et al.*, 1994b). The most common source of human infection is unpasteurized milk products. Dogs can be infected by several species of *Brucella*, including *Brucella abortus* and *B. melitensis* and play a role in the dispersion of these organisms between farms and potentially be a source of human contamination. Infection of dogs with *Brucella abortus* has been reported in experimental and field studies (Forbes, 1990). Evidence exists for transmission from cattle to dog by ingestion of infected reproductive tissues. Additionally, it seems likely that infected dogs can transmit *B. abortus* to naive cattle. At present, the zoonotic potential of *B. abortus* transmission between dog and man appears limited in most developed countries. Conversely, dogs are the main reservoir of *Brucella canis*, which is pathogenic to humans (Johnson and Walker, 1992; Kerwin *et al.*, 1992). In domestic and wild canids, *B. canis* is transmitted primarily by ingestion or inhalation of aerosolized post-abortion material, but venereal transmission is also reported (Johnson and Walker, 1992). Human infection by *B. canis* is not common, but at least 30 human cases have been reported (Lum *et al.*, 1985). Symptoms of *B. canis* infection in humans are largely non-specific including fever, splenomegaly, malaise, myalgia, headache, and anorexia (Lum *et al.*, 1985). Septicemia has been reported in 50% of patients (Rousseau, 1985). Though most cases respond well to antibiotic therapy, as many as 3% of treated patients may die from endocarditis or other complications (Rousseau, 1985).

In the dog, *B. canis* infection is characterized by prolonged bacteremia and reproductive failure in both males and females. Transient lymphadenopathy and fever are occasionally detected in early stages of infection (Johnson and Walker, 1992). In the pregnant bitch, *B. canis* causes embryonic or fetal death, or abortion by colonizing the placental epithelial cells. Live-born puppies, infected *in utero*, usually do not survive to weaning (Carmichael and Greene, 1990). In the male dog, *B. canis* causes epididymitis and infertility as a result of abnormal spermatogenesis (Johnson and Walker, 1992). In both genders, infection is largely asymptomatic and often remains undetected unless the animal is bred. Occasionally complications arise including diskospondylitis, uveitis, meningitis, glomerular nephritis, and draining skin lesions.

A diagnosis of brucellosis can be made by either blood culture or serology. In case of serology, specific *B. canis* antigen should be used, as serological tests for diagnosis of ruminant or swine brucellosis do not cross-react with this antigen (Polt *et al.*, 1982). Treatment is based on the use of doxycycline and an aminoglycoside (streptomycin, gentamycin, or netilmicin) for 4 weeks followed by doxycycline (200 mg per day) and rifampin (600-900 mg per day) orally for 4 to 8 weeks (Tan, 1997).

Leptospirosis

Leptospirosis is a spirochetal zoonosis that is ubiquitous and for which the human incidence is uncertain, but most likely underestimated (Levett, 1999), despite the high prevalence of the disease in wildlife and certain domestic species. The etiological agents of leptospirosis belong to the more than 200 pathogenic serovars within the 23 serogroups of *Leptospira interrogans* (André-Fontaine *et al.*, 1994). Many of these serovars are capable of causing disease in humans and dogs, but until recently the main serovars involved in zoonotic transmission between canid and humans were *Letopspira canicola* and *Letopspira icterohaemorrhagiae* (Farr, 1995). More recently, canine outbreaks caused by *Letopspira pomona* and *Letopspira grippothyphosa* have been reported in Europe (André-Fontaine *et al.*, 1994) and in the USA, and at a lesser extent by *Letopspira australis, Letopspira automnalis*, or some other serovars. The range of serovars common in temperate regions is much smaller than that found in tropical countries (Levett, 1999).

Leptospirosis is mainly a water-borne disease, and rodents are major reservoirs. Man is an accidental host that becomes infected through occupational or recreational exposure. Leptospirosis has a worldwide distribution, but human cases are more frequently reported from the tropics, such as Hawaii for the USA, where the average annual incidence is 1.08 per 100,000 population, while it is 0.05 per 100,000 population for the US as a whole (Sasaki *et al.*, 1993).

Dogs are the natural carrier host for *L. canicola*, but can also be infected with various other serovars and will shed these organisms in their urine for up to several weeks. Humans can become infected through licking from, or when petting, an infected dog. Recently, many cases of leptospirosis have been reported in dogs in the USA caused by *L. grippothyphosa*, especially in the northeastern states. The reservoirs are more likely to be racoons, opossums and skunks. The specific role of dogs as source of human infection is not well quantified, but is reported to be high. Human infection with *L. icterohaemorrhagiae* is associated with exposure to infected dogs and is the most commonly diagnosed leptospiral infection in humans (Heath and Johnson, 1994). As most dogs are vaccinated against *L. canicola* and *L. icterohaemorrhagiae* in developed countries, suspicion of leptospirosis is often ruled out in a differential diagnosis. However, dogs may be infected by other serovars, and be potential carriers and shedders of all serovars.

The course of infection caused by exposure to a leptospiral agent is largely dependent on host adaptation of the serovar. Infection of an animal with its species' host-adapted serovar usually results in a mild disease state and high likelihood of development of a chronic carrier and shedder state. Such individuals represent reservoir or maintenance hosts. Infection with a non-host-adapted serovar typically causes severe acute disease characterized by hepatitis, hemolytic crisis, and organ failure (Heath and Johnson, 1994). In dogs, leptospirosis can range from an acute septicemia, with hemolytic anemia, hepatorenal failure, uncontrollable vomiting and bloody diarrhea to a subacute form with fever and jaundice or to milder forms with chronic nephritis.

In humans, after an incubation period of 7 to 12 days, most persons will have a subclinical infection or anicteric febrile disease, often misdiagnosed as an influenza. In its initial febrile phase, which usually lasts for 4 to 7 days, fever, headache, myalgia, conjunctivitis, nausea, and vomiting are commonly seen (Acha and Szyfres, 1989). In severe cases, by the end of the first week, jaundice and renal failure may begin. By the third week, severe icterus with high levels of bilirubin are observed, usually associated with severe glomerulo or interstitial nephritis. The mortality rate may reach 10 to 20%. *Leptospira* may be isolated from the patient's blood or cerebrospinal fluid during the 10 days of infection or the urine after 21 days, and identified by dark-phase microscopy or culture. Recent molecular techniques, such as PCR or immunoblotting may reduce the time for diagnosis, as culture may require several weeks, but seems to be less sensitive than serological diagnosis (Levett, 1999). Laboratory diagnosis is still mainly based on serology, especially micro-agglutination. Agglutinins will appear between the 6 and 12 days of illness. A specific diagnosis is usually based on the demonstration of a fourfold rise in antibody titer. Several serological tests have been developed, including ELISA or IFA.

Leptospires are very sensitive to penicillin G and doxycycline, which are the most effective antibiotics in dogs and humans, especially when administered in the early phase of the disease. Prevention is based on rodent control and exposure reduction as well as dog vaccination.

Vector-borne zoonoses

Dogs are not usually the main source of human infection for vector-borne zoonoses. However, their role cannot be neglected as they either bring or attract in to the human environment the various vectors that can bite humans (fleas, ticks, phlebotomes) or can be a source of infection on which vectors feed upon and further transmit infectious agents to humans.

Lyme borreliosis

Lyme disease is a multisystemic, tick vectored, zoonotic disease associated with infection by spirochetes of the genus *Borrelia* (Levine, 1995). The disease was first characterized in the mid 1970s during an investigation of an outbreak of arthritis near Old Lyme, Connecticut (Spach *et al.*, 1993). Though the name Lyme disease was new, the syndrome was soon recognized to be similar to erythema chronicum migrans and acrodermatitis chronica atrophicans, disease entities recognized in Europe as early as 1883 (Levine, 1995). *Borrelia burgdorferi* is the etiological agent of Lyme disease in the US, while *Borrelia garinii* and *Borrelia afzelii* are also associated with borreliosis in Europe (Saint-Girons *et al.*, 1994).

Lyme disease is the most reported vector-borne disease of humans in the US with a mean of approximately 12,500 cases annually reported to the Centers for Disease Control and Prevention (CDC) from 1993 to 1997 (CDC, 1999). Lyme disease is common in children, with about one-fourth of all reported cases occurring in children < 14 years of age (Sood, 1999). The overall incidence in the US is about 5 cases per 100,000 population, with the greatest numbers of cases being reported from the northeastern and north-central states, the highest being 62.2 cases per 100,000 population in Connecticut (CDC, 1999). For comparison, in France, overall incidence is estimated to be 16.5 cases (range: 12-20 cases) per 100,000 population, with some areas like Alsace, where the incidence is above 30 cases per 100,000 population (Dournon *et al.*, 1989). Infection with *B. burgdorferi* has been demonstrated in several mammalian and avian species (Barbour and Fish, 1993; Levine, 1995). However, as Lyme disease is not a reportable disease in animals, reliable incidence data is not currently available for wild and domestic species.

The enzootic cycle of Lyme disease does not normally include humans or domestic animals (Mather *et al.*, 1989). Rather, maintenance of *B. burgdorferi* in the environment is dependent on a wildlife reservoir and a transmission vector. *B. burgdorferi* is exceptional amongst *Borrelia* species in that it is capable of infecting a wide range of tick and vertebrate hosts. Thus, different animals and vectors are responsible for perpetuating *B. burgdorferi* in different geographic regions in which Lyme disease is endemic. Several ticks of the genus *Ixodes* have been demonstrated to be competent in transmitting Lyme borreliosis. In the eastern and north-central US *Ixodes scapularis* is the main vector (more than 50% of the ticks can be found infected), while in the Pacific states transmission is primarily via *Ixodes pacificus* (for which 1-6% are infected). In Europe *Ixodes ricinus* is the main vector (Lane *et al.*, 1991; Barbour and Fish, 1993).

Transovarial passage of *B. burgdorferi* in *Ixodes* ticks is only 1-5% (Lane *et al.*, 1991), suggesting that ticks act as vectors rather than reservoirs for the spirochete. In the northeastern US, it has been shown that the white-footed mouse, *Peromyscus leucopus*, is the primary reservoir of *B. burgdorferi* (Mather *et al.*, 1989; Levine, 1995). Mice generally become infected when fed upon by nymph stage *I. scapularis* which acquire spirochetes during their larval feeding (Genchi, 1992). Adult *I. scapularis* feed primarily on white-tailed deer (*Odocoileus virginianus*). In northern California the life cycle of *B. burgdorferi* often involves two tick species. *Ixodes neotomae* is responsible for maintaining the spirochete in the dusky-footed wood rat (*Neotoma fuscipes*), the primary reservoir in that region (Lane *et al.*, 1991). However, the host range of *I. neotomae* is narrow so it is *I. pacificus* that is the vector responsible for spreading *B. burgdorferi* infection to other species including humans and dogs. All three stages of ticks can be found on humans and domestic animals (Kazmierczak and Sorhage, 1993). In Europe, Lyme borreliosis is mainly transmitted by *I. ricinus* (Genchi, 1992). The infection rate in these ticks varies from 4% to up to 40%. In France, Gilot *et al.* (1996) reported a prevalence of 5% of infection in nymphs and 11 to 12.5% in adult ticks.

A major concern of any zoonosis of the dog is the potential that contact with canines will increase the likelihood of humans contracting the disease. Recent studies have indicated that dogs are competent reservoirs of *B. burgdorferi* (Mather *et al.*, 1994). Thus, naive ticks that feed on infected dogs are likely to become infected. Such ticks are then capable of infecting other vertebrates including humans. By introducing infected ticks into the human environment, dogs are capable of increasing dog owners' exposure to *B. burgdorferi*.

Dogs infected with *B. burgdorferi* may manifest some of the clinical signs which are common in humans, including acute onset of recurrent lameness, fever, lethargy, and inappetence. Other symptoms that occur with lower frequency include generalized lymphadenopathy, central nervous system (CNS) disorders, uveitis, renal lesions, and cardiac disease (Kazmierczak and Sorhage, 1993).

In humans, Lyme disease manifests with a variety of dermatologic, rhumatologic, cardiac, and neurologic abnormalities (Steere, 1989; Levine,

1995). The CDC case definition of Lyme disease includes the characteristic erythema migrans (EM) lesion (> 5cm in diameter) or laboratory confirmation of *B. burgdorferi* infection, and at least one of the objective clinical signs of the disease (CDC, 1990). Erythema migrans is virtually pathognomonic when it occurs, but is only detected in approximately 60% of patients (Steere, 1989). In the early stages of the disease, EM is often accompanied by muscle pain, headache, and fatigue. Leukocytosis, increased RBC sedimentation rate, and hematuria may also occur. In Europe, the manifestations of Lyme borreliosis are slightly different, with nervous-system involvement being more common, especially facial palsy, meningitis and polyradiculoneuritis and are more common in children (17 to 38% of cases) than in adults (Sood, 1999). Chronic arthritis has been reported in up to one-third of German children with Lyme arthritis (Sood, 1999).

Diagnosis is mainly based on serological assays. A "two-step approach" has been widely adopted and has improved the diagnosis' specificity. It is based on an enzyme immunoassay or indirect immunofluorescence assay followed by an immunoblotting assay (Western blot). Detection of IgM is investigated in early stages of the infection.

Borreliosis is resolved in most patients with a 10 to 21 day course of treatment with doxycycline (100 mg x 2 per day) or amoxicillin (2 g x 3 per day) per os. Intravenous ceftriaxone (2 g per day for 2 to 3 weeks) may be indicated if the infection is not detected in the early stages or appears refractory to initial treatment protocols (Steere, 1989; Levine, 1995). For reasons that are poorly understood, some individuals are unable to overcome *B. burgdorferi* infection. These patients may experience chronic peripheral nervous system and CNS abnormalities including depression, fatigue, sleep disorders, and memory loss for months to years following the initial infection (Barbour and Fish, 1993; Leaven, 1995).

Prevention of Lyme disease in humans and domestic animals relies largely on minimizing exposure to ticks. Tick-infested areas should be avoided whenever possible. When traveling in areas of high tick density, exposure can be minimized by wearing long-sleeved shirts and long pants tucked into one's socks. Tick repellents and acaricides are available for human and animal use. Humans should inspect themselves and their pets regularly for ticks, and carefully remove ticks as soon as possible after contact (Barbour and Fish, 1993; Kazmierczak and Sorhage, 1993). Removal of ticks within 48 hours of attachment has been shown to significantly decrease the likelihood of transmission of *B. burgdorferi* from an infected tick (Shih and Spielman, 1993). In addition to vector control, the other method of preventing borreliosis in dogs and humans is by vaccination. There are currently two vaccines available for use in dogs in the USA. One is an inactivated whole organism bacterin while the other is a recombinant vaccine (Levine, 1995). Concern about residual pathogenicity has precluded development of whole-cell vaccines for human use (Barbour and Fish, 1993). A recombinant vaccine based on the *B. burgdorferi* OspA protein (31-kDa outer surface protein A) has been recently approved for human use (Sood, 1999).

Ehrlichiosis

Organisms of the genus *Ehrlichia* are pleomorphic, obligate intracellular bacteria of the family *Rickettsiacea* that parasitize the phagosomes of mononuclear or polymorphonuclear leukocytes (Eng *et al.*, 1990; Anderson *et al.*, 1991). Human ehrlichioses are recently recognized tick-borne infections (McQuiston *et al.*, 1999). In 1986, a clinically novel form of human monocytic ehrlichiosis (HME) was described and shown to induce an *Ehrlichia canis*-reactive humoral reaction (Maeda *et al.*, 1987). The advent of taxonomic determination based on 16S rRNA gene sequencing led to the discovery that *E. canis*-like human ehrlichiosis was actually caused by a previously undescribed species, subsequently named *Ehrlichia chaffeensis* (Anderson *et al.*, 1991). More recently, evidence of human infection with *E. canis*, the cause of canine monocytic ehrlichiosis, has been reported (Perez *et al.*, 1996). Finally, another agent causing granulocytic ehrlichiosis in dogs, *Ehrlichia ewingii*, was reported to cause human illness in four patients (Buller *et al.*, 1999). The main vector of *E. chaffeensis* and *E. ewingii* is the Lone Star tick, *Amblyomma americanum* and the dog tick, *Dermacentor variabilis* (Walker and Dumler, 1996). From 1986 through 1997 more than 700 human cases of HME have been reported to the CDC, mainly from the southeastern and south-central states (McQuiston *et al.*, 1999). In 1990, canine and human infections with granulocytic ehrlichiae were discovered in Minnesota and Wisconsin (Bakken *et al.*, 1994). Human granulocytic ehrlichiosis (HGE) is caused by an organism closely related to *Ehrlichia equi* and *Ehrlichia phagocytophila* (Chen *et al.*, 1994). The main vector of HGE agent is *I. scapularis* in the midwestern and northeastern states (Walker and Dumler, 1996). Since first identified, more than 450 human cases of HGE have been reported to the CDC, mainly from northeastern and upper midwestern states (McQuiston *et al.*, 1999). The zoonotic nature of the human ehrlichioses is supported by reports of natural infections with the same *Ehrlichia* species in dogs, deer, horses, and rodents (Buller *et al.*, 1999). Human, canine and equine cases of granulocytic ehrlichiosis have also been reported from Minnesota, Wisconsin and Sweden, caused by an agent closely related to *E. equi* (Johansson *et al.*, 1995; Greig *et al.*, 1996). Dogs likely contribute to the enzootic cycle and human infection. Dogs can also become infected with *E. chaffeensis* in experimental (Dawson and Ewing, 1992) and natural conditions (Breitschwerdt *et al.*, 1998).

Canine monocytic ehrlichiosis, caused by *E. canis*, has been described throughout most of the world, but is particularly prevalent in tropical and subtropical regions (Eng and Giles, 1989). This infection is mainly transmitted by *Rhipicephalus sanguineus*. In dogs, it manifests, in the acute phase, with fever, depression, anorexia, and weight loss. Typical laboratory findings include thrombocytopenia and hypergammaglobulinemia (Eng and Giles, 1989). Though most dogs recover uneventfully, some progress to a subclinical stage characterized by persistent hematological abnormalities and high antibody titers to *E. canis* (Codner and Farris-Smith, 1986). Chronic ehrlichiosis, characterized by pancytopenia and bone marrow hypoplasia, may develop weeks to years later. This chronic form has a high fatality rate attributed to hemorrhage and secondary infections (Eng and Giles, 1989).

Canine granulocytic ehrlichiosis, caused by *E. ewingii*, was first described in a dog from Arkansas (Ewing *et al.,* 1971) and has been reported since then from dogs in several southeastern states. In dogs, *E. ewingii* infection is usually milder than *E. canis* infection and responds to treatment with tetracycline (Buller *et al.,* 1999). In the series of cases reported by Buller *et al.* (1999), all four patients had been exposed to ticks and had had contact with dogs shortly before the onset of symptoms. One of the patient's dogs had asymptomatic infection, suggesting that dogs could act as a reservoir for *E. ewingii*.

Human monocytic and granulocytic ehrlichioses are nearly indistinguishable and are characterized by one or more of the following symptoms: fever, headaches, myalgia, chills, anorexia, rash in 20% of the patients (for HME, less common for HGE), leucopenia, thrombocytopenia, anemia, hypertension, coagulopathy, renal failure, pancytopenia, hepatocellular injury and elevated serum hepatic aminotransferase levels (Walker and Dumler, 1996; McQuiston *et al.*, 1999). The severity of the disease ranges from asymptomatic seroconversion to fatal infection. Case-fatality rates are as high as 5% for HME and 10% for HGE (Dumler and Bakken, 1995).

Human and animal ehrlichioses are mainly diagnosed by indirect immunofluorescence assay, although PCR assays are increasingly used (McQuiston *et al.*, 1999). Treatment of infections caused by *Ehrlichia* species is mainly based on the use of doxycycline at 100 mg twice a day for 5 to 7 days (Tan, 1997). Prevention is based on the same measures as reported for Lyme disease.

Spotted fever group rickettsioses

Spotted fever group *Rickettsiae* have been described throughout the world (Azad and Beard, 1998). Though the organisms are closely related, each causes a serologically and pathologically distinct disease. Most rickettsioses are considered zoonotic. Rocky Mountain spotted fever is caused by *Rickettsia rickettsii,* and occurs in the US, Canada, Mexico, and parts of Central and South America. In Japan, Oriental spotted fever is caused by *Rickettsia japonica*, while *Rickettsia conorii* causes Boutonneuse fever in several Mediterranean nations, southern Africa and the Middle East (Walker and Fishbein, 1991).

Rocky Mountain spotted fever

Rocky Mountain spotted fever (RMSF) is a tick-borne rickettsial disease caused by *R. rickettsii*, which affects several vertebrate species, including humans and dogs. It is certainly the most important and most severe disease in the spotted fever group (Chomel, 1997).

RMSF was first reported in 1896 when cases were identified in Idaho in the Snake River valley and in the Bitter Root valley of western Montana (Dalton *et al.*, 1995). Howard T. Ricketts first established the identity of the bacteria-like infectious particles seen in tick tissues and demonstrated the competence of the wood tick, *Dermacentor andersoni*, in acquiring and transmitting the infectious agent. Beginning in the 1930s, RMSF started to be reported from eastern states (Dalton *et al.*, 1995). RMSF is found all over the USA, the largest number of cases being reported from the southeastern, midwestern and south-central states. The disease exists also in Canada, Mexico, Central America and parts of South America (Colombia and Brazil). The natural history and distribution of RMSF in the USA are associated with the ecology of two ticks (Hibler *et al.*, 1985). *D. andersoni* is the principal vector of disease in the western US from the Cascade to the Rocky Mountains. Its larvae and nymphs feed on small mammals; the adults infest larger mammals. The wood tick is active primarily in the spring and early summer, when the disease incidence peaks. In the southeastern and eastern USA, the American dog tick, *D. variabilis* is the main vector. Its larvae and nymphs feed on wild rodents; adults feed on larger feral mammals, dogs and humans. In the eastern USA, the Lone Star tick, *A. americanum* is implicated in human infection. The rickettsiae are released from the salivary glands of feeding adult ticks during their 6 to 10 hours of attachment.

R. rickettsii initially infects the epithelial cells of the tick midgut, multiplies there, enters the hemocoel, and then invades all tick tissues, including the salivary glands and the ovaries. The organism can be found in the tick hemocytes as early as 3-5 days after the infective meal. When generalized infection occurs, all tick tissues can become infected within a 7-10 day period after feeding on a rickettsemic animal. Uninfected nymphs and adults may become infected with *R. rickettsii* when they feed on animals concurrently with infected nymphs or adults. Ticks mate while feeding. Female ticks transmit the infection through the eggs, but transfer through male spermatozoa is not efficient during mating (McDade and Newhouse, 1986). Acquisition of infection by ticks is limited to the rather short period of high rickettsemia (often 4-5 days only) in the small rodents.

The extensive range of mammals that are seropositive for *R. rickettsii* reflects the generalized feedings habits of the known tick hosts of *R. rickettsii*. The American dog tick (*D. variabilis*) feeds mainly on dogs for the adult form, but will also feed on many other domestic and wildlife mammals (cattle, sheep, horses, deer, raccoons, opossums, coyotes, foxes). Larvae and nymphs feed on various rodents, such as chipmunks, ground squirrels, voles and rabbits. *Rhipicephalus sanguineus*, a major vector in Mexico, is primarily associated with domestic dogs. Humans are an incidental host of the adults of all of these tick species, and therefore do not contribute to the transmission cycle (McDade and Newhouse, 1986). In both humans and dogs, the level of rickettsemia is low, and they do not serve to infect new ticks. Larvae and nymphs usually do not feed more than once before molting. Adult female ticks feed once before laying eggs, after which they die, and only adult males feed repetitively. Norment and Burgdorfer (1984) showed that dogs inoculated with 1000 to 10,000 egg infective doses of virulent *R. rickettsii* developed a rickettsemia that was detectable as early as 4 days after inoculation and as late as 10 days. No rickettsemia has been observed in dogs infected with *Rickettsia rhipicephali* or *Rickettsia montana*, two non-pathogenic rickettsiae. In dogs, rickettsemia lasts only for a few days. In the same experiment, Norment and Burgdorfer showed that a very limited number of ticks became infected after feeding on inoculated dogs.

Serologic information obtained since the 1930s indicated that dogs could be infected, but it is only since the late 1970s and early 1980s that clinical reports concerning naturally occurring RMSF in dogs have been made (Keenan *et al.*, 1977). Symptoms of RMSF vary considerably in dogs. Usually, fever (39°C to 41°C), anorexia, vomiting, diarrhea and depression can occur within 2 to 3 days after tick attachment (Greene *et al.*, 1985). Conjunctivitis, mucopurulent oculo-nasal discharge, and non-productive cough are often present. Weight loss, dehydration, lymphadenopathy and myalgia as well as joint tenderness may occur. Abdominal tenderness or paralumbar hyperesthesia can be observed. Early skin lesions include edema and hyperemia (lips, pinnae, prepuce, scrotum), followed by cutaneous petechiae and ecchymoses (only in 20% of the dogs, whereas it is in the majority of human cases), epistaxis and scleral injection. Hemorrhages are limited to the mucosae, rather than involving the skin. Necrosis of skin of the extremities has been seen as a complication of RMSF in dogs. Ocular lesions are characterized by subconjunctival hemorrhage, hyphema, anterior uveitis, retinal petechiae, focal retinal oedema (Davidson *et al.*, 1989).

Neurologic abnormalities, such as vestibular deficits, abnormal mental status, nystagmus, head tilt, circling, incoordination are also observed. Hematologic abnormalities include anemia (normocytic, normochromic), thrombocytopenia: platelet counts of less than 75,000 cells per µl (normal: 200,000 to 500,000), and mild leukopenia (at onset of fever), followed by: leukocytosis (> 20,000) with a left shift (normal: 6000 to 17,000). Biochemical abnormalities include increased glucose concentration, increased serum aspartate and alanine transaminases and alkaline phosphatase activity, hypoproteinemia.

In humans, 4 to 14 days after a tick bite, the patient suffering typical RMSF has an acute onset of fever, malaise, headache, and myalgia, followed a few days later (1 to 15 days after the onset of illness) by a petechial rash. Vomiting can be seen in 60% of the cases. The rash first appears as macules on the wrists and ankles, and subsequently spreads to involve the trunk, face, palms and soles. These cutaneous lesions often develop papular, petechial, or purpuric features. Acute renal failure, coagulopathy, and cerebral edema are common complications. Mortality, as high as 30% in the pre-antibiotic era, remains between 2% to 10% (4% between 1981-1992). In a review of human cases in the USA between 1981 and 1992, Dalton *et al.* (1995) reported more than 9,000 cases from 46 states, with an annual incidence of $5.2/10^6$ persons in 1981 to $2.0/10^6$ in 1992. In 90% of the confirmed cases, onset of symptoms occurred between April and September. Two-thirds of the confirmed cases reported tick attachment in the 14 days prior to illness. An additional 25.6% reported having been in a tick-infested area. Incidence was highest in children, peaking in those 5-9 years of age at $3.2/10^6$. Cases were more frequent in males than females (1.7:1), particularly in the age group 10-19 years of age (2.2:1). The case-fatality rate was 4.0% with a dramatic increase in people over 40 years of age. Fever was the most common symptom (94%) reported by patients with headache (86.2%) and myalgia (82.5%). 80% of the patients had a rash, but the classic triad of symptoms: fever, headache and rash were present in only 55.3% of the confirmed cases. Mortality was associated with delay in treatment and use of chloramphenicol rather than tetracycline. For all age groups, reported risk factors include exposure to dogs, residence in a wooded area, and being male.

Diagnosis of the infection is based on either isolation of the agent by inoculation to guinea-pigs, cell cultures, by direct immunofluorescence on skin biopsies, or by serological tests (IFA, ELISA, micro-agglutination) (Greene *et al.*, 1993). Testing by PCR of 17 KDa antigen has been developed more recently. In dogs, serodiagnosis based on detection of both IgM and IgG is also useful to identify acute infection (Breitschwerdt *et al.*, 1990).

The treatment of choice is tetracyclines (22 mg per kg every 8 hours, per os or chloramphenicol: 15 to 20 mg per kg, po, q 8 hours). Breitschwerdt *et al.* (1997) showed that prednisolone at anti-inflammatory or immunosuppressive dosages in conjunction with doxycycline does not potentiate the severity of *Rickettsia rickettsii* infection in dogs (rickettsemia was prolonged at immunosuppressive dose).

Mediterranean spotted fever or Boutonneuse fever

Boutonneuse fever, also called Mediterranean spotted fever (MSF), was first described by Connor and Bruch in Tunis in 1910. It is an acute infectious disease caused by *R. conorii* (Font-Creus *et al.*, 1985). The habitual reservoir and dominant vector is the brown dog tick, *R. sanguineus*, which very rarely feeds on humans. In 1930, Durand and Conseil produced the disease in man by injecting suspension of *R. sanguineus* taken from a dog. The disease is endemic along the Mediterranean coastline. The disease is also endemic in much of Africa, the Middle East, the Black and Caspian Seas, India and has also been reported in Southeast Asia. It is also the most common rickettsial disease in South Africa (Acha and Szyfres, 1989). In South Africa, the dog ticks, *Haemaphysalis leachi* and *R. sanguineus* are likewise the principal vectors of human infection. An increase in human cases has been reported in the last decade in several Mediterranean countries (Chomel, 1997).

In the Mediterranean countries, dogs seem to play an important role in the epidemiology of the disease as amplifiers of the reservoir and vector, the brown dog tick, in a domestic or peri-domestic cycle in urban or peri-urban areas. They also bring infected ticks into the vicinity of humans. Dogs are often considered to be the main source for infecting ticks, yet there are no quantitative data concerning susceptibility of dogs to this agent.

Senneville *et al.* (1991) reported the case of a 53-year-old man who presented a severe form of MSF 2 months after vacationing on the French Riviera. When tested, the pet dogs were found seropositive with very high titers. Three brown dog ticks found a few months later on the dogs were cultured and *R. conorii* was identified. The increase in human cases is related to the dispersion of *R. sanguineus* by dogs from southern Europe to more northern areas and also to the progressive adaptation of *R. conorii* to new tick species, such as *Dermacentor marginatus* or *Dermacentor reticulatus.* Dogs are exposed to infection, and, although clinical signs and symptoms have not been reported, they can be rickettsemic. Adult dogs can carry *R. conorii* without clinical signs, but they do not transmit it to their offspring. In Spain, Delgado and Carmenes (1995) and Segura-Porta *et al.* (1998) found that respectively 23.4% of 308 dogs and 26.1% of 138 dogs tested had significant antibody titer to *R. conorii*. The frequency of seropositive dogs increased during the summer months. Dogs from rural areas or heavily infested by ticks had a higher seroprevalence. It has been suggested to use dogs as sentinels to monitor the distribution of this zoonosis.

In other parts of the world, small rodents on which infected ticks feed upon, are the amplifiers on the infection. It is suspected that in the Mediterranean basin lagomorphs could play the role of amplifiers in the wildlife cycle. In a sero-survey, 76.5% of the wild rabbits tested had antibodies in the Salamanca Province, Spain (Ruiz-Beltran *et al.*, 1992).

In humans, MSF is characterized by a primary lesion at the site of the tick bite. It is a small reddish ulcer covered by a small black scab, called "tache noire", which may last throughout the course of the illness. Regional lymphadenopathy is often seen. Fever appears usually 5 to 7 days after the tick bite and is associated with severe cephalagia, muscular and joint pain. A generalized eruption, at first macular and then maculopapular, appears the fourth or fifth day of the fever and lasts about 1 week. Mortality is low. In a study of 227 cases in Spain, Font-Creus *et al.* (1985) reported a high fever and a generalized maculopapular rash in all patients. The *tache noire* was seen in 735 of the cases as well as myalgia. Other common signs were headaches (69%), conjunctivitis (32%), hepatomegaly (44%) and splenomegaly (19%). Contact with dogs was confirmed in 92% of the 170 cases analyzed. Seventy-two per cent of the cases were living in urban areas.

The epidemiology of MSF is determined by the biology of the tick and results in a consistent seasonal peak. Immature stages (larvae, nymphs) are generally the source of human contamination during the summer, while adult ticks are mainly active during the spring. The monthly distribution of human cases shows that the apparition of the disease parallels the maximal activity of the immature stage of *R. sanguineus* (Raoult *et al.*, 1992). *R. conorii* is transmitted transovarially from generation to generation. In their study, Raoult *et al.* (1992) found that incidence was positively correlated with preceding year spring and summer average temperatures and was negatively correlated with preceding year number of days with frost.

Raoult *et al.* (1993) also reported interesting data concerning prevalence of MSF and prevalence of infected ticks in the Marseille area. In northern

Marseille, the incidence of hospitalized patients with MSF was 24.2 per 10^5 persons compared with 9.8 and 8.8 per 10^5 for central and southeastern Marseille. Seroprevalence in blood donors, tested by microimmunofluorescence and confirmed by Western blot assays was higher in the northern area than the two other ones (6.7% versus 3.6 and 2.4). They indicated that this higher prevalence may be related to a greater tick exposure due to a higher number of dogs (32.6 per 100 inhabitants versus 28.4 and 27.2 per 100, respectively). About 9% to 15% of the ticks were infected in the various areas. For human infection, the brown tick needs to be attached for at least 20 hours. Dogs in northern Marseille are more frequently parasitized by ticks (51.4%) than in the two other areas (43.5% and 40%). Parasitized dogs are present in microfoci. In northern Marseille, a large percentage of the population has a low income and more than 25% are unemployed. It is therefore possible that such negative socioeconomic factors negate effects of adequate hygiene facilities on personal hygiene.

Diagnosis of the infection is performed usually by either isolation of the infectious agent (not done in regular practice) or serologically by microimmunofluorescence and Western blot assays (Teysseire and Raoult, 1992). The treatment is based on the use of tetracyclines (Doxycycline 100-200 mg per day for 7 to 15 days) and chloramphenicol.

Several other rickettsial spotted fevers have been reported from various parts of the world, but no data are available on the role of dogs in their epidemiology.

Plague

Plague, caused by *Yersinia pestis*, is an endemic disease of rodents in Asia, central and southern Africa and Madagascar, some areas of South America (Peru, Bolivia, Brazil) and the western US. It is maintained in nature by a flea-rodent cycle of transmission. In man, bubonic plague results from a flea bite, usually from a rodent flea, but sometimes from a cat or dog flea. In humans, infection with *Y. pestis* occurs through the bite of infected fleas, contact with bodily fluids of infected animals, or rarely through inhalation of aerosolized respiratory droplets of infected animals or other humans (Crook and Tempest, 1992). Inhalation infection results in pneumonic plague, the form associated with the greatest mortality. In the dog, infection is most likely to occur as a result of flea bites or ingestion of an infected rodent (Orloski and Eidson, 1995). In humans, clinical forms of plague present as bubonic, septicemic or pneumonic. Clinical signs for the bubonic form typically include fever, myalgia, lymphadenopathy (buboe), nausea, and vomiting (Crook and Tempest, 1992). The incubation period ranges from several hours to approximately one week.

In dogs, plague is usually a mild disease, characterized by a moderate fever, lethargy and enlarged lymph nodes (Orloski and Eidson, 1995). In endemic areas, plague antibody prevalence in pet dogs is usually low. In the USA, prevalence is less than 1% in pet dogs (Chomel *et al.*, 1994a) whereas rates of 4% to 6.5% have been reported in free-roaming dogs, especially on

Native Americans Reservations in California (Chomel *et al.*, 1994a) or Africa (Kilonzo *et al.*, 1992). However, rates of up to 16% have been reported in dogs from Navajo Reservations (Barnes and Poland, 1983). The frequency with which plague is transmitted from dog to human has not been thoroughly examined (Orloski and Eidson, 1995). Four cases of acquiring plague from skinning wild canids were documented between 1970 and 1993. Though 12 cases of human plague during this period were attributed to direct contact with an infected domestic cat, no analagous cases were confirmed to be due to interaction with a dog (Craven *et al.*, 1993). As with other arthropod-borne diseases, dogs potentially may act as a vehicle for introducing vectors infected with *Y. pestis* into the human environment. In this manner contact with dogs may increase the likelihood of humans contracting plague.

The plague bacillus is very sensitive to streptomycin, but tetracycline and doxycycline are also very effective. Major concern has been raised recently with the emergence of multiresistant plague bacilli from Madagascar (Galimand *et al.*, 1997). Dogs pose a risk to humans by transporting fleas and flea-infested animals or carcasses into or around the home. It is important that dogs and cats that roam outside be treated with appropriate insecticides to kill fleas.

Other uncommon bacterial zoonoses

Anthrax

Dogs are not very susceptible to anthrax and usually develop a subclinical or chronic form of anthrax, with moderate fever, pharyngeal and lingual edema, and enlarged lymph nodes (Acha and Szyfres, 1989). Direct infection of humans from dogs could potentially occur through a bite.

Chlamydiosis

Chlamydia psittaci, the agent of ornithosis in humans, is an obligate intracellular parasite that is capable of infecting a wide range of domestic and wild mammals and birds (Arizmendi *et al.*, 1992). In humans, *C. psittaci* infection is seen most often in exotic pet bird owners and poultry industry workers.

Reports of natural and experimentally induced chlamydiosis in dogs are rare. *C. psittaci* has been isolated in England from the feces of a dog that had ingested the carcasses of birds known to be infected with the same agent (Fraser and Norval, 1969). More recently, chlamydial conjunctivitis has been described in dogs (Krauss *et al.*, 1988). Additionally, experimental inoculations of dogs with the chlamydial agent of ovine polyarthritis support the notion that dogs are capable of supporting chlamydial infections (Maierhofer and Storz, 1969).

Seroprevalence of canine chlamydiosis has not been examined in the US. However, serosurveys have been conducted in Germany (Werth *et al.*, 1987) where 20% of the dogs tested had *C. psittaci* antibodies and in Japan (Fukushi *et al.*, 1985) where 9% of sampled dogs were seropositive. The role of dogs in transmission of *C. psittaci* to humans is still hypothetical, whereas a human case was acquired from a cat with *C. psittaci* pneumonia (Hugh-Jones *et al.*, 1995).

Conclusions

Bacterial disease transmission from dogs to humans is rather uncommon, especially if pet owners follow basic hygiene rules. Transmission by bites and by fecal shedding is among the main sources of human contamination from dogs. Special attention should be given to young children who may be more likely to be bitten by dogs or be in close contact with the pet and its environment. Regular vaccination of dogs and removal of ectoparasites are important preventive measures that a pet owner should follow carefully to prevent the occurrence of bacterial zoonoses.

References

Abedini, S. and Lester, A. (1997) *Erysipelothrix rhusiopathiae* bacteremia after dog bite. *Ugeskrift for Laeger* 159, 4400-4401.

Acha, P.N. and Szyfres, B. (1989) *Zoonoses and Communicable Diseases Common to Man and Animals*, 2nd edn. Scientific publication No. 503, P.A.H.O., Washington DC, pp. 963.

Alexander, C.J., Citron, D.M., Gerardo, S.H., Claros, M.C., Talan, D. and Goldstein, E.J. (1997) Characterization of saccharolytic *Bacteroides* and *Prevotella* isolates from infected dog and cat bite wounds in humans. *Journal of Clinical Microbiology* 35, 406-411.

Anderson, B.E., Dawson, J.E., Jones, D.C. and Wilson, K.H. (1991) *Ehrlichia chaffeensis*, a new species associated with human ehrlichiosis. *Journal of Clinical Microbiology* 29, 2838-2842.

André-Fontaine, G., Ruvoen-Clouet, N. and Ganière, J.P. (1994) Données récentes sur la leptospirose canine. *Receuil de Médecine Vétérinaire* 170, 663-668.

Angulo, F.J., Glaser, C.A., Juranek, D.D., Lappin, M.R. and Regnery, R.L. (1994) Caring for pets of immunocompromised persons. *Journal American Veterinary Medical Association* 205, 1711-1718.

Anonymous (1999) Tuberculosis [news]. *Journal of Small Animal Practice* 40, 145-147.

Aranaz, A., Liebana, E., Pickering, X., Novoa, C., Mateos, A. and Dominguez, L. (1996) Use of polymerase chain reaction in the diagnosis of tuberculosis in cats and dogs. *Veterinary Record* 138, 276-280.

Arizmendi, F., Grimes, J.E. and Relford, R.L. (1992) Isolation of *Chlamydia psittaci* from pleural effusion in a dog. *Journal of Veterinary Diagnostic Investigation* 4, 460-463.

Azad, A.F. and Beard, C.B. (1998) Rickettsial pathogens and their arthropod vectors. *Emerging Infectious Diseases* 4, 179-186.

Bakken, J.S., Dumler, J.S., Chen, S.M., Eckman, M.R., Van Etta, L.L. and Walker, D.H. (1994) Human granulocytic ehrlichiosis in upper midwest United States. A new species emerging? *Journal of the American Medical Association* 272, 212-218.

Barbour, A.G. and Fish, D. (1993) The biological and social phenomenon of Lyme disease. *Science* 260, 1610-1616.

Barnes, A.M. and Poland, J.D. (1983) Plague in the United States, 1982. *Morbidity Mortality Weekly Report* 32, 19SS-24SS.

Blaser, M., Cravens, J., Powers, B.W. and Wang, W.L. (1978) *Campylobacter* enteritis associated with canine infection. *Lancet* ii, 979-981.

Breitschwerdt, E.B., Levy, M.G., Davidson, M.G., Walker, D.H., Burgdorfer, W., Curtis, B.C. and Babineau, C.A. (1990) Kinetics of IgM and IgG responses to experimental and naturally acquired *Rickettsia rickettsii* infection in dogs. *American Journal of Vetererinary Research* 51, 1312-1316.

Breitschwerdt, E.B., Davidson, M.G., Hegarty, B.C., Papich, M.G. and Grindem, C.B. (1997) Predinisolone at anti-inflammatory or immunosuppressive dosages in conjunction with doxycycline does not potentiate the severity of *Rickettsia rickettsii* infection in dogs. *Antimicrobial Agents and Chemotherapy* 4, 141-147.

Breitschwerdt, E.B., Hegarty, B.C. and Hancock, S.I. (1998) Sequential evaluation of dogs naturally infected with *Ehrlichia canis, Ehrlichia chaffeensis, Ehrlichia equi, Ehrlichia ewingii*, or *Bartonella vinsonii*. *Journal of Clinical Microbiology* 36, 2645-2651.

Brook, I. (1987) Microbiology of human and animal bite wounds in children. *Pediatric Infectious Diseases Journal* 6, 29-32.

Buhariwalla, F., Cann, B. and Marrie, T.J. (1996) A dog-related outbreak of Q fever. *Clinical Infectious Diseases* 23, 753-755.

Buller, R.S., Arens, M., Hmiel, S.P., Paddock, C.D., Sumner, J.W., Rikhisa, Y., Unver, A., Gaudreault-Keener, M., Manian, F.A., Liddell, A.M., Schmulewitz, N. and Storch, G.A. (1999) *Ehrlichia ewingii*, a newly recognized agent of human ehrlichiosis. *New England Journal of Medicine* 341, 148-155.

Canton, P., May, T., Burdin, J. and Lion, C. (1987) Pasteurellosis and bacteria EF4, M5 and Iij: pathogenic role in man following animal bites and bacterial sensitivity. *Chemotherapia* 6, 26-28.

Carithers, H.A. (1985) Cat scratch disease. An overview based on a study of 1,200 patients. *American Journal of Diseases of Children* 139, 1124-1133.

Carmichael, L.E. and Greene, C.E. (1990) Canine brucellosis. In: Greene, C.E. (ed.) *Infectious Diseases of the Dog and Cat*. W.B. Saunders Co, Philadelphia, pp. 573-584.

C.D.C. (1990) Case definitions for public health surveillance. *Morbidity Mortality Weekly Report* 39, 19-21.

C.D.C. (1999) Lyme Disease: Epidemiology.www.cdc.gov/ncidod/dvbid/lymeepi.htm

Chen, S.M., Dumler, J.S., Bakken, J.S. and Walker, D.H. (1994) Identification of a granulocytic *Ehrlichia* species as the etiologic agent of human disease. *Journal of Clinical Microbiology* 32, 589-595.

Chomel, B.B. (1997) Rickettsial infections in dogs, cats and humans: an overview. International Forum on Ticks and Tick-Borne Diseases. Supplement to: *Compendium on Continuing Education for the Practicing Veterinarian* 19, 37-41.

Chomel, B.B., Jay, M.T., Smith, C.R., Kass, P.H., Ryan, C.P. and Barrett, L.R. (1994a) Serological surveillance of plague in dogs and cats, California, 1979-1991. *Comparative Immunology Microbiology and Infectious Diseases* 17, 111-123.

Chomel, B.B., DeBess, E.E., Mangiamele, D.M., Reilly, K.F., Farver, T.B., Sun, R.K. and Barrett, L.R. (1994b) Changing trends in the epidemiology of human brucellosis in California from 1973 to 1992: A shift toward foodborne transmission. *Journal of Infectious Diseases* 170, 1216-1223.

Citron, D.M., Hunt, C., Gerardo, S., Claros, M.C., Abrahamian, F., Talan, D. and Goldstein, E.J.C. (1996) Incidence and characterization of *Porphyromonas* species isolated from infected dog and cat bite wounds in humans by biochemical tests and PCR fingerprinting. *Clinical Infectious Diseases* 23, S78-S82.

Clercx, C., Coignoul, F., Jakovljevic, S., Mainil, J., Henroteaux, M. and Kaeckenbeeck, A. (1992) Tuberculosis in dogs: A case report and review of the literature. *Journal of the American Animal Hospital Association* 28, 207-211.

Codner, E.C. and Farris-Smith, L.L. (1986) Characterization of the subclinical phase of ehrlichiosis in dogs. *Journal of the American Veterinary Medical Association* 189, 47-50.

Craven, R.B., Maupin, G.O., Beard, M.L., Quan, T.J. and Barnes, A.M. (1993) Reported cases of human plague infections in the United States, 1970-1991. *Journal of Medical Entomology* 30, 758-761.

Crook, L.D. and Tempest, B. (1992) Plague: A clinical review of 27 cases. *Archives of Internal Medicine* 152, 1253-1256.

Dalton, M.J., Clarke, M.J., Holman, R.C., Krebs, J.W., Fishbein, D.B., Olson, J.G. and Childs, J.E. (1995) National surveillance for Rocky Mountain spotted fever, 1981-1992: epidemiologic summary and evaluation of risk factors for fatal outcome. *American Journal of Tropical Medicine and Hygiene* 52, 405-413.

Davidson, M.G., Breitschwerdt, E.B., Nasisse, M.P. and Roberts, S.M. (1989) Ocular manifestations of rocky mountain spotted fever in dogs. *Journal of the American Veterinary Medical Association* 194, 777-781.

Dawson, J.E. and Ewing, S.A. (1992) Susceptibility of dogs to infection with *Ehrlichia chaffeensis*, the causitive agent of human ehrlichiosis. *American Journal of Veterinary Research* 53, 1322-1327.

Decker, G.R., Lavelle, J.P., Kumar, P.N. and Pierce, P.F. (1991) Pneumonia due to *Bordetella bronchiseptica* in a patient with AIDS. [letter]. *Reviews of Infectious Diseases* 13,1250-1251.

Delgado, S. and Carmenes, P. (1995) Canine seroprevalence of *Rickettsia conorii* infection (Mediterranean spotted fever) in Catilla y Leon (northwest Spain). *European Journal of Epidemiology* 11, 597-600.

Demers, D.M., Bass, J.W., Vincent, J.M., Person, D.A., Noyes, D.K., Staege, C.M., Samlaska, C.P., Lockwood, N.H., Regnery, R.L. and Anderson, B.E. (1995) Cat-scratch disease in Hawaii: etiology and seroepidemiology. *Journal of Pediatrics* 127, 23-26.

Dournon, E., Villemot, S. and Hubert, B. (1989) La maladie de Lyme en France: enquête réalisée auprès d'un réseau sentinelle de médecins généralistes. *Bulletin Epidémiologique Hebdomadaire* 45, 185-186.

Dumler, J.S. and Bakken, J.S. (1995) Ehrlichial diseases of humans: emerging tick-borne infections. *Clinical Infectious Diseases* 20, 1102-1110.

Dworkin, M.S., Sullivan, P.S., Buskin, S.E., Harrington, R.D., Olliffe, J., MacArthur, R.D. and Lopez, C.E. (1999) *Bordetella bronchiseptica* infection in human immunodeficiency virus-infected patients. *Clinical Infectious Diseases* 28, 1095-1099.

Eng, T.R. and Giles, R. (1989) Ehrlichiosis. *Journal of the American Veterinary Medical Association* 194, 497-499.

Eng, T.R., Harkess, J.R., Fishbein, D.B., Dawson, J.E., Greene, C.N., Redus, M.A. and Satalowich F.T. (1990) Epidemiologic, clinical, and laboratory findings of human ehrlichiosis in the United States, 1988. *Journal of the American Medical Association* 264, 2251-2258.

Ewing, S.A., Robertson, W.R., Buckner, R.G. and Hayat, C.S. (1971) A new strain of *Ehrlichia canis*. *Journal of the American Veterinary Medical Association* 159, 1771-1774.

Fantasia, M., Mingrone, M.G., Martini, A., Boscato, U. and Crotti, D. (1993) Characterisation of *Yersinia* species isolated from a kennel and from cattle and pig farms. *Veterinary Record* 132, 532-534.

Farr, W. (1995) Leptospirosis. *Clinical Infectious Diseases* 21, 1-8.

Fenwick, S.G., Madie, P. and Wilks, C.R. (1994) Duration of carriage and transmission of *Yersinia enterocolitica* biotype 4, serotype 0:3 in dogs. *Epidemiology and Infection* 113, 471-477.

Ferry, N.S. (1910) A preliminary report of the bacterial findings in canine distemper. *American Veterinary Revue* 37, 499-503.

Foley, J.E., Marks, S.L., Munson, L., Melli, A., Dewhirst, F.E., Yu, S., Shen, Z. and Fox, J.G. (1999) Isolation of *Helicobacter canis* from a colony of bengal cats with endemic diarrhea. *Journal of Clinical Microbiology* 37, 3271-3275.

Font-Creus, B., Bella-Cueto, F., Espejo-Arenas, E., Vidal-Sanahuja, R., Munoz-Espin, T., Nolla-Salas, M., Casagran-Borrell, A., Mercade-Cuesta, J. and Segura-Porta, F. (1985) Mediterranean spotted fever: A cooperative study of 227 cases. *Revue of Infectious Diseases* 7, 635-642.

Forbes, L.B. (1990) *Brucella abortus* infection in 14 farm dogs. *Journal of the American Veterinary Medical Association* 196, 911-916.

Ford, R.B. (1995) *Bordetella bronchiseptica* has zoonotic potential. *Topics in Veterinary Medicine* 6, 18-22.

Fraser, G. and Norval, J. (1969) A case history of psittacosis in the dog. *Veterinary Record* 85, 54-58.

Fukushi, H., Ogawa, H., Minamoto, N., Hashimoto, A., Yagami, K., Tamura, H., Shimakura, S. and Hirai, K. (1985) Seroepidemiological surveillance of *Chlamydia psittaci* in cats and dogs in Japan. *Veterinary Record* 117, 503-504.

Galimand, M., Guiyoule, A., Gerbaud, G., Rasoamanana, B., Chanteau, S., Carniel, E. and Courvalin, P. (1997) Multidrug resistance in *Yersinia pestis* mediated by a transferable plasmid. *New England Journal of Medicine* 337, 677-680.

Ganière, J.P., Escande, F., André, G. and Larrat, M. (1993) Characterization of *Pasteurella* from gingival scrapings of dogs and cats. *Comparative Immunology, Microbiology and Infectious Diseases* 16, 77-85.

Genchi, C. (1992) Arthropoda as zoonoses and their implications. *Veterinary Parasitology* 44, 21-33.

Gilot, B., Degeilh, B., Pichot, J., Doche, B. and Guiguen, C. (1996) Prevalence of *Borrelia burgdorferi* (*sensu lato*) in *Ixodes ricinus* (L.) populations in France, according to a phytoecological zoning of the territory. *European Journal of Epidemiology* 12, 395-401.

Glaser, C.A., Angulo, F.J. and Rooney, J.A. (1994) Animal-associated opportunistic infections among persons infected with the human immunodeficiency virus. *Clinical Infectious Diseases* 18, 14-24.

Greene, C.E., Burgdorfer, W., Cavagnolo, R., Philip, R.N. and Peacock, M.G. (1985) Rocky Mountain spotted fever in dogs and its differentiation from canine ehrlichiosis. *Journal of the American Veterinary Medical Association* 186, 465-472.

Greene, C.E., Marks, M.A., Lappin, M.R., Breitschwerdt, E.B., Wolski, N.A. and Burgdorfer, W. (1993) Comparison of latex agglutination, indirect immunofluorescent antibody, and enzyme immunoasay methods for serodiagnosis of Rocky Mountain spotted fever in dogs. *American Journal of Veterinary Research* 54, 20-28.

Greig, B., Asanovich, K.M., Armstrong, P.J. and Dumler, J.S. (1996) Geographic, clinical, serologic, and molecular evidence of granulocytic ehrlichiosis, a likely zoonotic disease, in Minnesota and Wisconsin dogs. *Journal of Clinical Microbiology* 34, 44-48.

Griego, R.D., Rosen, T., Orengo, I.F. and Wolf, J.E. (1995) Dog, cat, and human bites: a review. *Journal of the American Academy of Dermatology* 33, 1019-1029.

Hald, B. and Madsen, M. (1997) Healthy puppies and kittens as carriers of *Campylobacter* spp., with special reference to *Campylobacter upsaliensis*. *Journal of Clinical Microbiology* 35, 3351-3352.

Heath, S.E. and Johnson, R. (1994) Leptospirosis. *Journal of the American Veterinary Medical Association* 205, 1518-1523.

Hibler, S.C., Hoskins, J.D. and Greene, C.E. (1985) Rickettsial infections in dogs. Part I. Rocky Mountain spotted fever and *Coxiella* infections. *Compendium of Continuing Education* 7, 856-868.

Hugh-Jones, M.E., Hubbert, W.T. and Hagstad, H.V. (1995) *Zoonoses. Recognition, Control, and Prevention.* Iowa State University Press, Ames, Iowa, pp. 369.

Hurvell, B. (1981) Zoonotic *Yersinia enterocolitica* infection: host range, clinical manifestations, and transmission between animals and man. In: Bottone, E.J. (ed.) Yersinia enterocolitica. CRC Press, Boca Raton, Florida, pp. 145-159.

Johansson, K.E., Pettersson, B., Uhlen, M., Gunnarsson, A., Malmqvist, M. and Olsson, E. (1995) Identification of the causative agent of granulocytic ehrlichiosis in Swedish dogs and horses by direct solid phase sequencing of PCR products from the 16S rRNA gene. *Research in Veterinary Sciences* 58, 109-112.

Johnson, C.E. and Walker, R.D. (1992) Clinical signs and diagnosis of *Brucella canis* infection. *Compendium on Continuing Education for the Practicing Veterinarian, Small Animal Practice* 14, 763-772.

Kapperud, G. (1994) *Yersinia enterocolitica* infection. In: Beran, G. (ed.) *Handbook of Zoonoses, second edition, Section A: Bacterial, Rickettsial, Chlamydial, and Mycotic.* CRC Press, Boca Raton, Florida, pp. 343-353.

Kazmierczak, J.J. and Sorhage, F.E. (1993) Current understanding of *B. burgdorferi* infection with emphasis on its prevention in dogs. *Journal of the American Veterinary Medical Association* 203, 1524-1528.

Keenan, K.P., Buhles, W.C., Jr., Huxsoll, D.L., Williams, R.G. and Hildebrandt, P.K. (1977) Studies on the pathogenesis of *Rickettsia rickettsii* in the dog: clinical and clinicopathologic changes of experimental infection. *American Journal of Veterinary Research* 38, 851-856.

Kerwin, S.C., Lewis, D.D., Hribernik, T.N., Partington, B., Hosgood, G. and Eilts, B.E. (1992) Diskospondylitis associated with *Brucella canis* infection in dogs: 14 cases (1980-1991). *Journal of the American Veterinary Medical Association* 201, 1253-1257.

Kiehn, T.E., Hoefer, H., Bottger, E.C., Ross, R., Wong, M., Edwards, F., Antinoff, N. and Armstrong, D. (1996) *Mycobacterium genavense* infections in pet animals. *Journal of Clinical Microbiology* 34, 1840-1842.

Kilonzo, B.S., Makundi, R.H. and Mbise, T.J. (1992) A decade of plague epidemiology and control in the western Usambara mountains, north-east Tanzania. *Acta Tropica* 50, 323-329.

Krauss, H., Schmeer, N. and Wittenbrink, M.M. (1988) Significance of *Chlamydia psittaci* infection in animals in the F.R.G. *Proceedings of the European Society of Chlamydia Research* Bologna, Italy, May 30-June 1, pp. 65.

Krol-van Straaten, M.J., Landheer, J.E. and de Maat, C.E.M. (1990) *Capnocytophaga canimorsus* (formerly DF-2) infections: review of the literature. *Netherlands Journal of Medicine* 36, 304-309.

Lane, R.S., Piesman, J. and Burgdorfer, W. (1991) Lyme borreliosis: relation of its causitive agent to its vector and host in North America and Europe. *Annual Review of Entomology* 36, 587-609.

Laughlin, T., Waag, D., Williams, J. and Marrie, T. (1991) Q fever: from deer to dog to man. *Lancet* 337, 676-677.

Levett, P.N. (1999) Leptospirosis: re-emerging or re-discovered disease? *Journal of Medical Microbiology* 48, 417-418.

Levine, J.F. (1995) *Ixodes*-borne *Borrelia* spp. infections. *Journal of the American Veterinary Medical Association* 207, 768-775.

Lion, C., Escande, F. and Burdin, J.C. (1996) *Capnocytophaga canimorsus* infections in human: review of the literature and cases report. *European Journal of Epidemiology* 12, 521-533.

Lum, M.K., Pien, F.D. and Sasaki, D.M. (1985) Human *Brucella canis* infection in Hawaii. *Hawaii Medical Journal* 44, 66-68.

Maeda, K., Markowitz, N., Hawley, R.C., Ristic, M., Cox, D. and McDade, J.E. (1987) Human infection with *Ehrlichia canis*. *New England Journal of Medicine* 316, 853-856.

Maierhofer, C.A. and Storz, J. (1969) Clinical and serological responses in dogs inoculated with the Chlamydial (psittacosis) agent of ovine polyarthritis. *American Journal of Veterinary Research* 30, 1961-1966.

Margileth, A.M. (1993) Cat scratch disease. *Advances in Pediatric Infectious Diseases* 8, 1-21.

Marrie, T.J., Van Buren, J., Fraser, J., Haldane, E.V., Faulkner, R.S., Williams, J.C. and Kwan, C. (1985) Seroepidemiology of Q fever among domestic animals in Nova Scotia. *American Journal of Public Health* 75, 763-766.

Mather, T.N., Wilson, M.L., Moore, S.I., Ribeiro, J.M. and Spielman, A. (1989) Comparing the relative potential of rodents as reservoirs of the Lyme disease spirochete. *American Journal of Epidemiology* 130, 143-150.

Mather, T.N., Fish, D. and Coughlin, R.T. (1994) Competance of dogs as reservoirs for Lyme disease spirochetes (*B. burgdorferi*). *Journal of the American Veterinary Medical Association* 205, 186-188.

Mayer, G. and Van Ore, S. (1983) Recurrent pharyngitis in family of four. Household pet as reservoir of group A streptococci. *Postgraduate Medicine* 74, 277-279.

McDade, J.E. and Newhouse, V.F. (1986) Natural history of *Rickettsia rickettsii*. *Annual Review of Microbiology* 40, 287-309.

McDonough, P.L. and Simpson, K.W. (1996) Diagnosing emerging bacterial infections: salmonellosis, campylobacteriosis, clostridial toxicosis, and helicobacteriosis. *Seminars in Veterinary Medicine and Surgery (Small Animal)* 11, 187-197.

McQuiston, J.H., Paddock, C.D., Holman, R.C. and Childs, J.E. (1999) The human ehrlichioses in the United States. *Emerging Infectious Diseases* 5, 635-642.

Mollaret, H.H. and Affre, P. (1981) *Le Bestiaire Médical, Bactéries, Virus, Parasites et Mycoses Transmis à l'Homme Par Ses Animaux Familiers*. Editions Médicales Fournier frères, Paris, France.

Norment, B.R. and Burgdorfer, W. (1984) Susceptibility and reservoir potential of the dog to spotted fever group rickettsiae. *American Journal of Veterinary Research* 45, 1706-1710.

Orloski, K.A. and Eidson, M. (1995) *Yersinia pestis* infection in three dogs. *Journal of the American Veterinary Medical Association* 207, 316-318.

Perez, M., Rikihisha, Y. and Wen, B. (1996) *Ehrlichia canis*-like agent isolated from a man in Venezuela: antigenic and genetic characterization. *Journal of Clinical Microbiology* 34, 2133-2139.

Polt, S.S., Dismukes, W.E., Flint, A. and Shaefer, J. (1982) Human brucellosis caused by *Brucella canis*: clinical features and immune response. *Annals Internal Medicine* 97, 717-719.

Raoult, D., Tissot-Dupont, H., Caraco, P., Brouqui, P., Drancourt, M. and Charrel, C. (1992) Mediterranean spotted fever in Marseille: descriptive epidemiology and the influence of climatic factors. *European Journal of Epidemiology* 8, 192-197.

Raoult, D., Tissot-Dupont, H., Chicheportiche, C., Peter, O., Gilot, B. and Drancourt, M. (1993) Mediterranean spotted fever in Marseille, France: correlation between prevalence of hospitalized patients, seroepidemiology, and prevalence of infected ticks in three different areas. *American Journal of Tropical Medicine and Hygiene* 48, 249-256.

Rousseau, P. (1985) *Brucella canis* infection in a woman with fever of unknown origin. *Postgraduate Medicine* 78, 249-257.

Ruiz-Beltran, R., Herrero-Herrero, J.I., Martin-Sanchez, A.M. and Criado-Gutierrez, L.A. (1992) Role of *Lagomorpha* in the wild cycle of *Rickettsia conorii* in Salamanca (Spain). *European Journal of Epidemiology* 8, 136-139.

Saeed, A.M., Harris, N.V. and DiGiacomo, R.F. (1993) The role of exposure to animals in the etiology of *Campylobacter jejuni/coli* enteritis. *American Journal of Epidemiology* 137, 108-114.

Saint-Girons, I., Old, I.G. and Davidson, B.E. (1994) Molecular biology of the *Borrelia*, bacteria with linear replicons. *Microbiology* 140, 1803-1816.

Salfield, N.J. and Pugh, E.J. (1987) Campylobacter enteritis in young children living in households with puppies. *British Medical Journal* 294, 21-22.

Sasaki, D.M., Pang, L., Minette, H.P., Wakida, C.K., Fujimoto, W.J., Manea, S.J., Kunioka, R. and Middleton, C.R. (1993) Active surveillance and risk factors for leptospirosis in Hawaii. *American Journal of Tropical Medicine and Hygiene* 48, 35-43.

Segura-Porta, F., Diestre-Ortin, G., Ortuno-Romero, A., Sanfeliu-Sala, I., Font-Creus, B., Munoz-Espin, T., de Antonio, E.M. and Casal-Fabrega, J. (1998) Prevalence of antibodies to spotted fever group rickettsiae in human beings and dogs from an endemic area of mediterranean spotted fever in Catalonia, Spain. *European Journal of Epidemiology* 14, 395-398.

Senneville, E., Ajana, F., Lecocq, P., Chidiac, C. and Mouton, Y. (1991) *Rickettsia conorii* from ticks introduced to northern France by a dog. *Lancet* 337, 676.

Shih, C. and Spielman, A. (1993) Accelerated transmission of Lyme disease spirochetes by partially fed vector ticks. *Journal of Clinical Microbiology* 31, 2878-2881.

Sood, S.K. (1999) Lyme disease. *Pediatric Infectious Disease Journal* 18, 913-925.

Spach, D.H., Liles, W.C., Campbell, G.L., Quick, R.E., Anderson, D.E. Jr. and Fritsche, T.R. (1993) Tick-borne diseases in the United States. *New England Journal of Medicine* 329, 936-947.

Steere, A.C. (1989) Lyme disease. *New England Journal of Medicine* 321, 586-596.

Stehr-Green, J.K. and Schantz, P.M. (1987) The impact of zoonotic diseases transmitted by pets on human health and the economy. *Veterinary Clinics of North America: Small Animal Practice* 17, 1-15.

Stolte, M., Wellens, E., Bethke, B., Ritter, M. and Eidt, H. (1994) *Helicobacter heilmannii* (formerly *Gastrospirillum hominis*) gastritis: an infection transmitted by animals? *Scandinavian Journal of Gastroenterology* 29, 1061-1064.

Talan, D.A., Citron, D.M., Abrahamian, F.M., Moran, G.J. and Goldstein, E.J.C. (1999) Bacteriologic analysis of infected dog and cat bites. *New England Journal of Medicine* 340, 85-92.

Tan, J.S. (1997) Human zoonotic infections transmitted by dogs and cats. *Archives of Internal Medicine* 157, 1933-1943.

Teysseire, N. and Raoult, D. (1992) Comparison of Western immunoblotting and micro-immunofluorescence for diagnosis of Mediterranean spotted fever. *Journal of Clinical Microbiology* 30, 455-460.

Thomson, M.A., Storey, P., Greer, R. and Cleghorn, G.J. (1994) Canine-human transmission of *Gastrospirillum hominis*. *Lancet* 343, 1605-1607.

Tsukahara, M., Tsuneoka, H., Lino, H., Ohno, K. and Murano, I. (1998) *Bartonella henselae* infection from a dog. *Lancet* 352, pp. 1682.

Underman, A.E. (1987) Bite wounds inflicted by dogs and cats. *Veterinary Clinics of North America: Small Animal Practice* 17, 195-207.

Walker, D.H. and Dumler, J.S. (1996) Emergence of the ehrlichioses as human health problems. *Emerging Infectious Diseases* 2, 18-29.

Walker, D.H. and Fishbein, D.B. (1991) Epidemiology of rickettsial diseases. *European Journal of Epidemiology* 7, 237-245.

Werth, D., Schmeer, N., Muller, H.P., Karo, M. and Krauss, H. (1987) Demonstration of antibodies against *Chlamydia psittaci* and *Coxiella burnetii* in dogs and cats: comparison of the enzyme immunoassay, immunoperoxidase technic, complement fixation test and agar gel precipitation test. *Zentralblatt fur Veterinarmedizin. Reihe B* 34, 165-176.

Willard, M.D., Sugarman, B. and Walker, R.D. (1987) Gastrointestinal zoonoses. *Veterinary Clinics of North America: Small Animal Practice*, 17, 145-178.

Williberg, P., Ruppanner, R., Behymer, D.E., Haghighi, S., Kaneko, J.J. and Franti, C.E. (1980) Environmental exposure to *Coxiella burnetii*: A sero-epidemiologic survey among domestic animals. *American Journal of Epidemiology* 111, 437-443.

Wilson, K.S., Maroney, S.A. and Gander, R.M. (1995) The family pet as an unlikely source of group A beta-hemolytic streptococcal infection in humans. *Pediatric Infectious Disease Journal* 14 , 372-375.

Woodard, D.R., Cone, L.A. and Fosvedt, K. (1995) *Bordetella bronchiseptica* in HIV-infected persons [letter]. *Clinical Infectious Diseases* 20, 193-199.

Chapter Five

Dogs and Protozoan Zoonoses

Richard W. Ashford and Karen F. Snowden

The protozoan parasites of the dog

In general, carnivores are poorer than herbivores as hosts to protozoa. This is due in part to the low population density of carnivores in nature. Direct transmission of any parasite is difficult between hosts, such as most carnivores, which live at low population densities; whereas many parasites of herbivores can be transmitted directly from one host to another by contamination. Most of the parasites of carnivores have complex life histories by which they overcome the vanishingly small chance of direct transmission. Complex life cycles are best developed in the helminths, which partly explains the scarcity of protozoa and abundance of helminths among the parasites of carnivores.

Many of the coccidian protozoa, however, have exceptionally complex life histories by which they can be transmitted up the food chain, using herbivorous intermediate hosts to gain access to carnivorous final hosts. Examples include the genus *Sarcocystis* which is particularly well represented (at least experimentally) in the dog, and *Toxoplasma gondii*, a parasite of the cat rather than the dog, which has an extraordinarily complex and flexible life history. Alternatively, parasites of carnivores may be vector-borne. Transmission between carnivores by a free-flying vector is very unlikely; the vectors of host-specific dog parasites are mostly ticks; just a few filarial worms and *Leishmania infantum* are transmitted by free-flying vectors. Many of these protozoa with complex life histories tend to depend on specific final hosts so are unlikely to infect humans zoonotically. The few dog protozoa which have simple life histories tend to be much less host-specific but, while these are the ones shared with man, the dog is not usually one of the most important hosts. In contrast to the helminths, then, only relatively few of the protozoa of dogs are important as agents of human disease. Some of these few, however, are of considerable significance in human health. The most significant of these are Chagas' disease, caused by *Trypanosoma cruzi*, for which dogs and humans are both important sources of infection, and *L. infantum* infection, which is normally transmitted to man from dogs. The latter disease is the one for which the dog is most important from the point of view of the reduction of public health problem, and this chapter will emphasize the role of the dog as a reservoir host of *L. infantum*.

Any consideration of the importance of zoonotic sources of human infections depends greatly on precise taxonomic information on the causative organisms (Ashford and Crewe, 1998). If parasites of man and animals form part of a single gene pool it is likely that transmission between the two hosts, in one direction or the other, occurs with some frequency; if the two gene pools are different, inter-host transmission is rare at best. Insufficient is known as yet of the genetics of most of the parasites apparently shared between man and dog to be able to determine the rate or direction of gene flow, but there are some remarkable exceptions. Most notable success has been in the *Leishmania* species, in which taxonomy based on isoenzyme analysis has solved many of these questions, but has raised many more. Despite much study, the situation with *Giardia* spp. and *Cryptosporidium* spp. is still open (Xiao *et al.*, 2000; Thompson *et al.*, 2000), while other minor parasites such as the non-pathogenic amoebae and flagellates have hardly been studied with modern techniques. Of course, the mere presence of identical parasites in both man and dog gives no indication of the direction of any transmission between them (Table 5.1). It would be all to easy to blame the dog as the source of the many parasites shared by dogs and people, but it is quite probable that at least as many parasitic infections are passed from people to dogs as the other way round. It is not a trivial matter, requiring considerable ecological study to determine which, if any, is the 'source' host and which the 'sink' host.

Table 5.1. Protozoan parasites of the dog, their origins and host specificity. References (Levine, 1983; Dubey *et al.*, 1989) and other references in text. *Species shared with man. Note: *Sarcocystis* spp. can rarely be identified to the species level in natural infections; most of those listed are from experimental feeding of dogs on infected meat.

Parasite	Transmission	Intermediate/ final host	Normal maintenance hosts
*Encephalitozoon cuniculi	Urine/feco-oral transplacental		Many species
*Giardia duodenalis	Feco-oral		Dog, human
*Pentatrichomonas hominis	Feco-oral		Human
Tetratrichomonas canistomae	Direct-oral contact		Cat
Tetratrichomonas sp.	Feco-oral		??
Tritrichomonas sp.	Feco-oral		??
*Trypanosoma brucei	Vector borne	Tsetse fly	Human, ungulates

Parasite	Transmission	Intermediate/ final host	Normal maintenance hosts
Trypanosoma evansi	Vector borne	Tabanid diptera	Ungulates
Trypanosoma congolense	Vector borne	Tsetse fly	Ungulates
*Trypanosoma cruzi	Vector borne	Reduviid bug	Human, many others
Trypanosoma rangeli	Vector borne	Reduviid bug	Many species
Leishmania tropica	Vector borne	Sandfly	Human
Leishmania major	Vector borne	Sandfly	Rodents
Leishmania infantum	Vector borne	Sandfly	Dog
Leishmania braziliensis	Vector borne	Sandfly	Dog and others??
Leishmania peruviana	Vector borne	Sandfly	Human? Dog?
Acanthamoeba spp.	Free living		Free living
Entamoeba coli	Feco-oral		Human
Entamoeba gingivalis	Feco-oral		Human
Entamoeba hartmanni	Feco-oral		Human
Entamoeba histolytica	Feco-oral		Human
Hartmanella sp.			Free living
Blastocystis hominis	Feco-oral?		Many species
Babesia canis	Vector borne	Tick	Dog
Babesia gibsoni	Vector borne	Tick	Dog (but see text)
Babesia vogeli	Vector borne	Tick	
Hepatozoon canis	Vector borne	Tick	Dog
Eimeria canis	Feco-oral		Probably pseudoparasite from prey
Eimeria rayii	Feco-oral		Probably pseudoparasite from prey
Cryptosporidium parvum	Feco-oral		Ungulates
Isospora bahiensis	Carnivory		
Isospora burrowsi	Feco-oral/ carnivory		
Isospora canis	Feco-oral/ carnivory		Dog

Parasite	Transmission	Intermediate/ final host	Normal maintenance hosts
Isospora neorivolta	Feco-oral/ carnivory		Dog
Isospora ohioensis	Feco-oral/ carnivory		
Toxoplasma gondii	Carnivory	Cat	Cat, numerous intermediate hosts
Hammondia spp.			Toxoplasma-like oocysts of unknown identity are occasionally found in dogs
Neospora caninum	Carnivory	Unknown, Dog?	Cow?
Sarcocystis alceslatrans	Carnivory	Moose	Canids/moose
Sarcocystis arieticanisi	Carnivory	Sheep	Canids/sheep
Sarcocystis bertrami	Carnivory	Horse	Canids/horse
Sarcocystis cameli	Carnivory	Camel	Canids/camel
Sarcocystis capracanis	Carnivory	Goat	Canids/goat
Sarcocystis cervicanis	Carnivory	Wapiti	Canids/deer
Sarcocystis cruzi	Carnivory	Cow	Canids/cow
Sarcocystis equicanis	Carnivory	Horse	Canids/horse
Sarcocystis fayeri	Carnivory	Horse	Canids/horse
Sarcocystis hemionilatrantis	Carnivory	Deer	Canids/deer
Sarcocystis hircicanis	Carnivory	Goat	Canids/goat
Sarcocystis levinei	Carnivory	Water buffalo	Canids/buffalo
Sarcocystis miescheriana	Carnivory	Pig	Canids/pig
Sarcocystis odocoleocanis	Carnivory	White-tailed deer	Canids/deer
Sarcocystis sybillensis	Carnivory	Wapiti	Canids/deer
Sarcocystis tenella	Carnivory	Sheep	Canids/sheep
Sarcocystis wapiti	Carnivory	Wapiti	Canids/deer
Sarcocystis spp.	Carnivory	Gazelle, chicken, pheasant	Canids/various intermediate hosts
*Balantidium coli	Feco-oral		Pig, primates

Intestinal parasites: flagellates

The intestinal flagellates generally have simple life histories with direct transmission. As noted above, such forms are unlikely to be specialist parasites of carnivores. Although several species may be shared by man and dog, the importance of the dog as a reservoir host of human infection is probably negligible.

Pentatrichomonas hominis

Most veterinary clinical texts simply use the imprecise term "trichomonads" when referring to this group of intestinal flagellates. Although data based on careful isolation and species identification are not readily available, the identity of the organisms found in dogs is usually given as *Pentatrichomonas hominis*, the same species found in humans (Barr, 1998). Typically, intestinal trichomonads are considered to be non-pathogenic, incidental findings that are occasionally seen in fresh liquid diarrheas caused by some other pathogen.

Since trichomonads have no environmentally resistant cyst stages, probably there is minimal risk of transmission between dog and man. From a veterinary diagnostic standpoint the importance of these organisms is to differentiate trichomonads from the more important and diarrhea-associated species, *Giardia duodenalis* which also has a motile flagellated stage.

According to Levine, (1983) *Tetratrichomonas canistomae*, which is occasionally found in the mouth of dogs, is apparently different from *Tetratrichomonas tenax* of the human mouth, but possibly the same as *Tetratrichomonas felistomae* of the cat.

Giardia duodenalis

Giardia is one of the commonest protozoan pathogens of the human intestine. Although infections are usually self-limiting, they may cause prolonged diarrhea with offensive stools and general nausea and malaise. In highly endemic areas most infections are in very young children, older people being immune.

The taxonomy and nomenclature of the genus *Giardia* is still in some confusion which makes it difficult to know whether or not human infections are caused by the same parasites as those in other animals (Thompson *et al.*, 2000). The name *Giardia lamblia* is the most commonly used combination for the human parasite, but *G. duodenalis* is used for morphologically similar forms from whatever host. Diverse names such as *Giardia canis*, *Giardia cati*, *Giardia bovis*, *Giardia equi* etc. were given in the early 1920s, and some references continue to use *G. canis* for parasites found in dogs. However, isolates from dogs are no longer generally considered to belong to a separate species (Soulsby, 1982).

Lewis (1988) listed only 15 studies including his own, showing the prevalence of canine *Giardia* infection, nine from North America, five from Western Europe, and one from Australia. Different sampling methods preclude reliable comparison, but crude prevalence varied between 1% in Louisiana and 68% in Ohio. More recent surveys in the USA report prevalences of 2.5% and 4.7% (Nolan and Smith, 1995; Barr, 1998).

The two morphologically different forms in mammals are conveniently called *G. duodenalis* and *Giardia muris*. Infections in humans are of the *G. duodenalis* type and are conventionally named *Giardia intestinalis* or *G. lamblia*. The dog is commonly infected with parasites of this type. A recent study amongst aboriginal communities in Australia found that the genotyping of *G. intestinalis* from human and dog isolates found differences in the small subunit ribosomal RNA, indicating that zoonotic infection between dogs and humans does not appear to commonly occur (Hopkins *et al.*, 1997).

As implied by the old nomenclature, *Giardia* infections have been documented in a number of animal hosts as well as humans. However, it is still controversial whether animal to human transmission occurs commonly or even at all under natural conditions. A number of cross-transmission studies attempting infections using a variety of parasite isolates in several rodent hosts have reported contradictory results. Biochemical techniques have not been much more helpful than cross-transmission experiments. More recently, three studies used different molecular techniques to compare parasite isolates from humans and several different animal hosts. In one study, two human and three dog isolates differed significantly (Hay *et al.*, 1990). By contrast, in two other studies, animal and human isolates segregated into three molecular types with human and animal hosts represented in each group (Baruch *et al.*, 1996; Ey *et al.*, 1996).

According to Erlandsen (1994), "it is clear that despite the isolation of *Giardia* from [dogs], no natural human infection attributable to these animals has been reported". It would be difficult to design epidemiological studies to assess the importance of the dog as an actual as well as potential source of human infection. In communities where people defecate promiscuously and dogs constitute the solid waste removal system, dogs must constantly be exposed to any feces-borne parasites which are immediately infective.

Whether or not the parasites in dogs are the same as those in humans, it is generally considered that infections in humans are derived from humans, or occasionally from rodents, and that the dog is epidemiologically irrelevant. Recently a *Giardia* vaccine has become commercially available in the USA which reduces cyst shedding in dogs and cats and prevents clinical signs of infection in these animals (Olson *et al.*, 2000). The relevance of this development for human health is as yet unclear.

Intestinal parasites: amoebae

Like the intestinal flagellates, amoebae are mostly transmitted directly from host to host, usually by means of a resistant cyst. In many countries nearly all humans are infected with amoebae, and the domestic dog is the main sewage system. In towns and villages where people defecate promiscuously, the dogs feed hungrily on this relatively rich source of nutrients.

Entamoeba coli

This is the commonest of all human amoebae. The distinctive cysts are frequently found in nearly all people in the community. The occasional records of this parasite in dogs are likely to be the result of dogs eating human feces.

Entamoeba histolytica

According to Beaver *et al.* (1984), natural infections of *Entamoeba histolytica* occur in dogs but there is no evidence that any animal is more than a minor source of human exposure compared with man himself. In fact, since, in dogs, these amoebae do not readily produce the environmentally resistant cyst stage that is responsible for transmission, it is more likely that dogs become infected from ingestion of cysts from human feces rather than vice versa (Barr, 1998).

Acanthamoeba spp.

The *Acanthamoebae* are free-living forms which occasionally become parasitic. Human infection may reach the brain, or may be restricted to the cornea. The species which infect humans are sometimes found in dogs, but there is little likelihood that infection is passed from one host to the other. All infections are presumably acquired independently from free-living populations.

Entamoeba gingivalis

This amoeba lives in the mouth of humans and is transmitted from person to person by direct oral contact or, possibly on shared feeding implements. There is no cyst stage in the life history, and the amoebae have only limited ability to survive in the environment. Although it is commoner in people with unhealthy mouths, there is no indication that it is harmful. According to Levine (1983), *Entamoeba gingivalis* can be transmitted to dogs with gingivitis, but not to dogs with healthy gums, and natural infections are occasionally found in dogs. Doubtless the natural transmission from humans to dogs is by direct or indirect oral contact.

Entamoeba hartmanni

This is yet another non-pathogenic amoeba, which lives commensally in the gut of humans and other primates, and is occasionally reported from dogs. In all probability the parasites in dogs were ingested with human feces.

Intestinal parasites: sporozoa

Cryptosporidium parvum

Cryptosporidium parvum is a relatively newly discovered human pathogen which, under normal conditions, produces at most a short-lived diarrhea. In immunocompromised people, especially AIDS victims, it produces severe, untreatable diarrhea, which is normally fatal. The minute oocysts are passed in huge numbers by infected hosts and are immediately infective. From a veterinary perspective, the parasite is most frequently identified as a cause of neonatal diarrhea in dairy calves. The few cases of infection in dogs probably originate from cattle or humans rather than the other way round.

Infection with *C. parvum* causing clinical diarrheas is rarely diagnosed in dogs. In one prevalence study, four of 200 stray dogs (2%) were passing oocysts, while 20 of 664 human fecal samples (3%) were positive (El-Ahraf *et al.*, 1991). Similarly, experimentally infected puppies shed oocysts for as long as 80 days, but numbers of oocysts were very low (Lloyd and Smith, 1997). Most human infections are now thought to be of human origin, and the importance of dogs as reservoirs of infection or as sources of transmission to humans is minimal (Current, 1998).

Although the dog is probably not a reservoir host in the sense that *Cryptosporidium* populations can be maintained indefinitely in dog populations, the close relationship between dogs and people potentially leads to occasional transfer of infection from dogs to humans. In view of the devastating consequences for immunocompromised individuals, contact between AIDS victims and dogs or other pets should be regarded as a mixed blessing.

Cyclospora cayetanensis

This parasite was first described in 1979 as a rare cause of human diarrhea in Papua New Guinea. It was recognized as a coccidian but was not named as the generic identity was uncertain (Ashford, 1979). What seems to have been the same organism was next seen in New York, in travellers from Haiti and Mexico. Soave *et al.* (1986) thought it looked like a coccidian oocyst but could not rule out a fungal spore. The same organism was variously described as resembling *Cryptosporidium muris* in Peru or a "Cyanobacterium-like body" which was found in 1991 to cause seasonal outbreaks of diarrhea in the American Embassy clinic in Nepal. The Peruvian parasite was eventually shown to be a species of *Cyclospora* by the presence of two sporozoites in each oocyst, and named, in 1994, in honour of the Cayetano University in Lima. Only in 1993 was it recognized that the parasites from Papua New Guinea, Nepal and Peru are one and the same thing (Ashford *et al.*, 1993). *Cyclospora cayetanensis* is now being recognized more and more as a cause of sporadic, sometimes epidemic diarrhea worldwide. It is intriguing to speculate on how it was missed until so recently, or from where it might have suddenly emerged. The facts that the original description was missed by subsequent authors, and that it was so comprehensively misidentified are clear indications that it could have been overlooked.

It has even been suggested that this is "the *Cryptosporidium* of the nineties" but there are good reasons to think that *C. cayetanensis* is much less of a potential problem. The fact that the oocysts require nearly 2 weeks at high temperature to sporulate probably limits the parasite to warm climates, and rules out the possibility of autoinfection. Further, unlike *C. parvum*, *C. cayetanensis* infection is treatable, and does not seem to be particularly dangerous to AIDS patients.

C. cayetanensis has also been described in non-human primates, baboons and possibly chimpanzees. More recently, Yai *et al.* (1997) found two dogs infected with coccidia resembling *C. cayetanensis*, and suggest that the dog may also harbour this parasite. These authors found two diarrheic dogs passing coccidian oocysts about the same size as those of *C. cayetanensis*, which produced two sporocysts. However, their illustration shows a collapsed oocyst which could equally well be a *Hammondia* species, such as is occasionally found in the feces of canids. Clearly there is still a lot to learn about this "new" parasite.

Other intestinal protozoans

Blastocystis hominis

Blastocystis has intrigued parasitologists since it was first described late in the 19th century. The parasite is found in an extraordinarily wide range of both vertebrate and invertebrate hosts, in which its morphology is remarkably uniform, yet no close relative is known which might indicate its relations with other organisms. It has been described as a yeast, a sporozoan protozoan, an amoeba and a stramenopile. The great French zoologist Grassé included one of the best reviews of the subject in his PhD study of flagellates because of the possibility that it might be either a degenerate form or a cyst of one of these. In man, *Blastocystis* is one of the most commonly seen parasites. The pattern of its occurrence in settled communities is identical to that of certain non-pathogenic protozoa but, in visitors, it may be closely associated with intractable chronic traveller's diarrhea (Ashford and Atkinson, 1992). The life history is poorly described, some of the stages being of unpredictable occurrence, and the transmission mechanism, though presumably by contamination, is not fully known.

In view of the ubiquity of *Blastocystis* it would be surprising not to find it in the dog and, indeed, it has been reported. In one of the few studies, 43 of 60 dogs tested in an Australian pound were found to be infected (Boreham and Stenzel, 1998). In a further study, 70.8% of dogs surveyed were positive for parasites in feces (Duda *et al.*, 1998). No biochemical or molecular comparison between human and canine isolates has been reported to date, but there is no reason to believe that the dog is an important source of human infection with *Blastocystis hominis*.

Balantidium coli

Balantidium coli is a large ciliated protozoan typically found in the large bowel of pigs, primates, and occasionally man, dogs and other mammalian hosts (Barr, 1998). These organisms usually act as commensals, but may occasionally become invasive into intestinal mucosa causing enteric disease. The environmentally resistant cyst stage passed in feces is infective when ingested by a susceptible host. Although the organisms have been occasionally identified in both man and dog, the potential for transmission between those hosts is negligible.

Parasites of the blood and other tissues

The leishmaniases

One of the main consequences of recent advances in the taxonomy of the genus *Leishmania* has been the demonstration that each species has distinctive epidemiological features, which may vary geographically with different vectors or reservoir hosts. With reliable and repeatable methods of identification, vectors and reservoir hosts can be accurately associated with given parasites even when several forms are sympatric. One of the many generalizations which have emerged is that transmission tends to be focalized in both space and time. The complete spectrum of zoonotic systems, from purely animal infection though purely human infection to secondary animal infection in new areas is illustrated by the various *Leishmania* species.

The genus *Leishmania* contains around 20 described species. These are morphologically similar, but can be distinguished by their biological or biochemical properties. Extensive study by isoenzyme analysis has allowed a useful classification of the species into the following groups: *L. tropica*, *L. aethiopica*, *L. major*, *L. donovani*, *L. braziliensis* and *L. mexicana*. Each of these groups is diverse, containing several species or subspecies, and numerous distinct strains. The taxonomic differences are only vaguely related to differences in the associated human disease, but there is generally a strong relation between their taxonomy and their ecology, vectors and reservoir hosts. Unfortunately, strains referable to *L. donovani* and *L. infantum* may differ only at a single genetic locus, and are occasionally sympatric so, while their ecology is usually markedly different, they are taxonomically very close.

The diseases caused in humans by this group of parasites, the leishmaniases, form a complex spectrum ranging from the simple cutaneous lesions of oriental sore which self-cure, to the potentially fatal visceral leishmaniasis known as kala-azar and grossly disfiguring espundia or mucocutaneous leishmaniasis which may erode the mucous membranes destroying much of the patient's face.

In 1992 leishmaniasis was known or suspected to occur in 97 countries, with 100,000 visceral cases and 400,000 cases of cutaneous disease reported annually

(Ashford *et al.*, 1992). Only a small proportion of cases are ever reported, and the figure of 12 million cases annually is sometimes estimated.

Morphology and life history of Leishmania *species*

All *Leishmania* species have basically similar life histories and are morphologically difficult to distinguish. In the mammal host the parasites are spherical or fusiform bodies between 2 and 5 µm in length, termed amastigotes. In the phlebotomine sandfly vector they become elongate, motile, flagellate bodies termed promastigotes. Both amastigotes and promastigotes divide repeatedly by longitudinal binary fission. Transmission depends on the uptake of amastigotes by a feeding sandfly and their inoculation to a new host at a subsequent meal.

Amastigotes contain two concentrations of DNA, in the nucleus and in a modified mitochondrion, the kinetoplast which is characteristic of this group of flagellates. A rudimentary flagellum occupies an indentation of the surface, the flagellar pocket. Amastigotes are intracellular, and are restricted to cells of the macrophage-monocyte series. Disruption of the host cell, which may contain as many as 50 organisms, allows the parasites to be phagocytosed, thereby infecting new cells. Infected cells may be restricted to the dermis, where they may or may not be restricted to a discrete lesion. Alternatively they may circulate throughout the body in lymph or blood, and infect the spleen, liver, bone marrow, lymph nodes, or mucosa. In these organs they are distributed throughout, not restricted to discrete lesions. Restriction to the skin may be explained in part by the temperature sensitivity of certain species.

On being ingested by a sandfly and released from the host cell the amastigotes continue to divide, at the same time elongating, and the flagellum extends greatly. These motile promastigotes divide repeatedly in the mid-gut of the sandfly as the blood-meal is digested. After a series of morphological, behavioral and biochemical changes they congregate in the cardiac valve, where the chitinous fore-gut projects into the mid-gut. The attachment of hundreds of parasites in this area impedes ingestion of a subsequent blood-meal. A possibly distinct series of parasites become free-swimming infective forms with short bodies and long flagella. These metacyclic promastigotes may enter the fore-gut and mouthparts, and are inoculated into a new mammalian host when the sandfly next feeds on blood.

Leishmania infantum

Without doubt, infantile visceral leishmaniasis caused by *L. infantum* is the most important protozoan zoonosis for which the domestic dog is the reservoir host. The disease in humans was known as *ponos* in Greece, or infantile splenomegalic anemia in Italy for long before Nicolle discovered the parasite, first in humans, then in dogs, in Tunisia. Similar infection was found in Brazil where Convit initially thought the parasite was different so named it *Leishmania chagasi*. Although he later withdrew this name, and although the parasite cannot reliably be distinguished from

Old World forms, some authors prefer to use, incorrectly, this junior synonym for the parasite causing canine and infantile visceral leishmaniasis in the New World.

Parasites termed *L. infantum* are very close to *L. donovani*, especially in southern Sudan, but are consistently distinguishable by certain isoenzyme patterns and generally have very different ecological features. Ashford (1998) has suggested that *L. donovani* and *L. infantum* were once indistinguishable, and originated as a pure zoonosis in an as yet unknown host, in East Africa, probably in southeastern Sudan, western Ethiopia and northern Kenya. With the influence of humans, one group of strains, which infect man only with difficulty and depend on the dog for their maintenance, expanded northwards through West Asia to Europe and North Africa and thence, quite recently, to South America, and also through Central Asia to China. This group became *L. infantum*. In all these countries the various vectors are opportunistic feeders. A second group of strains, *L. donovani*, would have been exported, probably via the port of Sawakin on the Red Sea coast, in the late 18th or early 19th century, to Bengal, where the parasites could survive without dogs, being transmissible from man to man. The vector, *Phlebotomous argentipes*, rarely feeds on dog blood. In India the parasites spread widely in those areas where the vector is synanthropic, causing repeated devastating epidemics, especially in the newly opened tea gardens of Assam. A third group of strains emerges occasionally from the heartland of the parasite, southward into Kenya where, again, important epidemics have occurred.

The dog is thus important for the maintenance of those strains which infect man with difficulty, and for spreading them, possibly from Africa to Europe and Asia and, more certainly, from Europe to South America.

L. infantum is widely distributed in the Mediterranean basin both in southern Europe and North Africa as well as West Africa. The distribution includes southern Saudi Arabia and Yemen and extends through Iraq, Iran and Pakistan to northwest India. Foci in the deserts of Central Asia are now largely inactive and the disease has almost completely disappeared from China where it was a major problem till the 1950s. Canine visceral leishmaniasis is widely distributed in South and Central America.

The ecological distribution of *L. infantum* infection is closely associated with the distribution of the vector sandflies. *Phlebotomus ariasi* in southwest France is concentrated in mixed oakwoods of *Quercus ilex* and deciduous *Quercus* species, which occur mainly between 300 m and 800 m above sea level; in this region transmission is therefore concentrated at this level. *Phlebotomus perniciosus* is more widespread, in drier regions mainly with natural or artificial outcrops of limestone. This explains the transmission of *L. infantum* in much of southern Europe and North Africa, where it is concentrated in suburbs and villages close to the coast, with dry stone walls and terraces frequently protecting olive or fig trees. Other Mediterranean vectors such as *Phlebotomus major* are less well known but no doubt each has its own story. The vector throughout South America is *Lutzomyia longipalpis* chiefly known as a synanthropic species in semi-arid areas. *L. infantum* in South America is concentrated in the degraded lands of northeast Brazil.

Semiao-Santos (1996) reviewed 35 serological studies on dogs in the Mediterranean basin other than Portugal. The overall average of these admittedly disparate studies was 12.5% prevalence of seropositivity. According to these authors, the rates in 13 studies in Portugal averaged 6.4%. By comparison, five studies of foxes averaged 9.3%. In view of the scarcity of foxes compared with dogs in the Mediterranean basin, clearly the bulk of the parasite suprapopulation resides in dogs.

There is no evidence that *L. infantum* is transmitted from man to man other than by syringe. The predominant reservoir host is the domestic dog and transmission among dogs may be very intense. In an experiment, in southern France, where 50 naive beagles were held in open-air pens for 2 years, 39 showed signs of infection after one transmission season, and 49 after two. Many of the dogs apparently self-cured but were not then resistant to reinfection. In highly enzootic areas more than 20% of dogs may be seropositive at any one time, and in some places it is very difficult to maintain dog populations.

L. infantum has been isolated from many species of wild canid, rats and opossums. The role of these animals in maintaining the parasite suprapopulations is controversial. Generally, carnivores live at densities which are too low for the maintenance of parasites transmitted by free-flying vectors. On Marajao Island in Brazil, a large proportion of the foxes *Cerdocyon thous* are infected but even there, it seems probable that it is the foxes which visit farmyards with infected dogs and *Leishmania longipalpis* which become infected. Circumstantial evidence has been presented in favor of various other reservoir host systems but none of these is fully substantiated. Courtenay *et al.* (1996) show that, in all probability, the records of *L. infantum* infection in the "fox" *Dusicyon vetulus* "were instances of mistaken identity", and the only wild canine host of this parasite in South America is *Cerdocyon thous*.

Canine visceral leishmaniasis

The experiment in France mentioned above gives important insight into the early natural history of natural infection. The first indication of infection was sometimes a small chancre on the ear or nose which reached almost 1 cm in diameter then cured after a few weeks. Alternatively, serological (ELISA) positivity developed in the absence of any initial chancre. Seropositivity titers generally increased gradually over a period of 2-3 months then either declined below the threshold of positivity or continued to increase. Those dogs which "cured" serologically during the winter remained healthy till the following transmission season. Those dogs whose serological titer continued to rise became sick and died or were sacrificed 2 to 12 months later. The apparently resistant dogs which became reinfected in the second year were similarly divided in two groups: some recovered a second time and some became progressively sicker. There was no clear correlation between the occurrence of an initial chancre and the eventual outcome.

More generally, visceralization of the parasites follows infection, and the parasites are concentrated in lymph nodes and bone marrow; there is less sign of splenomegaly than in human visceral leishmaniasis. The parasites later invade the skin where they may be very numerous but cause no necrosis or ulceration. The skin becomes dry and hypertrophic; there is considerable depilation which starts round the eyes as "spectacles", wasting, lethargy and lymph node enlargement. The alopecia together with the cachexia gives the appearance of a very sick animal. The dermal hypertrophy is particularly marked in the claws which become excessively elongate, adding to the sorry sight.

The disease may have an insidious onset and progress slowly with regression and relapse, or may proceed rapidly to death. Recent evidence shows that dogs may self-cure following early stages of infection but the fully developed disease is fatal and treatment can only delay death. Anomalously, the development of greatly elevated antibody levels indicates a poor prognosis. The humoral response to infection is clearly not effective in protection.

Diagnosis by serology is specific and sensitive in fully developed cases but can only be confirmed by aspiration of infected material and microscopic examination of slides or cultures for the presence of parasites. The popliteal lymph nodes are a useful source of aspirate; alternatively sternal bone marrow may be taken.

Treatment, as with humans, is with pentavalent antimony compounds which, however, do not produce complete cure and may require repetition on at least an annual basis for the remaining life of the dog.

Human visceral leishmaniasis

The principal signs of infantile visceral leishmaniasis are intermittent mild fever, hepatosplenomegaly, anemia with leucopenia, and highly elevated serum proteins with reversed albumin/globulin ratio, but none of these is pathognomonic. The fully developed disease is fatal if not treated.

For diagnosis, serological tests are useful from an early stage, especially a direct agglutination test (DAT) which is positive at very high dilutions. However, diagnosis can only be confirmed by demonstration of the parasites. Rapidly executed spleen puncture with a biopsy needle is widely practiced in Africa but rarely in India. Only a minute amount of material is aspirated but this is sufficient to demonstrate parasites in a Giemsa-stained smear or in culture. Bone marrow or lymph node aspirates are also used but are less reliable.

Treatment involves daily injections of pentavalent antimony compounds over a long period, normally 30 days and is usually supported by a rich diet and antibiotics. The diarrhea may be a problem.

Human infection with *L. infantum* is nowhere common and epidemics are unknown. Infantile visceral leishmaniasis caused by *L. infantum* was classically a disease of children aged less than 2 years, but in some areas the age profile has changed considerably. In southern Europe, where it has become very rare in children, the age distribution has also changed, and adult cases are now the majority. The causes of the former restriction to infants and the subsequent changes are unclear but must have little to do with selective exposure to infection or to acquired immunity: Even in areas where transmission among dogs remains intense, and people are frequently bitten by the sandfly vector, human infection is very rare, and still restricted to infants. Further, among visitors from northern Europe to the Mediterranean, who are less likely than residents to have acquired immunity, the age pattern of infection is similar (Ashford, 1988). It seems that, in endemic areas, people of all ages are frequently exposed to infection but only a small (and declining) fraction of children are susceptible; in addition, a very small (but increasing) proportion of older people are susceptible. The decline in susceptibility of infants may be due to improved living standards. In Brazil undernourished children are particularly susceptible; many otherwise healthy children develop serological changes indicating infection, but develop little or no disease. The increase in incidence in adults is due to immunodepression caused by concomitant HIV infection, by transplant surgery or by chemotherapy for malignant disease, which may reactivate latent infection or promote susceptibility to new infection. The fact that most HIV/*L. infantum* co-infection is in drug abusers raises the question of possible needle-transmission (Alvar and Jimenez, 1994).

In many parts of its range, particular strains of *L. infantum* cause a simple cutaneous lesion in humans resembling that of *L. tropica*. HIV infection sometimes causes these dermotropic strains to visceralize.

The enormous variation in prepatent period is illustrated by the occasional occurrence of visceral leishmaniasis in people who only visited the enzootic areas many years previously.

Prevention and control

The World Bank, UNDP, WHO Special Programme for Tropical Diseases has highlighted the public health importance of the leishmaniases but this is still not fully recognized by national health services in many endemic nations. This is in part due to the locality of the diseases in both space and time and also to their generally rural distribution. Increasing health expectations among rural people as well as improvements in potential control measures are changing this attitude.

The control of *L. infantum* infection should be considered both for the protection of the numerous dogs at risk, and for the small number of human patients. Prevention and control depend on the collection and maintenance of good records. In many countries this is the responsibility of malaria departments eager to diversify their activities in the aftermath of failed or completed malaria control programs. Because of the diverse expertise required for leishmaniasis control, WHO has recommended the establishment of a multidisciplinary committee of public health officers, entomologists and veterinarians to co-ordinate activities. In some countries the treatment of canine leishmaniasis is so important as a source of income to veterinarians that they need convincing of the benefits of control measures.

There is as yet no fully effective vaccine available against any of the leishmaniases. Trials are in progress for vaccines against cutaneous leishmaniasis in Iran, and a product is available in Brazil whose effectiveness is in question. The latter product is also being tried against visceral leishmaniasis in dogs. Prophylactic chemotherapy is not feasible due to the toxicity and expense of available products.

Experimentally, collars and topical insecticide application have been tried for the protection of individual dogs.

Personal protection may be achieved by avoiding the bites of phlebotomine sandflies. As these almost invariably occur at night, small-mesh window screens or bed nets are effective against infection transmitted by endophagic sandflies. Chemical repellents on skin or clothing are effective for nocturnal activities out of doors; usually these are used to prevent the irritation of insect bites in general rather than leishmaniasis. These measures are not practical, or would require modification, for the protection of dogs.

Phlebotomine sandflies are susceptible to most insecticides so spraying of houses is very effective for endophilic species. Many vector species are, however, exophilic and are difficult to control. Fogging with ultra low volume insecticides in the period of still air at dusk is sometimes used to control *Phlebotomus papatasi* in small towns where it is a serious nuisance. This is not applicable in sylvatic sites, where no form of sandfly control is readily available. Pheromone traps or the destruction of larval sites are potential methods at an early stage of development.

Control of *L. infantum* infection by the elimination of infected dogs has been tried, and may be an option in certain circumstances. In China in the 1950s, elimination of dogs appeared to be highly effective. More usually, attempts to identify infected dogs and destroy them selectively have largely failed due either to popular antagonism or to the inefficiency of diagnostic methods. The elimination of symptomatic dogs only would have little effect on transmission since many dogs are infected and infective, but are asymptomatic.

From the time when leishmaniasis largely disappeared from many places in the 1950s, few if any control programs have been accompanied by effective evaluation. Methods of evaluation have not been developed to any degree of sophistication. The idea of a controlled experiment on a scale larger than that of a small pilot trial is inconceivable and the aggregation of cases in both space and time tends to invalidate the use of historic data.

With the exception of the compulsory reporting of cases, which applies in an increasing number of countries on the recommendation of WHO, legislation is inappropriate in leishmaniasis. Transportation of infected dogs between countries is unlikely to carry great risk of introducing canine leishmaniasis to new areas. It is probable that the infection already exists wherever it can. However, occasional infections have been recorded in dogs which have never been in endemic areas. On at least one occasion there was good circumstantial evidence that the infection was acquired in the UK from an imported dog, which must have been transmitted without the assistance of a sandfly (Guy *et al.*, 1993; Harris, 1994). The sporadic occurrence of the disease in extralimital areas in the USA may be similarly explained. Such occasions are sufficiently rare that they should not be used to limit travelling with dogs. On the other hand, it is not uncommon for dogs visiting endemic areas to become infected and for the disease to become apparent after their return home. In non-endemic areas the disease is likely to be misdiagnosed and inappropriately treated. The removal of quarantine restrictions in the UK would certainly lead to large numbers of British dogs holidaying on the Mediterranean coast, and to the importation of canine leishmaniasis into that country. It is important that veterinarians in the UK be aware of this potentially important problem, but the risk is to dogs rather than humans.

Leishmania tropica

L. tropica is much less widely distributed than was originally thought, being largely restricted to the densely populated cities of central and West Asia from Northwest India to Syria. The human disease is called oriental sore, or is named after localities where the risk of infection, especially in visitors, is high, such as Baghdad boil, Aleppo boil, Delhi boil, Sart sore, Balkh sore.

Although *L. tropica* has recently been found to cause zoonotic cutaneous leishmaniasis in Kenya, where the reservoir host is the rock hyrax *Procavia johnstoni*, there is no evidence that *L. tropica* in Asia depends on zoonotic sources. Domestic dogs have been found infected in India, Afghanistan and Iran, but the density of infected dogs is far less than that of humans and it is more likely that humans are the source of canine infection.

Leishmania major

L. major has been identified from dogs in Saudi Arabia, but only very rarely. This is a parasite of desert rodents which causes epidemics of cutaneous leishmaniasis in man. The dog is not an important host.

Leishmania braziliensis *and* Leishmania peruviana

L. braziliensis is a heterogeneous species with many local variants, widely distributed, mainly in primary forest areas of Brazil and surrounding countries including Bolivia, Ecuador and Colombia. *Leishmania peruviana* is closely similar, but has very different ecology, being distributed in the high arid valleys of the western slopes of the Andes of Peru and probably Ecuador. Stocks isolated from the northern limits of *L. peruviana*, in the wetter, forested highlands of Ecuador are difficult to distinguish from *L. braziliensis*.

L. braziliensis causes severely disfiguring disease in humans: initially an ulcer develops at the site of the infective bite; this usually cures even if untreated, though cure may take several years. It is after the cure of the initial lesion that more serious problems arise. After an indeterminate period, sometimes as long as 40 years, the parasites reappear in the mucosa of the mouth or nose, where they slowly cause the tissue to die, so that large areas of the face may be destroyed. This condition is known as mucocutaneous leishmaniasis or espundia. *L. peruviana* rarely if ever causes this devastating condition, the disease is usually limited to the initial lesion.

In view of the seriousness of both diseases and the considerable investment in research on them, it is surprising that the ecology of the parasites remains so poorly known. This is partly due to the difficulty of growing the parasites in culture. Human infection is classically associated with life in rainforest, where miners, settlers and military expeditions are affected. Indigenous people are much less severely affected, possibly because they are infected mildly at an early age, but they may be seriously affected if they move from their native lands. In recent years there have been alarming increases in the numbers of cases of *L. braziliensis* infection in towns and cities.

Throughout their range both species are probably at least partially zoonotic; both species have been isolated from various wild animals as well as domestic dogs, but the primary reservoir hosts remain unknown. The altitudinal range of vectors of *L. peruviana*, *Lutzomyia verrucarum* and *Lutzomyia peruensis* is coincident of that of the human infection, between 500 and 2800 m above sea level. The vectors of *L. braziliensis* are less well known; *Lutzomyia* (*Psychodopygus*) *wellcomei* is fully incriminated in sylvatic transmission in Serra dos Carajas, Brazil, and various species are provisionally incriminated in peridomestic transmission.

Reithinger and Davies (1999) have given a comprehensive review of the evidence that the dog may be a reservoir host for American cutaneous leishmaniasis. They conclude that, though infection with both of these important *Leishmania* species is found in dogs throughout the areas where domestic transmission is suspected, the evidence that the dog is more than an incidental host is circumstantial and inconclusive. Beaver *et al.* (1984) speculate that *L. peruviana* was probably once transmitted in an enzootic cycle involving some unknown wild animal. With increasing aridity and/or clearing of vegetation for agriculture, the original host has disappeared, and the reservoir host today is the domestic dog. It is possible that a similar process is actively occurring with the urbanization of *L. braziliensis* infection, so detailed studies of the dynamics of transmission and of the role of the dog are urgently needed. At present there is no justification for destruction of dogs for the control of these diseases.

Trypanosoma brucei

In popular consciousness, sleeping sickness or African trypanosomiasis is one of the best known of all the tropical diseases, and the vector tsetse flies are almost as well known as mosquitoes. The 25,000 cases reported annually (Gibson, 1998) are probably only a fraction of those which occur, and epidemics have devastated populations. The species of trypanosome which cause the disease nagana in cattle are generally not the same as those causing human disease.

The dog is susceptible to infection with most of the African trypanosome species, some of which cause severe disease (reviewed by Steven, 1986). *Trypansoma brucei* is generally regarded as being composed of three subspecies, *T. b. brucei* which is not infective to humans but is lethal to dogs, *T. b. rhodesiense* which is zoonotic in wild ungulates and causes sporadic or epidemic acute disease in humans, and *T. b. gambiense* which is largely anthroponotic and causes less acute disease in humans.

Much effort has been expended on the description of the foci of infection of all these parasites, especially on vector and reservoir host studies. *T. b. rhodesiense* seems not to have been isolated from the dog, and its epidemiology is readily explained by infections in ungulates. *T. b. gambiense* has been isolated from ungulates, pigs and dogs (Zilmann *et al.*, 1984). Of these hosts, it is not possible to determine which if any is able to maintain populations of the parasite, and there is insufficient evidence to incriminate the dog as a reservoir host. Rather, it seems probable that dogs may acquire their infections from humans or other animals.

Trypanosoma cruzi

Trypanosoma cruzi infection is widely distributed in South America, extending into the southern US, where it has been found in dogs in Texas, Oklahoma, Louisiana, South Carolina and Virginia (Barr *et al.*, 1995). The parasite is transmitted between its mammal hosts by triatomine bugs. When these feed on blood they defecate; the feces contains infective trypanosomes which may be rubbed into the wound, or may actively penetrate the mucous membranes. In humans the infection may pass unnoticed, may cause acute life-threatening disease or may produce chronic changes in the heart predisposing the patient to cardiac failure, or to the intestine causing severe malfunction. There is no satisfactory treatment, so prevention of infection is a major public health priority. Some 16-18 million people are estimated to be infected.

The most remarkable feature of *T. cruzi* is the extraordinarily large number of host species from which it has been isolated. More than 150 species of mammal have been found infected. This makes it particularly difficult to assess the relative importance of any one in the maintenance of the parasite. There are numerous morphologically similar forms, including parasites of bats in the Old World, which can only be identified by biochemical methods.

A presumably ancient cycle of transmission exists in sylvatic foci, in which man is rarely infected. At the other extreme are strains which seem only to be transmitted in peridomestic conditions, where man probably shares a major role in the maintenance of the parasite. It is in the peridomestic foci that the dog and cat may play a major role. According to Steven (1986) dogs and cats have been found infected with *T. cruzi* throughout Latin America and must constitute an important reservoir of infection for man. In northern Argentina, Gurtler *et al.* (1991) showed that the infection rate in the vector *Triatoma infestans* was closely related to the presence of infected dogs, but not to the presence of infected people. They later showed (Gurtler *et al.*, 1996) that seropositive dogs were 12 times more infective to bugs than were seropositive children, and 100 times more infective than adults. Taking into account the different infection rates between people and dogs, a bug was 500 times more likely to become infected by biting a dog than by biting a human. Given the preference of *T. infestans* for dog blood, the dog is clearly much more important than humans as a source of source of transmitted infection in this area.

According to Miles (1998), although 150 species of mammal, from 24 families have been found infected, dogs are especially important as reservoir hosts because of their close association with man, and their high infection rate. It is possible, however, that opossums *Didelphis* spp. are even more important, as these may become infected by eating triatomine bugs and may transmit the infection through glandular secretions.

Chagas' disease has been controlled in much of Brazil, and an ambitious program is underway in the "Southern Cone" countries of Argentina, Bolivia, Brazil, Chile, Paraguay, and Uruguay. Control measures are based on the elimination of the peridomestic vector, *T. infestans*, and are unaffected by the fact that the dog may be an important host. The infection of dogs occurs in the same place as humans, so reducing the rate of transmission will affect both hosts simultaneously (reviewed by Schofield and Dias, 1998).

Toxoplasma gondii

The cat rather than the dog is the natural definitive host for *Toxoplasma gondii*. The dog shares with man and almost every other mammal the role of intermediate host, and it seems most unlikely that one could serve as a source of infection for the other. Nevertheless, Frenkel *et al.* (1996), who knew more about the subject than most, did ascribe a possible role to the dog as a source of human infection. The habit, he suggested, of dogs to roll in the feces of other animals, would allow their fur to be contaminated with oocyst-bearing cat feces which might then contaminate a doting pet lover.

Babesia gibsoni

Babesia gibsoni is a parasite of dogs and a *B. gibsoni*-like parasite, WA1, infects humans throughout a broad area along the Pacific coast of the USA. However, the parasite isolated from humans fails to infect dogs but will infect rodents of many species (Telford and Spielman, 1998). The vector is unknown, but the ticks, *Ixodes pacificus*, *Dermacentor variabilis*, and *Ornithodoros coriaceus* are frequent in the areas where human infection has been reported, so are candidates.

According to Cox (1998), the first of these cases, from California, was described in 1966 and the parasite resembled *B. equi* of horses or *B. canis* of the dog. More recent isolates from Washington State resembled *B. gibsoni*.

Microsporidia

Members of the phylum Microspora, commonly known as the microsporidia, are obligate, intracellular, single-celled organisms found in a wide range of vertebrate and invertebrate hosts. Not many years ago the microsporidia were studied primarily for their potential use as biological control agents against insects, and their major importance in mammals was as parasites of laboratory rodents and rabbits. This situation has changed dramatically, so that at the latest count, more than a dozen species have been recorded in humans (reviewed by Didier *et al.*, 1998). Since the HIV virus results in immunosuppression of its human host, numerous hitherto unknown parasites have been documented in AIDS patients and other immunocompromised people, and microsporidia are important among these emerging infections. It is intuitively logical that many of these infections must be of zoonotic origin, but the epidemiology has not yet been satisfactorily described for any of these organisms. At least one species, *Encephalitozoon cuniculi*, is possibly shared by man and dog.

The microsporidia are intracellular parasites which replicate asexually. The final product is a spore which is remarkable for its small size and internal complexity. Although the spores are usually only between 2 and 5 μm long, each contains a coiled hollow filament or polar tubule which may reach 100 μm length. When the filament is explosively expelled from the spore, the sporoplasm is extruded through it, and is directly injected into a new host cell.

Encephalitozoon cuniculi

E. cuniculi was the first microsporidian species to be described in mammals, in the 1920s, and it is the type-species of its genus. *E. cuniculi* has a wide host range including rodents and rabbits; and occasionally it is reported in dogs, foxes, wild carnivores, and primates including man (reviewed in Snowden and Shadduck, 1999). The first confirmed reports of microsporidial infections in dogs were published in the 1950s (Plowright and Yeoman, 1952), and the first *in vitro* culture of the parasite from canine tissues was reported by Shadduck *et al.* (1978). The largest number of investigations and experimental infections in dogs have been conducted by researchers in South Africa, but canine infections have also been reported in England, Germany, USA, Tanzania and Zimbabwe (reviewed by Botha *et al.*, 1979; VanDellen *et al.*, 1989).

The prevalence of infection in canine populations varies depending on the survey method and the population selected for study. In a Swiss study, 212 dogs were serologically negative and 102 fecal specimens were parasitologically negative (Deplazes *et al.*, 1996). In contrast, 13.3% of 248 adult dogs in a London pound (Hollister *et al.,* 1989), and 18% of 220 random dog sera in South Africa (Stewart *et al.*, 1981) were seropositive. Generally it is believed that infections in adult carnivores are usually subclinical, so the relevance of seropositivity is difficult to define.

The most common clinical manifestation of canine microsporidial infection is an encephalitis-nephritis syndrome in puppies under 10 weeks of age, often resulting in death (reviewed by Snowden and Shadduck, 1999). Progressive neurologic disease is most frequently described, but chronic renal disease has also been reported in young adult dogs. Parasites replicate in parasitophorous vacuoles in macrophages, epithelial cells and kidney tubule cells, and are most easily demonstrated histologically in the brain and kidney, although infection in other organs has been reported. Both oral and transplacental routes of transmission have been described. Dogs exposed by feeding infected tissues from naturally infected dogs established infections but developed no clinical disease (Botha *et al.*, 1979). It is probable that young puppies with disease became infected *in utero* from their asymptomatic dams (McInnes and Stewart, 1991).

Spore shedding in feces and in urine has been reported from clinically ill puppies (Botha *et al.*, 1986). Parasites have been histologically identified in the kidney of asymptomatic dogs (McInnes and Stewart, 1991), and in urine and/or feces from dams and asymptomatic littermates of symptomatic puppies (Snowden *et al.*, unpublished observation).

The duration and intensity of spore shedding in symptomatic or clinically normal dogs has not generally been well documented. Early descriptions of *E. cuniculi* in dogs were based on morphologic and ultrastructural descriptions of the parasite in tissues. Recently, molecular analysis of the small subunit ribosomal RNA genes have confirmed the identity of dog isolates (Didier *et al.*, 1996). Furthermore, molecular sequencing of the internal transcribed spacer region (ITS region) between large and small subunits of the ribosomal RNA genes of *E. cuniculi* has shown subtle differences based on the number of repeats of a 4-base (GTTT) sequence. Rabbit and mouse isolates of *E. cuniculi* had two or three repeats respectively, while dog and human isolates were identical with four repeats of the sequence. The epidemiological significance of these observations and the potential for zoonotic transmission of *E. cuniculi* between man and dog needs further study. However, these data suggest that dogs may be an unrecognized reservoir of *E. cuniculi* infection for potential human exposure.

Conclusions

It is frequently stated, not least by scientists seeking research support, that the domestic dog is a source of numerous diseases of humans. As far as protozoal diseases are concerned, this is an overstatement. Although it is true that the dog shares with us various parasitic protozoa, many of these are maintained in humans and the dog is an incidental host. Very few of these shared parasites are maintained in dogs. Only with *T. cruzi* and *L. infantum* has the dog been shown to be an important source of human disease and, for the former, there are other sources including humans themselves. These two, and particularly *L. infantum*, are by far the most important human protozoan pathogens whose source is the dog.

Complacency is not justified, however: as the response to infection of humans in Western society has been altered by our changing lifestyles, new infections have emerged and more can be expected to do so. Veterinary and medical scientists must be ever on the alert to new dangers.

References

Alvar, J. and Jimenez, M. (1994) Could infected drug users be potential *Leischmania infantum* reservoirs? *AIDS* 8, 84.

Ashford, R.W. (1979) Occurrence of an undescribed coccidian in man in Papua New Guinea. *Annals of Tropical Medicine and Parasitology* 73, 497-500.

Ashford, R.W. (1988) Leishmaniasis in Europe. In: *International Development Research Center Research on Control Strategies for the Leishmaniases.* International Development Research Center - MR 184e Ottawa, pp. 172-177.

Ashford, R.W. (1998) The leishmaniases. In: Palmer, S.R., Lord Soulsby and Simpson, D.I.H. (eds) *Zoonoses.* Oxford University Press, Oxford, pp. 528-543.

Ashford, R.W. and Atkinson, A. (1992) Epidemiology of *Blastocystis* infection in Papua New Guinea. *Annals of Tropical Medicine and Parasitology* 86, 129-136.

Ashford, R.W. and Crewe, W. (1998) *The Parasites of* Homo sapiens: *an* Annotated Checklist of the Protozoa Helminths and Arthropods for Which *We are Home.* Liverpool, pp. 128.

Ashford, R.W., Desjeux, P. and de Raadt, P. (1992) Estimation of population at risk of infection and numbers of cases of Leishmaniasis. *Parasitology Today* 8, 104-105.

Ashford, R.W., Warhurst, D.C. and Reid, G.D.F. (1993) Human infection with cyanobacterium-like bodies. *Lancet* 341, 1034.

Barr, S.C. (1998) Enteric protozoal infections. In: Greene, C.E. (ed.) *Infectious Diseases of the Dog and Cat.* WB Saunders Company, Philadelphia, pp. 482-490.

Barr, S.C., Van-Beek, O., Carlisle-Nowak, M.S., Lopez, J.W., Kirchhoff, L.V., Allison, N., Zajac, A., de-Lahunta, A., Schlafer, D.H. and Crandall, W.T. (1995) *Trypanosoma cruzi* infection in Walker hounds from Virginia. *American Journal of Veterinary Research* 56, 1037-1044.

Baruch, A.C., Isaac-Renton, J. and Adam, R.D. (1996) The molecular epidemiology of *Giardia lamblia*: a sequence-based approach. *Journal of Infectious Diseases* 174, 233-236.

Beaver, P.C., Jung, R.C. and Cupp, E.W. (1984) *Clinical Parasitology,* 9th edition. Lea and Febiger, Philadelphia, pp. 825.

Boreham, P.F.L. and Stenzel, D.J. (1998) Blastocystosis. In: Palmer, S.R., Lord Soulsby and Simpson, D.I.H. (eds) *Zoonoses.* University Press, Oxford, pp. 625-634.

Botha, W.S., VanDellen, A.F. and Stewart, C.G. (1979) Canine encephalitozoonosis in South Africa. *Journal of the South African Veterinary Medical Association* 50, 135-144.

Botha, W.S., Dormehl, I.C. and Goosen, D.J. (1986) Evaluation of kidney function in dogs suffering from canine encephalitozoonosis by standard clinical pathological and radiopharmaceutical techniques. *Journal of the South African Veterinary Medical Association* 57, 79-86.

Courtenay, O., Santana, E.W., Johnson, P.J., Vasconcelos, I.A.B. and Vasconselos, A.W. (1996) Visceral leishmaniasis in the hoary zorro *Dusicyon vetulus*: a case of mistaken identity. *Transactions of the Royal Society of Tropical Medicine and Hygiene* 90, 498-502.

Cox, F.E.G. (1998) Babesiosis and malaria. In: Palmer, S.R., Lord Soulsby and Simpson, D.I.H. (eds) *Zoonoses*. Oxford University Press, Oxford, pp. 599-608.

Current, W.L. (1998) Cryptosporidiosis. In: Cox, F.E.G., Kreier, J.P. and Wakelin, D. (eds) *Topley & Wilson's Microbiology and Microbial Infections, Vol. 5, Parasitology*. Arnold, London, pp. 329-348.

Deplazes, P., Mathis, A., Muller, C. and Weber, R. (1996) Molecular epidemiology of *Encephalitozoon cuniculi* and first detection of *Enterocytozoon bieneusi* in faecal samples from pigs. *Journal of Eukaryotic Microbiology* 43, 93S.

Didier, E.S., Visvesvara, G.S., Baker, M.D., Rogers, L.B., Bertucci, D.C., DeGroote, M.A. and Vossbrinck, C.R. (1996) A microsporidian isolated from an AIDS patient corresponds to *Encephalitozoon cuniculi* III, originally isolated from domestic dogs. *Journal of Clinical Microbiology* 34, 2835-2837.

Didier, E.S., Snowden, K.F. and Shadduck, J.A. (1998) Biology of microsporidian species infecting mammals. In: Baker, J.R., Muller, R. and Rollinson, D. (eds) *Advances in Parasitology* Vol. 40. Academic Press, San Diego, California, pp. 281-320.

Dubey, J.P., Speer, C.A. and Fayer, R. (1989) *Sarcocystosis of Animals and Man*. CRC Press, Boca Raton, pp. 215.

Duda, A., Stenzel, D.J. and Boreham, P.F. (1998) Detection of *Blastocystis* sp. in domestic dogs and cats. *Veterinary Parasitology* 76, 9-17.

El-Ahraf, A., Tacal, J.V., Sobih, M., Amin, M., Lawrence, W. and Wilcke, B.W. (1991) Prevalence of cryptosporidiosis in dogs and human beings in San Bernadino County, California. *Journal of the American Veterinary Medical Association* 198, 631-634.

Erlandsen, S.L. (1994) Biotic transmission - is giardiasis a zoonosis? In: Thompson, R.C.A., Reynoldson, J.A. and Lymbery, A.J. (eds) *Giardia, from Molecules to Disease*. CAB International, Wallingford, pp. 87-93.

Ey, P.L., Bruderer, T., Wehrli, C. and Köhler, P. (1996) Comparison of genetic groups determined by molecular and immunologic analyses of *Giardia* isolated from animals and humans in Switzerland and Australia. *Parasitology Research* 82, 52-60.

Frenkel, J.K., Dobesh, M., Parker, B.B. and Lindsay, D.S. (1996) Xenosmophilia of dogs: a habit favoring the mechanical transmission of *Toxoplasma gondii* and other fecal microbes. *Programme Guide and Abstracts for the Joint Meeting of the American Society of Parasitologists and the Society of Protozoologists*. pp. 110.

Gibson, W. (1998) African trypanosomosis. In: Palmer, S.R., Lord Soulsby and Simpson, D.I.H. (eds) *Zoonoses*. Oxford University Press, Oxford, pp. 501-512.

Gurtler, R.E., Cecere, M.C., Rubel, D.N., Petersen, R.M., Schweigmann, N.J., Lauricella, M.A., Bujas, M.A., Segura, E.L. and Wisnivesky-Colli, C. (1991) Chagas disease in north-west Argentina: infected dogs as a risk-factor for the domestic transmission of *T. cruzi*. *Transactions of the Society of Tropical Medicine and Hygiene* 85, 741-745.

Gurtler, R.E., Cecere, M.C., Castanera, M.B., Canale, D., Lauricella, M.A., Chu, R., Cohen, J.E. and Segura, E.L. (1996) Probability of infection with *Trypanosoma cruzi* of the vector *Triatoma infestans* fed on infected humans and dogs in northwest Argentina. *American Journal of Tropical Medicine and Hygiene* 55, 24-31.

Guy, M., Bailey, W. and Snowden, K. (1993) Canine leishmaniasis (Letter). *Veterinary Record* 132, 396.

Harris, M.P. (1994) Suspected transmission of leishmaniasis (Letter). *Veterinary Record* 133, 339.

Hay, D.C., Savva, D. and Nowell, F. (1990) Characterisation of *Giardia* species of canine and human origin using RFLPs. *Veterinary Record* 126, 274.

Hollister, W.S., Canning, E.U. and Viney, M. (1989) Prevalence of antibodies to *Encephalitozoon cuniculi* in stray dogs as determined by an ELISA. *Veterinary Record* 124, 332-336.

Hopkins, R.M., Meloni, B.P., Groth, D.M., Wetherall, J.D., Reynoldson, J.A. and Thompson, R.C.A. (1997) Ribosomal RNA sequencing reveals differences between the genotypes of *Giardia* isolates recovered from humans and dogs living in the same locality. *Journal of Parasitology* 83, 44-51.

Levine, N.D. (1983) *Veterinary Protozoology*. Iowa State University Press, Ames, pp. 414.

Lewis, P.D. (1988) Prevalence of *Giardia* sp. in dogs in Alaska. In: Wallis, P.M. and Hammond, B.R. (eds) *Advances in* Giardia *Research*. University of Calgary Press, Calgary, pp. 61-64.

Lloyd, S. and Smith, J. (1997) Pattern of *Cryptosporidium parvum* oocyst excretion by experimentally infected dogs. *International Journal of Parasitology* 27, 779-801.

McInnes, E.F. and Stewart, C.G. (1991) The pathology of subclinical infection of *Encephalitozoon cuniculi* in canine dams producing pups with overt encephalitozoonosis. *Journal of the South African Veterinary Medicine Association* 62, 51-54.

Miles, M.A. (1998) New World trypanosomes. In: Cox, F.E.G., Kreier, J.P. and Wakelin, D. (eds) *Topley and Wilson's Microbiology and Microbial Infections Vol 5, Parasitology*. Arnold, London, pp. 283-302.

Nolan, T.J. and Smith, G. (1995) Time series analysis of the prevalence of endoparasitic infections in cats and dogs presented to a veterinary teaching hospital. *Veterinary Parasitology* 59, 87-96.

Olson, M.E., Ceri, H. and Morck, D.W. (2000) *Giardia* vaccination. *Parasitology Today* 16, 213-217.

Plowright, W. and Yeoman, G. (1952) Probable *Encephalitozoon* infection of the dog. *Veterinary Record* 64, 3871-3883.

Reithinger, R. and Davies, C.R. (1999) Is the domestic dog (*Canis familiaris*) a reservoir host of American cutaneous leishmaniasis? A critical review of the evidence. *American Journal of Tropical Medicine and Hygiene* 61, 530-541.

Schofield, C.J. and Dias, J.C.P. (1998) The Southern Cone initiative against Chagas' disease. *Advances in Parasitology* 42, 1-27.

Semiao-Santos, S.J. (1996) *Canine Visceral Leishmaniasis in Evora District, Portugal: a Sero-Epidemiological Study.* Den Haag: Gegevens Koninklijke Bibliotheek, pp. 174.

Shadduck, J.A., Benedele, R. and Robinson, G.T. (1978) Isolation of the causitive organism of canine encephalitozoonosis. *Veterinary Pathology* 15, 449-460.

Snowden, K.F. and Shadduck, J.A. (1999) Microsporidia in higher vertebrates. In: Wittner, M. (ed.) *Microsporidia and Microsporidiosis.* ASM Press, Washington, DC, pp. 393-417.

Soave, R., Dubey, J.P., Ramos, L.J. and Tummings, M.A. (1986) A new intestinal pathogen? *Clinical Research* 34, 533A.

Soulsby, E.J.L. (1982) *Helminths, Arthropods and Protozoa of Domesticated Animals,* 7th edn. Baillière Tindall, London.

Steven, L.E. (1986) *Trypanosomiasis a Veterinary Perspective.* Pergamon, Oxford pp. 551.

Stewart, C.G., VanDellen, A.F. and Botha, W.S. (1981) Antibodies to a canine isolate of *Encephalitozoon* in various species. *South African Journal of Science* 77, 572.

Telford, S.R. and Spielman, A. (1998) Babesiosis of humans In: Cox, F.E.G., Kreier, J.P. and Wakelin, D. (eds) *Topley and Wilson's Microbiology and Microbial Infections Vol 5, Parasitology,* Arnold, London pp. 349-360.

Thompson, R.C.A., Hopkins, R.M. and Homan W.L. (2000) Nomenclature and genetic groupings of *Giardia* infecting mammals. *Parasitology Today* 16(5), 210-213.

Van Dellen, A.F., Steward, C.G. and Botha, W.S. (1989) Studies of encephalitozoonosis in vervet monkeys (*Cercopithecus pygerythrus*) orally inoculated with spores of *Encephalitozoon cuniculi* isolated from dogs (*Canis familiaris*). *Onderstepoort Journal of Veterinary Research* 56, 1-22.

Xiao, L., Morgan, U.M., Fayer, R., Thompson, R.C.A. and Lal, A.A. (2000) *Cryptosporidium* systematics and implications for public Health. *Parasitology Today* 16(7), 287-292.

Yai, L.E., Bauab, A.R., Hirschfeld, M.P., de Oliveira, M.L., Damaceno, J.T. (1997) The first two cases of *Cyclospora* in dogs. *Revista do Instituto de Medicina Tropical de São Paulo* 39, 177-179.

Zilmann, U., Mehlitz, D. and Sachs, R. (1984) Identity of *Trypanozoon* stocks isolated from man and a domestic dog in Liberia. *Tropenmedicine und Parasitologie* 35, 105-108.

Chapter Six

Dogs and Trematode Zoonoses

Ralph Muller

The trematodes or flukes belong to the phylum Platyhelminthes. They are all endoparasites and characteristically are flat and leaf-like, or occasionally globular, hermaphroditic organisms (except for one group, the schistosomes, which have a male folded about its long axis and a cylindrical female). Adults have a blindly ending bifurcate intestine without an anus and two suckers, an anterior oral sucker surrounding the mouth, and a more posterior ventral sucker or acetabulum by which the worm attaches itself to the host. All organs are surrounded by parenchyma as there is no coelom and the outer tegument, which often contains spines, is composed of a syncytial cytoplasmic layer which secretes enzymes and is of great importance in nutrition; it is thus an antigenically active site.

Trematodes have an indirect life cycle which always involves a snail as first intermediate host. Most are freshwater species of snails but a few utilize terrestrial snails (e.g. *Dicrocoelium dendriticum*) or, for sea birds, marine species. Inside the snail all trematodes undergo asexual reproduction and most which parasitize both humans and dogs have a cystic stage in a secondary intermediate host such as a fish or edible crustacean (again except for the schistosomes in which larvae penetrate the skin). Thus infection depends very much on the dietary habits of the hosts. Adult trematodes are very catholic in their choice of definitive host, although almost all are very specific in which snails they can develop. There are over 60 trematode species which have been reported from both humans and dogs (listed in Table 6.1), but for many trematodes they are occasional hosts only and dogs are not the most important reservoir hosts of human infection.

The trematode parasites of dogs are considered in standard textbooks (Dunn, 1978; Euzeby, 1982; Georgi and Georgi, 1992; FAO, 1994; Bowman, 1999; Kassai, 1999) and zoonotic trematode parasites in general in various monographs (Malek, 1980; Hillyer and Hopla, 1982; Schultz, 1982; Geerts *et al.*, 1987; Hugh-Jones *et al.*, 1995; WHO, 1995; Hinz, 1996).

The Schistosomes

Superfamily Schistosomatoidea: Family Schistosomatidae

Three species of schistosomes (*Schistosoma japonicum, Schistosoma mansoni* and *Schistosoma haematobium*) are the cause of what is undoubtedly the most important human helminthic disease of schistosomiasis. There are about 20 million severely ill sufferers from schistosomiasis world wide and another 120 million have symptomatic disease. Its distribution has been recently reviewed by Savioli *et al.* (1997). Schistosomiasis in humans is primarily a rural disease, particularly effecting agricultural communities and, in Africa, fishermen. Schistosomiasis in humans is primarily a rural disease, particularly effecting agricultural communities and, in Africa, fishermen.

Of the primarily human species, *S. japonicum* is a true zoonosis and dogs as well as bovines are often infected and act as reservoir hosts. Human infection is principally confined to China, Sulawesi and the Philippines (there were estimated to be 1.52 million cases in China in 1987, with currently a 1% infection rate in Indonesia and a 3.6% infection rate in the Philippines). In China many animals can act as reservoir hosts but the most important are bovines (with up to 90% infection rates in cattle and buffalo) and dogs (10% infected) (Jordan *et al.*, 1993). An increasing challenge in China is likely to follow the building of the Gorges Super Dam Project on the Yangtze river. A very similar species, *Schistosoma mekongi*, is an important human parasite in the Mekong Delta region of Laos and Cambodia and dogs are the only reservoir hosts.

S. mansoni is widely distributed in Africa and also occurs in foci in the Middle East, South America and the Caribbean (principally Puerto Rico and the Dominican Republic). Reservoir hosts are of little epidemiological significance although primates and rodents may be of local importance. Dogs can be infected but often do not pass eggs (Jordan *et al.*, 1993).

The other widespread human species, *S. haematobium*, is not a zoonosis and so is not considered here.

Adult *S. mansoni* and *S. japonicum* worms live in the posterior mesenteric veins, the smaller and thinner female residing permanently in a canal formed by the fleshy ventral folds of the male which measures about 12 mm. Eggs (those of *S. japonicum* and *S. mekongi* measuring 85 x 60 µm with a small knob and those of *S. mansoni* measuring 140 x 60 µm and with a lateral spine) laid in the small venules, penetrate through the wall of the large intestine and are passed out in feces. On reaching fresh water a larva, known as a miracidium, emerges and penetrates into a suitable species of snail (see Table 6.1), multiplies inside the snail, and a few weeks later the next free-living, fork-tailed larval stage, the cercaria, emerges and can survive for a few days in water. If it comes into contact with a susceptible mammal it penetrates through the skin by means of histolytic glands, reaches the lungs, and then migrates to its final site via the pulmonary veins.

The adult worms do little damage, but in chronic infections more and more eggs get trapped in the tissues producing an inflammatory response leading to the formation of granulomas and eventually extensive fibrosis. This phase of infection may be symptomless or accompanied by bloody intermittent diarrhea and headache. However, in heavy infections eggs get carried the wrong way in the veins to the liver and granulomas formed around them there (Figure 6.1) lead in 5-15 years to extensive fibrosis surrounding the branches of the portal vein. This causes portal hypertension with enlargement of the liver and spleen and compensatory enlargement of the minor veins from the liver which sometimes burst (Rollinson and Simpson, 1987; Guttierez, 1990; Jordan *et al.*, 1993). In Taiwan, infection occurs only in these hosts and humans are refractory. Diagnosis is by finding eggs in the feces or by newer serological methods such as ELISA with monoclonal antibodies, and effective treatment is possible with praziquantel.

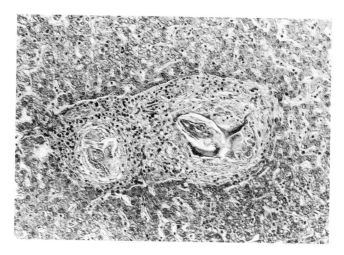

Figure 6.1. Microscope section of liver with trapped eggs of *Schistosoma mansoni* surrounded by a mixed leucocytic infiltrate and multinuclear giant cells.

The epidemiology of schistosomiasis is determined by the habits of the snail intermediate hosts. Those of *S. japonicum* live either in the muddy margins of streams and rivers (in China) or in rice paddies (in the Philippines), while snails transmitting *S. mansoni* inhabit slow-flowing streams, irrigation canals or large ponds or lakes. The distribution of *S. mansoni* is increasing in Africa because of many new irrigation schemes, particularly the large-scale ones in Egypt and Sudan. Prevention is by avoiding contact with water in which transmission may be occurring. Possible control measures have been recently reviewed by Savioli *et al.* (1997).

Heterobilharzia americana is a parasite of dogs and other mammals in the southwest US. In humans the penetrating cercariae cannot develop further and cause a dermatitis, similar to that caused by many bird schistosomes and known as "swimmer's itch". Dogs get infected by paddling in swampy areas or swimming in canals in areas where racoons are present, and suffer from chronic intermittent dysentery, loss of weight, anemia and inflammation of the lymph nodes (lymphadenopathy). Fenbendazole is effective in treatment.

The Opisthorchids

Superfamily Opisthorchioidea: Family Opisthorchiidae

Members of this family are typically flattened, elongate, hermaphroditic flukes, measuring 5-15 mm in length. The adults are found in the hepatic and pancreatic ducts of fish-eating mammals or birds and the cercariae encyst in freshwater fish (Table 6.1).

Table 6.1. Trematodes reported from both humans and dogs. * = rare. So far as possible the authorities quoted are recent, accessible publications which review the infection.

Parasite	Intermediate hosts	Final hosts	Distribution and location in host (reference)
Family Cathycotylidae			
Prohemistomum vivax	1. *Cleopatra* 2. Brackish water fishes	Kite, dog*, cat, man (once)*	Egypt **small intestine** (Nasr, 1941)
Family Diplostomatidae			
Alaria alata	1. *Planorbis* (?) 2. Frogs	Dog, cat, fox, man (larvae)*	USA, Canada, Europe, Mid. East **small intestine** (Dalimi and Mobedi, 1992)
A. americana	1. *Planorbis* 2. Frogs and snakes	Cat, dog, fox, man (larvae)*	SW USA, Canada **small intestine** (Freeman *et al.*, 1976)
A. marcianae	1. *Planorbis* 2. Frogs and snakes	Cat, dog, coyote, fox, man (larvae)*	SW USA, Canada **small intestine** (Shoop and Corkum, 1983a, b)

Parasite	Intermediate hosts	Final hosts	Distribution and location in host (reference)
Family Echinostomatidae			
Echinochamus fujianensis	1. *Bellamya*	Dog, cat, pig	China **small intestine** (Yu and Mott, 1994)
E. japonicus	1. *Parafossarulus* 2. Fw fish and frogs	Heron, dog, cat, man	China, Japan, Taiwan **small intestine** (Lin, 1985)
E. liliputanus	1. Snails 2. Fw fish or none	Dog, man	China **small intestine** (Xiao *et al.*, 1994)
E. perfoliatus	1. *Lymnaea, Bithynia* 2. Fw fish	Dog, cat, fox, pig, man	Japan, Taiwan, Europe **small intestine** (Lu, 1996)
Echinoparyphium recurvatum	1. *Lymnaea, Planorbis* 2. As above	Domestic birds, man (exper. dog, cat)	Taiwan **small intestine** (Lu, 1982)
Echinostoma angustitestis	1. Snail 2. Fw fish	Dog (exper.), man*	China **small intestine** (Chen *et al.*, 1992)
E. cinetorchus	1. *Segmentina* 2. Snails, frogs	Domestic birds, dog, cat, man	Japan, Korea, Taiwan **small intestine** (Ryang *et al.*, 1986)
E. hortense	1. *Lymnaea* 2. Fw fish	Cat, rats, dog, man	China, Japan, Korea **small intestine** (Tani, 1976)
E. ilocanum	1. *Hippeutis* 2. Snails	Dog, cat, man	Philippines, Malaysia China, Indonesia **small intestine** (Geerts *et al.*, 1987)

Parasite	Intermediate hosts	Final hosts	Distribution and location in host (reference)
E. malayanum	1. *Lymnaea* 2. Snails, fish	Pig, rat, man (exper. dog)	China, India, Indonesia **small intestine** (Lie-Kian and Virik, 1963)
E. revolutum	1. *Helisoma* 2. Snails	Domestic birds, man, muskrat (exper. dog)	Indonesia, Taiwan **small intestine** (Lu, 1982)
Episthmium caninum	1. Snails? 2. Fw fish	Dog, man*	Thailand **small intestine** (Radomyos et al., 1991)
Family Dicrocoeliidae			
Dicrocoelium dendriticum	1. *Helicella* 2. Ants	Most herbivores, dog*, man*	Europe, Asia, Africa, Americas **bile ducts** (Petithory and Ardoin, 1990)
Family Fasciolidae			
Fasciolopsis buski	1. *Hippeutis* 2. On plants	Pig, man, dog	Bangladesh, India Cambodia, China, Vietnam, Laos, Malaysia, Taiwan, Thailand **small intestine** (Kumar, 1987)
Family Heterophyidae			
Apophallus donicus	1. *Flumenicola* 2. Fw fish	Heron, fox, dog, cat (exper. man)	East Europe, Canada **small intestine** (Niemi and Macy, 1974)
Centrocestus armatus	1. *Semisulcos- pira* 2. Fw fish	Fish-eating birds, dog, cat (exper. man)	Japan **small intestine** (Hubbert *et al.*, 1975)

Parasite	Intermediate hosts	Final hosts	Distribution and location in host (reference)
C. formosanus	1. *Semisulcos-pira, Melania* 2. Fw fish, frogs	Fish-eating birds, dog, cat, rat, man	China, Japan **small intestine** (Cheng *et al.*, 1991)
Cryptocotyle lingua	1. *Tantoglabrus* 2. Marine fish	Fish-eating birds and mammals, dog, cat, man*	Greenland **small intestine** (Rausch *et al.*, 1967)
Haplorchis pumilio	1. *Melania* 2. Fish (*Puntius*)	Fish-eating birds, dog, cat, man	Philippines, Laos, Egypt **small intestine** (Giboda *et al.*,1991)
H. tachui	1. *Melania* 2. Fish	Cattle, dog, cat, man	Philippines, Laos, Egypt **small intestine** (Tadros and El-Mokkadem, 1983)
H. yokogawai	1. *Stenomelania* 2. Fish	Fish-eating birds, cattle, dog, cat, man	Philippines, Indonesia, Hawaii, Egypt **small intestine** (Kwo En Hoa and Lie Kian Joe, 1953)
Heterophyes dispar	1. *Pirenella* 2. Marine fish	Fish-eating mammals, fox, dog, cat, man	Korea **small intestine** (Chai and Lee, 1990)
H. heterophyes	1. *Pirenella, Cerithidea* 2. Brackish w fish	Fish-eating mammals, fox, dog, cat, man	Egypt, Japan, Korea, France **small intestine** (Murrell, 1995)
Heterophyopsis continua	1. *Cerithidea?* 2. Marine fish	Dog, cat, man	Japan, Korea **small intestine** (Chai and Lee, 1990)
Metagonimus yokogawai	1. *Semisulcosp-ira* 2. Fw fish	Fish-eating birds, dog, cat, rat, man	China, Japan, Korea, Philippines, **small intestine** (Murrell, 1995)

Parasite	Intermediate hosts	Final hosts	Distribution and location in host (reference)
Phagicola longa	1. Snails? 2. Mullet	Fish-eating birds, dog*, man*	Brazil **small intestine** (Chieffi *et al.*, 1992)
P. ornamentata	1. Snails? 2. *Tilapia*	Man? (exper. dog)	Egypt **small intestine** (Shalaby and Trenti, 1994)
P. ornata	1. Snails? 2. *Tilapia*	Man? (exper. dog)	Egypt **small intestine** (Shalaby *et al.*, 1994)
Pharyngostomum flapi	1. Snails? 2. *Tilapia*	Man? (exper. dog)	Egypt **small intestine** (Shalaby *et al.*, 1994)
Procerovum calderoni	1. *Melania, Thiara* 2. Fw fish	Man (exper. dog, cat, chicken)	Philippines, Egypt **small intestine** (Shalaby and Trenti, 1994)
P. varium	1. Snails? 2. Fish	Heron, man* (exper. dog)	Japan **small intestine**
Pygidopsis summa	1. *Tympanotus* 2. Brackish w fish	Fish-eating birds, dog, cat, man*	Korea **small intestine** (Chai and Lee, 1990)
Stellantchasmus falcatus	1. *Stenomelania* 2. Brackish w fish	Fish-eating birds, dog, cat, rat, man	Hawaii, Philippines, Thailand, Korea, Japan **small intestine** (Radomyos *et al.*, 1994)
Stictodora manilensis	1. *Pirenella*? 2. Mullet, goby	Dog, man (once)*	Korea, Thailand **small intestine** (Chai *et al.*, 1988)

Parasite	Intermediate hosts	Final hosts	Distribution and location in host (reference)
Family Lecithodendriidae			
Moedlingeria amphoraeformis	1. Snails? 2. *Tilapia*	(Exper. dog) man?	Egypt **small intestine** (Shalaby and Trenti, 1994)
Phaneropsolus bonnei	1. *Bithynia*? 2. Insect larvae, fw fish	Man, dog	Indonesia, Thailand **small intestine** (Bhaibulaya, 1982; Radomyos *et al.*, 1994)
P. spinicirrus	1. ? 2. Insect larvae	Primates, man*, dog?	Thailand **small intestine** (Hinz, 1996)
Prosthodendrium glandulosum	1. *Bithynia*? 2. Insect larvae	Rat, bat, dog*, cat, man*	Thailand **small intestine** (Bhaibulaya, 1982; Hinz, 1996)
P. molenkampi	1. *Bithynia*? 2. Insect larvae	Primates, man, dog?	Thailand, Indonesia **small intestine** (Bhaibulay, 1982; Radomyos *et al.*, 1994)
P. obtusum	1. *Bithynia* 2. Insect larvae	Rat, bat, dog*, cat, man*	Thailand **small intestine** (Hinz, 1996)
Family Microphallidae			
Microphallus minutus	1. Snails? 2. Shrimp	Dog, rat (exper. man*)	Japan **small intestine** (Smales *et al.*, 1990)
Family Opisthorchidae			
Amphimerus pseudofelineus (=*Opisthorchis quayaquiensis*)	1. Snails? 2. Fw fish?	Coyote, dog, cat, man*	Brazil, Ecuador, Panama, USA **bile and pancreatic ducts** (Dill, 1993)

Parasite	Intermediate hosts	Final hosts	Distribution and location in host (reference)
Metorchis albidus	1. *Bithynia* 2. Fw fish	Fish-eating mammals, dog, cat, man	Alaska, Russia, France, Turkey Iran **bile ducts?** (Dalimi and Mobedi, 1992)
M. conjunctus	1. *Amnicola* 2. Fish	Fish-eating mammals, dog, cat, man	Canada, Greenland **bile ducts?** (Maclean *et al.*, 1996)
Clonorchis (= *Opisthorchis*) *sinensis*	1. *Bulimus, Parafoss- arulus* 2. Cyprinid fish	Man, cat, dog, pig, fish-eating carnivores	Vietnam, Japan, Korea, China, Taiwan **bile and pancreatic ducts** (Kumar, 1987)
Opisthorchis felineus	1. *Bithynia* 2. Fw fish	Cat, dog, pig, fox, man	Russia, Siberia, Central Europe **bile ducts?** (Lebedev, 1990)
O. noverca	1. ? 2. ?	Pig, dog*, man*	India **gall bladder** (Leiper, 1913)
O. viverrini	1. *Bythnia* 2. Fw fish	Civet cat, dog, man	Thailand, Laos **bile ducts** (Hinz, 1996)
Pseudamphisto- mum truncatum	1. Snails 2. Fw fish	Fish-eating mammals, dog, cat, man	Italy, Russia, Portugal, Germany **bile ducts** (Semenova and Ivanov, 1990)
Family Paragonimidae			
Paragonimus africanus	1. Snails? 2. Crabs	Civet cat, dog, man, mongoose	Cameroon, Gabon, Nigeria, E. Guinea **lungs** (Khalil, 1991)

Parasite	Intermediate hosts	Final hosts	Distribution and location in host (reference)
P. heterotremus	1. *Tricula* 2. Crabs	Cat, dog, rat, man	Thailand, China, Laos **lungs** (Kino *et al.*, 1995; Hinz, 1996)
P. hueit'ungensis	1. *Tricula* 2. Crabs	Cat, dog, man*	China **lungs** (Chung *et al.*, 1977)
P. kellicotti	1. *Pomatiopsis* 2. Crayfish	Wild carnivores, cat, dog, pig, man*	Canada, USA **lungs** (Dubey, 1979)
P. mexicanus	1. *Araopyrgus* 2. Crabs	Wild carnivores, opossum, cat, dog, man	Mexico, Peru, Central America, Ecuador **lungs** (Argumedo, 1989)
P. miyazakii	1. *Bythinella* 2. Crabs (*Potamon*)	Wild carnivores, cat, dog, man*	Japan **lungs** (Nishida, 1989; Sugano *et al.*, 1989)
P. philippinensis	1. *Antemelenia* 2. Crabs (*Sesarma*)	Man (exper. dog, rat)	Philippines **lungs** (Ito *et al.*, 1979)
P. pulmonalis	1. Semisulcos-pira 2. Crabs, etc.	Cat, dog, man*	Taiwan, Korea, Japan **lungs** (Miyazaki, 1978)
P. skrjabini	1. *Tricula* 2. Crabs	Palm civet, cat, dog, man*	China **lungs** (Wang *et al.*, 1985)
P. uterobilateralis	1. *Afropomus*? 2. Crabs (*Liberonautes*)	Primates, wild carnivores, dog, man	Cameroon, Nigeria, Liberia **lungs** (Sachs and Cumberlidge, 1990)

Parasite	Intermediate hosts	Final hosts	Distribution and location in host (reference)
P. westermani	1. Semisulcos-pira 2. Crabs and crayfish	Man, dog, cat, pig, wild carnivores	Asia, Russia **lungs** (Yokogawa, 1965, 1969)
Family Plagiorchidae			
Plagiorchis muris	1. Lymnaea 2. Snails, midge	Rodents, birds, dog, sheep, man*	Japan, China, Korea, Nigeria **small intestine** (Asada et al., 1962)
Family Schistosomatidae			
Heterobilharzia americana	1. Lymnaea, Pseudosucc-nea 2. None	Dog, wild carnivores, man (larvae)	SW USA **mesenteric blood vessels** (Lee, 1962; Thrasher, 1964)
Schistosoma incognitum	1. Radix 2. None	Pig, sheep, dog, man (once)*	India, Thailand, Indonesia **mesenteric blood vessels** (Agrawal and Shah, 1989)
S. japonicum	1. Oncomelania 2. None	Man, cattle, buffalo, dog	Indonesia, China, Philippines, Japan, Malaysia, Thailand **mesenteric blood vessels** (Jordan et al., 1993)
S. mansoni	1. Biomphalaria 2. None	Man, primates, rodents, dog	Africa, Caribbean, S. America **mesenteric blood vessels** (Jordan et al., 1993)

Parasite	Intermediate hosts	Final hosts	Distribution and location in host (reference)
S. mekongi	1. *Neotricula* 2. None	Man, dog	Cambodia, Thailand, Laos **mesenteric blood vessels** (Bruce and Sornmani, 1980)
S. rodhaini	1. *Biomphalaria* 2. None	Rodents, dog*, man (once)*	Congo, Burundi, Uganda **mesenteric blood vessels** (Rollinson and Simpson, 1987)
Family Troglotrematidae			
Nanophyetus salmincola	1.*Goniobasis oxytrema* 2. Salmon	Fish-eating mammals, fish-eating birds, dog, cat, man	USA **small intestine** (Milleman and Knapp, 1970)
N. salmincola schikhobalowi	1. *Semisulco-spira* 2. Fw fish	Badger, mink, fox, dog, cat, man	Siberia **small intestine** (Milleman and Knapp, 1970)

Clonorchis sinensis is the only species which can be regarded as primarily a human parasite and it is estimated that 19 million people are infected worldwide, although 9 million are infected with *Opisthorchis viverrini* and 1.2 million with *Opisthorchis felineus* (Haswell-Elkins and Elkins, 1998). Both genera are very similar in morphology and life cycle, the main difference being that in *Clonorchis* the testes are in tandem and have long branched lobes (Figure 6.2), while in *Opisthorchis* the testes are semi-adjacent and are lobate. The life cycle of *C. sinensis* is shown in detail in Figure 6.2 and is typical of most trematodes apart from the schistosomes. Because of the multiplication of various larval stages in the snail, many thousands of cercaria emerge over the life of the snail for each miracidium which penetrated.

All the liver flukes have similar clinical manifestations. The majority of infections are symptomless and the presence of worms is only diagnosed at necropsy. Heavier infections (over 100 worms in humans) result in diarrhea, fever, edema, and some swelling of the liver (hepatomegaly) and spleen (splenomegaly); there is also a high eosinophilia (up to 40%). There can also be recurrent gall-bladder colic with loss of weight (see Georgi and Georgi, 1992 for effects in dogs). Pathologically the adult flukes cause proliferation of the bile duct epithelium (Figure 6.3). Stones in the bile ducts and gall bladder are a common finding in cases of *C. sinensis* sometimes with recurrent cholangitis. Cancer of the bile ducts is strongly associated with *O. viverrini* infection and is a major cause of death in endemic areas, and very probably occurs with other species, in humans, dogs and cats. *O. felineus* is a common parasite of cats, and to a lesser extent dogs, in Russia and East Europe, but human infection only occurs occasionally except for areas of Siberia, where salted or smoked fish is habitually eaten raw. Human infection with this species is often accompanied by acute symptoms of high fever and abdominal pain.

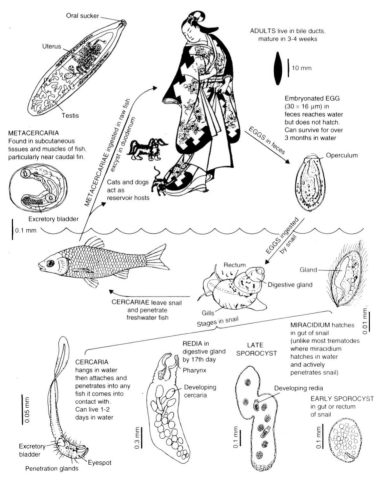

Figure 6.2. The life cycle stages of *Clonorchis sinensis* (modified from Muller, 1975).

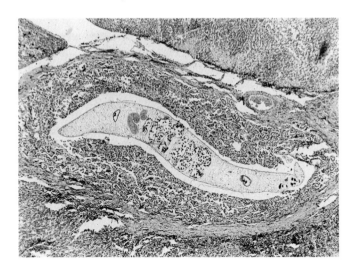

Figure 6.3. Microscope section of liver with adult of *Clonorchis sinensis* (containing numerous small dark eggs). The bile duct epithelium has proliferated greatly.

Two liver flukes normally parasitic in fish-eating mammals, *Metorchis albidus* and *Metorchis conjunctus*, occasionally occur in humans if they eat raw fish. The latter species was responsible for infection in 19 people in Canada who suffered from upper abdominal pain, low grade fever, and a high eosinophilia, lasting up to 4 weeks, who had all eaten sashimi in a restaurant. Praziquantel was very effective in treatment (Maclean *et al.*, 1996).

Amphimerus pseudofelineus causes cholangitis, pancreatic neoplasms and abdominal distension in cats, treatable with high doses of praziquantel, but there is little information on its effect in dogs or humans.

The Heterophids

Superfamily Opisthorchioidea: Family Heterophyidae

The heterophyids are a group of minute hermaphroditic flukes usually measuring less than 2.5 mm in length, with a body covered in spines. The adults live among the crypts of the small intestine attached to the epithelial cells and can be easily missed at necropsy. They are all very similar morphologically and have almost indistinguishable, small (26 x 15 μm), operculate eggs, containing a miracidium when passed out in feces. In fresh water the miracidia hatch and penetrate and develop in appropriate species of snails where they multiply and after a few weeks release cercariae. These encyst in several species of fresh water or brackish water fish which, when eaten raw or undercooked, pass on the infection. Because the eggs are difficult or impossible to differentiate, reliable data on infection with the different species are lacking. Most species are parasites of fish-eating carnivores or birds in Southeast Asia and have almost identical life cycles. Twenty infections have been reported from both humans and dogs (Table 6.1) and many more from one or the other.

Heterophyes heterophyes and the very similar Metagonimus yokogawai are the most common species which infect humans and dogs. They both measure 1.0 to 1.7 mm in length and differ mainly in that the former species has an accessory genital sucker near the ventral sucker. The adults live in the mucosal crypts of the duodenum and jejunum and produce superficial inflammation and necrosis with excessive secretion of mucus. In light infections they are usually asymptomatic but in heavier infections there may be diarrhea, nausea and intense griping pains. However, occasionally worms penetrate very deeply into the crypts close to large lymphatics and blood vessels. Eggs have been found in the central nervous system and heart valves of humans dying of congestive heart failure. An adult Heterophyes has also been recovered from the heart (Collomb et al., 1960). Eggs of another species, Haplorchis pumilis, have been recovered from the spinal cord, producing transverse myelitis, with loss of motor and sensory function (see Guttierez, 1990). In the Nile Delta region of Egypt, human infection with Heterophyes is associated with eating pickled mullet at the feast of Sham-al-Nessim and there is a high infection rate in children and young adults. Other species are common in areas of Southeast Asia from fecal examinations for eggs but it is not known whether they are pathogenic.

The Paragonimids

Superfamily Plagiorchioidea: Family Paragonimidae

The paragonimids are almost globular hermaphroditic trematodes, most measuring about 12 mm in length and 6 mm in width, with small suckers and symmetrical lobed testes in the posterior part of the body. They live in pairs in cysts in the lung and crustaceans act as second intermediate hosts. Many species occur in carnivores throughout the world but most of the estimated 22 million human infections are caused by Paragonimus westermani in Southeast Asia (Toscano et al., 1995), as this is the main part of the world where crustaceans are eaten uncooked. Many other species which can also infect humans (Table 6.1) can be distinguished by (often slight) morphological and life cycle differences.

Eggs of paragonimids, measuring about 100 x 55 μm, are produced by the adult worms in the lungs and are conveyed up the trachea and passed out in the sputum or are swallowed and escape in the feces. Once an egg reaches fresh water a miracidium larvae develops inside it in a few weeks, emerges and enters a suitable species of snail. After the usual multiplicative stages in the snail, the cercariae emerge and enter freshwater crabs or crayfish. When the infected crustacean is eaten raw, the metacercarial larvae excyst and reach the lungs after penetrating through the intestinal wall, the diaphragm and lung capsule. In China "drunken crabs" are steeped in rice wine before eating, in the Philippines crab juice is a delicacy, while in Korea crayfish juice is used as a cure for measles in children.

The developing worm pairs in the lung provoke inflammatory and granulomatous reactions around them to form a cyst with an opening into the bronchiole. Fully formed cysts measure about 20 mm in diameter. Eventually the contained worms die and the cysts become fibrotic and calcify. The most serious effects follow when worms migrate out of the lungs, along the soft tissues to the brain, and become foci for abscesses, giving rise to symptoms resembling epilepsy, a cerebral tumor or an embolism and possibly leading to paralysis. *Paragonimus mexicanus*, a New World species (Table 6.1), is particularly prone to cause cerebral paragonimiasis, a condition more common in children. In general, human infection caused by the rarer more clearly zoonotic species tends to have worms occupying ectopic locations outside the lungs, often in organs in, or the wall of, the abdominal cavity. Infection in the lungs is often mistaken for tuberculosis (Toscano *et al.*, 1995), although the patient appears to be much healthier than in the latter infection, and the condition usually resolves spontaneously after a few years. Treatment is with praziquantel and diagnosis by finding the eggs in sputum or feces.

Susceptible species of crabs and crayfish live in fast-flowing mountain streams, and in most parts of the world these are not eaten raw and so human infections in Africa and the Americas are rare and sporadic and occurs only in individuals from remote areas. *P. westermani* and *Paragonimus heterotremus* can also infect rodents and these can act as paratenic hosts for cats and dogs, since the worms do not usually develop fully in them.

Paragonimus kellicotti is a parasite of dogs in North America and X-rays showed saccular bronchial dilatations after 2-3 weeks, often with pneumothorax and distinct air-filled cavities measuring 20-30 mm after 4 weeks. These conditions sometimes resolved but treatment with fenbendazole, albendazole or praziquantel were all effective (Dubey, 1979). A cough is typical of infections with paragonimids in dogs.

The Troglotrematids

Superfamily Plagiorchioidea: Family Troglotrematidae

This group is related to the paragonimids and most do not inhabit the alimentary tract (occupying body sinuses, kidney and liver), although the one species occasionally found in man is intestinal. They differ from the paragonimids in that the genital pore is posterior to the ventral sucker and there is a cirrus sac.

Nanophyetus salmincola is an intestinal parasite of wild carnivores, birds and domestic dogs in Siberia and the Pacific Northwest of the US (Table 6.1). Eggs are passed out in the feces and the miracidia which develop inside hatch in fresh water and penetrate suitable species of snails. Asexual multiplication occurs in the snail and the cercariae which emerge form cysts in various tissues, particularly the kidney, of salmonid fishes. Infection is non-pathogenic in wild bears and racoons, but in dogs in the USA results in a hemorrhagic enteritis with high fever, anorexia, vomiting and lymphadenopathy; there is a high mortality occurring 10-14 days after infection. This is known as "salmon poisoning" of dogs and is caused by a rickettsial organism, *Neorickettsia helminthoeca*, which is transmitted by the trematode (Milleman and Knapp, 1970). The rickettsia has not been reported from humans who ate raw or insufficiently cooked salmon but it is possible they may be susceptible. In Russia and the US some patients suffered from diarrhea with weight loss, nausea, vomiting, fatigue, anorexia and a high eosinophilia (43%). Symptoms usually resolved after a few months. One case also had a high fever but the possible role of a rickettsia was not investigated (Eastburn *et al.*, 1987). Diagnosis in both hosts is by finding the characteristic unembryonated eggs in the feces, measuring about 80 x 45 μm.

Prevention is by not eating raw or smoked salmon and not feeding it to dogs. There has also been one case of infection through handling fish (Harrell and Deardorff, 1990). A 4.2% human infection rate has been reported from a focus on the lower Amur River in Siberia (Bernshtein *et al.*, 1992). Treatment with praziquantel is effective (Fritsche *et al.*, 1989). Wild carnivores act as reservoir host for both humans and dogs.

Lecithodendriids (Superfamily Plagiorchioidea: Family Lecithodendriidae) are usually intestinal parasites of insect eating mammals, particularly bats. They are minute flukes recognizable by the fact that the gonads and vitelline body are in the forebody region. *Phaneropsolus* is the only genus regularly found in man and dogs, although there are other occasional parasites (Table 6.1). In a region of Thailand, adults of *Phaneropsolus bonnei* were recovered from 15% of inhabitants, and adults of *Prosthodendrium molenkampi* from 19% (Radomyas *et al.*, 1994). Larvae, particularly those of dragonflies, act as second intermediate hosts. Pathogenicity is unknown, nor is it known how the final hosts are infected; presumably the parasites infect humans in areas where insects are eaten as delicacies or by accidentally ingesting insect larvae in water or on edible vegetation. It appears unlikely that dogs are the normal definitive hosts for *P. bonnei*.

Only one plagiorchid (Superfamily Plagiorchioidea: Family Plagiorchidae), *Plagiorchis muris*, has been reported from the intestine of man in Japan and Korea. It is a natural parasite of wild mice and it and other species have very occasionally been recovered from dogs (Dalimi and Mobedi, 1992). The second intermediate hosts for humans and dogs are probably freshwater fish, although the usual hosts were stated to be snails and midges (Coombs and Crompton, 1991).

The Fasciolids

Superfamily Echinostomatoidea: Family Fasciolidae

These are large spiny trematodes with a flattened body and deeply lobed testes. The best known member of this family, the cattle and sheep liver fluke, *Fasciola hepatica*, can be an important human parasite in some parts of the world. The only member found in both humans and dogs is the giant intestinal worm, *Fasciolopsis buski*. The most important reservoir host for this trematode is the pig, dogs only rarely becoming infected. This is primarily because there is no second animal intermediate host, the cercariae forming metacercarial cysts on water plants, some of which, including the water chestnut and water caltrop, are eaten by people in many parts of Asia: others are fed to pigs. The large adult worms, measuring up to 70 mm, attach by their suckers to the wall of the small intestine. The eggs, measuring 130 x 80 μm, pass out in the feces and on reaching fresh water a miracidium develops inside in about 1 month. Light infections are often asymptomatic but large numbers of worms, which can be many hundreds, cause inflammation and ulceration of the intestinal mucosa with excessive production of mucus. Clinically, there is anorexia, nausea, acute abdominal pain and possible facial edema. Children in particular get infected by removing the outer covering of the fruits or nuts with their teeth. Treatment is by praziquantel or albendazole.

The Echinostomatoidea

Superfamily Echinostomatoidea: Family Echinostomatidae

Echinostomes are all parasites of the small intestine, measuring a few millimeters in length. They have an oval or elongate body and the tegument is covered with spines. The most characteristic feature is the presence of a collar behind the oral sucker with a single or double crown of longer spines. Both suckers are well developed. Most species are parasites of birds but some are natural parasites of mammals and most also have a wide host range.

The characteristic eggs of echinostomes are relatively large, measuring about 100 x 65 μm, although it is difficult to tell them apart. The second intermediate hosts (in addition to the snail first intermediate host) are large edible types of snail, amphibians, or fish (Table 6.1). In the definitive host, heavy infections with mature worms produce an inflammatory reaction of the mucosa and ulceration at the site of attachment and there may be diarrhea, nausea and intestinal colic in the morning relieved by food. Treatment is with praziquantel.

Echinostoma ilocanum is a common parasite of dogs in Canton and was first reported from prisoners in jail in Manila in 1907. Occasional human cases have been reported since from the Philippines, China, Malaysia and Indonesia. Infection is contracted from eating uncooked large edible snails (e.g. *Pila* or *Vivipara*) containing metacercariae.

The Diplostomes

Superfamily Diplostomoidea: Family Diplostomatidae

In this group the body is divided into two regions, with a wide flattened, concave, anterior portion and a cylindrical posterior portion. Most are parasites of birds but members of the genus *Alaria* parasitize mammals. The cercariae form metacercarial cysts in fish or amphibians.

Alaria americana and *Alaria marcianae* are two very similar species which are intestinal parasites of carnivores in North America, where they are found in racoons, weasels, red foxes, badgers, cats, and occasionally dogs. They both have very similar, unusual, life cycles and are often considered as the same species but Pearson and Johnson (1988) regarded them as distinct. Thus in the older literature it is not always clear which species is being referred to.

The life cycle of (presumably) *A. marcianae* has been elucidated from experimental infections in carnivores and rodents (Shoop and Corkum, 1983a, b; Smyth, 1995). If eggs from feces reach water, the miracidia hatch out and penetrate and multiply in suitable species of snails (probably including *Heliosoma* spp.). Cercariae which emerge develop in amphibian tadpoles where they develop into an unusual larval stage known as a mesocercaria. Basically this is an enlarged cercaria with the penetration glands but a more complex excretory system. Adult frogs and snakes act as carrier or paratenic hosts by ingesting tadpoles. When these are ingested by young carnivores, mesocercariae penetrate through the intestinal wall and diaphragm to reach the lungs. After developing into metacercariae in the lungs they are coughed up and become adults in the small intestine producing eggs in about 20 days. The adults attach to the villi in the small intestine but cause little damage. However, in pregnant cats and dogs, the mesocercariae migrate to the mammary glands and infect suckling kittens or puppies. They can continue to infect subsequent litters until the larvae are all finished. In the neonates the parasites develop into adults (Figure 6.4).

The process was termed "amphiparatenesis" by Shoop (1994). A pregnant callitrichid monkey has been infected experimentally and a similar situation ensued. This has serious implications for zoonotic human infections (Shoop, 1990).

While *A. americana* and *A. marcianae* are rare parasites in both dogs and humans they are potentially very dangerous ones. A fatal case in Canada occurred

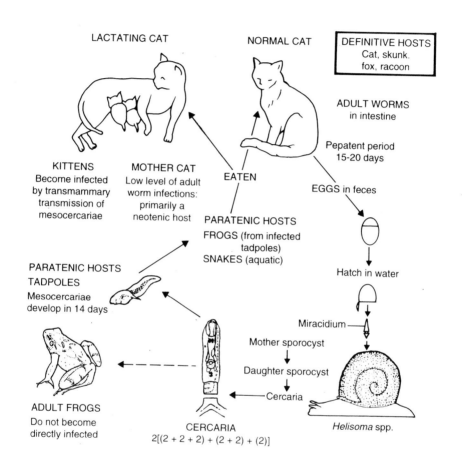

LACTATING CAT

NORMAL CAT

DEFINITIVE HOSTS
Cat, skunk.
fox, racoon

ADULT WORMS
in intestine

Pepatent period
15-20 days

KITTENS
Become infected
by transmammary
transmission of
mesocercariae

MOTHER CAT
Low level of adult
worm infections:
primarily a
neotenic host

EATEN

EGGS in feces

PARATENIC HOSTS
FROGS (from infected
tadpoles)
SNAKES (aquatic)

Hatch in water

PARATENIC HOSTS
TADPOLES
Mesocercariae
develop in 14 days

Miracidium

Mother sporocyst

Daughter sporocyst

Cercaria

ADULT FROGS
Do not become
directly infected

CERCARIA
2[(2 + 2 + 2) + (2 + 2) + (2)]

Helisoma spp.

Figure 6.4. The life cycle of *Alaria marcianae* in the cat - or dog (from Smyth, 1995).

in a man who ingested frogs' legs while hiking (Freeman *et al.*, 1976). He was thought to be suffering from gastric flu but died 9 days later from extensive pulmonary hemorrhage and at autopsy was found to have mesocercariae in many tissues. They probably penetrated the stomach wall and migrated to the lungs and other tissues both directly and by the circulatory system. Mesocercariae have also lodged in the eyes of both humans and dogs, causing neuroretinitis (at least in the former).

Alaria alata is a European species with a similar life cycle and larvae have been found in humans although not causing the serious effects mentioned above (Shoop, 1994), and *Alaria nasuae* from wild carnivores has been found recently in domestic dogs in Mexico although, so far, not in humans (Shoop, 1989; Shoop *et al.*, 1989).

The Dicrocoelioidea

Superfamily Dicrocoelioidea: Family Dicrocoeliidae

Dicrocoelium dendriticum is a cosmopolitan parasite of the biliary ducts of sheep and cattle. Herbivores become infected by ingesting ants containing metacercariae which alter the ants' behavior so that they attach to grass leaves and increase the chances of ingestion. It is probable that most reported cases in humans and particularly in dogs are spurious, the eggs having been found in the feces following ingestion of infected liver. Genuine human cases result in disturbed liver function, biliary tree disease and a high eosinophilia (Mohamed and Mummery, 1990).

Prohemistomum vivax (Superfamily Strigeoidea: Family Cathycotylidae) is a parasite of fish-eating birds in Egypt. There has been one reported human case, when 2000 adults were recovered from the small intestine (M.J. Ulmer in Hubbert *et al.*, 1975), and it has been found a few times in dogs.

Conclusions

It is clear that infection with all trematodes apart from the schistosomes is based on dietary habits and human prevention is by thorough cooking of fish, crustaceans, snails, amphibians or snakes and possibly by avoidance of eating insects. Dogs are not nearly so important as reservoir hosts for most of these parasites as are cats because they are not so likely to eat these intermediate hosts. Avoidance of schistosome infections is by not entering ponds, canals or streams containing cercariae released from snails: not an easy task for humans living in endemic regions, particularly children, fishermen and farmers, or for dogs.

References

Agrawal, M.C. and Shah, H.L. (1989) A review of *Schistosoma incognitum* Chandler 1926. *Helminthological Abstracts* 58, 239-251.

Argumedo, R.L. (1989) *Paragonimus mexicanus* y paragonimiasis en Mexico y America. Thesis Universidad Nacional Autonomia de Mexico DF 04510, Mexico.

Asada, J.L., Otagaki, H., Morita, D., Takeuchi, T., Sakai, Y., Kojishi, T. and Okahashi, K. (1962) A case report on the human infection with *Plagiorchis muris* Tanabe, 1922. *Japanese Journal of Parasitology* 11, 512-516.

Bernshtein, A.M., Karablev, V.N. and Yavotskii, C.S. (1992) Intestinal trematode infections (*Metagonimus, Nanophyetus*): clinical and parasitological study and first trial of Azinox in the lower River Amur focus [Eng. summary]. *Meditsinkaya Parazitologiya I Parazitarnye Bolezni* 2, 25-27.

Bhaibulaya, M. (1982) Zoonotic helminths of Thailand. *Molecular and Biochemical Parasitology* (supp.), 627.

Bowman, D.D. (1999) *Georgi's Parasitology for Veterinarians,* 7th edn. W.B. Saunders, Philadelphia.

Bruce, J.I. and Sornmani, S. (eds) (1980) *The Mekong Schistosome.* White Lake, Michigan.

Chai, J.Y. and Lee, S.H. (1990) Intestinal trematodes of humans in Korea: *Metagonimus,* heterophyids and echinostomes. *Korean Journal of Parasitology* 28, 103-122.

Chai, J.Y., Hong, S.J., Lee, S.H. and Seo, B.S. (1988) *Stictodora* (Trematoda: Heterophidae) recovered from a man in Korea. *Korean Journal of Parasitology* 26, 127-132.

Chen, X.Q., Lin, J.X., Fang, Y.Y., Lin, A.Q., Chen, B.J. and Zhunag, H.J. (1992) Discovery of human infection with *Echinostoma angustitestis* [In Chinese]. *Chinese Journal of Zoonoses* 8, 7-8.

Cheng, Y.Z. [*et al.*] (1991) First report of human *Centrocestus formosanus* infection. *Chinese Journal of Parasitology and Parasitic Diseases* [in Chinese] 9, 275.

Chieffi, P.P., Gorla, M.C.O., Torres, D.M.A.G.U., Dias, R.M.D.S., Mangini, A.C.S., Monteira, A.V., Woiciechovski, E., Vieira-Torres, M.A.G. and Souza-Dias, R.M.D. (1992) Human infection by *Phagicola* sp. (Trematoda: Heterophyidae) in the municipality of Registro, Sao Paulo State, Brazil. *Journal of Tropical Medicine and Hygiene* 95, 346-348.

Chung, H.L., Hsu, C.P., Ho, L.Y., Kao, P.C., Lan, S. and Chiu, F.H. (1977) Studies on a new pathogenic lung fluke *Paragonimus hueit'ungensis* sp nov. *Chinese Medical Journal* 3, 374-394.

Collomb, H., Deschiens, R.E.A. and Demarchi, J. (1960) Sur deux cas de distomase cerebrale a *Heterophyes heterophyes. Bulletin de la Societé de Pathologie Exotique* 53, 144-147.

Coombs, I. and Crompton, D.W.T. (1991) *A Guide to Human Helminths.* Taylor and Francis, London.

Dalimi, A. and Mobedi, I. (1992) Helminth parasites of carnivores in northern Iran. *Annals of Tropical Medicine and Parasitology* 86, 395-397.

Dill, M.E. (1993) Pancreatic diseases of cats. *Compendium on Continuing Education for the Practising Veterinarian* 15, 596-598.

Dubey, J.P. (1979) Experimental *Paragonimus kellicotti* infection in dogs. *Veterinary Parasitology* 5, 325.

Dunn, A.M. (1978) *Veterinary Helminthology*, 2nd edn. Heinemann Medical, London.

Eastburn, R.L., Fritsche, T.R. and Terhume, C.A. Jr. (1987) Human intestinal infection with *Nanopyetus slamincola* from salmonid fishes. *American Journal of Tropical Medicine and Hygiene* 36, 586-591.

Euzeby, J. (1982) *Diagnostic Expérimental des Helminthoses Animales.* Ministerè de l'Agriculture, Paris, Tome 2, pp. 110-113.

FAO (1994) *Diseases of Domestic Animals Caused by Flukes.* FAO, Rome.

Freeman, R.S., Stuart, P.F., Cullen, J.B., Ritchie, A.C., Mildon, A., Fernandes, B.J. and Bonin, R. (1976) Fetal human infection with mesocercariae of the trematode *Alaria americana. American Journal of Tropical Medicine and Hygiene* 25, 803-807.

Fritsche, J.R., Eastburn, R.L., Wiggins, L.H. and Terhune, C.A. Jr. (1989) Praziquantel for treatment of human *Nanophyetus salmincola* (*Troglotrema salmincola*) infection. *Journal of Infectious Diseases* 160, 896-899.

Geerts, S., Kumar, V. and Brandt, J. (eds) (1987) *Helminth Zoonoses.* Nijhoff, Dordrecht.

Georgi, J.R. and Georgi, M.E. (1992) *Canine Clinical Parasitology.* Lea and Febiger, Philadelphia.

Giboda, M., Dilrich, O., Scholtz, T., Viengsay, T. and Bouaphanh, S. (1991) Human *Opisthorchis* and *Haplorchis* infections in Laos. *Transactions of the Royal Society of Tropical Medicine and Hygiene* 85, 438-540.

Guttierez, Y. (1990) *Diagnostic Pathology of Parasitic Infections with Clinical Correlations.* Lea and Febiger, Philadelphia.

Harrell, L.W. and Deardorff, J.L. (1990) Human nanophyetiasis: transmission by handling infected coho salmon (*Oncorhynchus kisutch*). *Journal of Infectious Diseases* 161, 146-148.

Haswell-Elkins, M.R. and Elkins, D.B. (1998) Lung and liver flukes. In: Cox, F.E.G., Kreier, J.P. and Wakelin, D. (eds) *Topley and Wilson's Microbiology and Microbial Infections*, 9th edn. Arnold, London 5, 508-520.

Hillyer, G.V. and Hopla, C.E. (1982) *CRC Handbook Series in Zoonoses. Section C, Parasitic Zoonoses III.* CRC Press, Boca Raton, Florida.

Hinz, E. (1996) *Helminthiasien des Menschen in Thailand.* Peter Lang, Frankfurt-am-Main.

Hubbert, W.T., McCulloch, D.V.M. and Schnurrenberger, P.R. (eds) (1975) *Diseases Transmitted from Animals to Man,* 6th edn. Thomas, Springfield, Illinois.

Hugh-Jones, M.E., Hubbert, W.T. and Hagstad, H.V. (1995) *Zoonoses: Recognition, Control and Prevention.* Iowa State University Press: Ames, Iowa.

Ito, J., Yokogawa, M., Araki, K. and Kobayashi, M. (1979) Further observations on the morphology of adult lung fluke, *Paragonimus philippinensis* Ito, Yokogawa, Araki and Kobayashi 1978. *Japanese Journal of Parasitology* 28, 253-259.

Jordan, P., Webbe, G. and Sturrock, R.F. (1993) *Human Schistosomiasis.* CAB International, Wallingford.

Kassai, T. (1999) *Veterinary Helminthology.* Butterworth Heinemann, Oxford.

Khalil, L.F. (1991) Zoonotic helminths of wild and domestic animals in Africa. In: Macpherson, C.N.L. and Craig, P.S. (eds) *Parasitic Helminths and Zoonoses in Africa.* Unwin Hyman, London, pp. 260-272.

Kino, H., Nguyen Van de, Ha Viet Vien, Li Thi Chuyen and Sano, M. (1995) *Paragonimus heterotremus* Chen et Hsia 1964 from a dog in Vietnam. *Japanese Journal of Parasitology* 44, 470-472.

Kumar, V. (1987) Zoonotic trematodiasis in south-east and far-east Asian countries. In: Geerts, S., Kumar, V. and Brandt, J. (eds) *Helminth Zoonoses.* Nijhoof, Dordrecht, pp. 106-118.

Kwo En Hoa and Lie Kian Joe (1953) Occurrence in man in Indonesia of trematodes commonly found in animals. *Journal of the Indonesian Medical Association* 3, 131-136.

Lebedev, V.P. (1990) The role of *Opisthorchis* infection in the development of gastroduodenal pathology in young men. Prophylaxis and rehabilitation. *Terapevticheskii Arkhiv* [Eng. summary] 62, 46-49.

Lee, H.F. (1962) Susceptibility of mammalian hosts to experimental infection with *Heterobilharzia americana. Journal of Parasitology* 48, 740-745.

Leiper, R.T. (1913) Observations on certain helminths of man. *Transactions of the Royal Society of Tropical Medicine and Hygiene* 6, 265-297.

Lie-Kian, J. and Virik, H. (1963) Human infection with *Echinostoma malayanum* Leiper 1911 (Trematoda: Echinostomidae). *Journal of Tropical Medicine and Hygiene* 66, 77-82.

Lin, J.X. (1985) Epidemiological investigation and experimental infection of *Echinochasmus japonicus. Journal of Parasitology and Parasitic Diseases* 3, 89-91.

Lu, Sen-Chi (1982) Echinostomiasis in Taiwan. *International Journal of Zoonoses* 9, 33-38.

Lu, Y.J. [*et al.*] (1996) A case of *Echinochasmus perfoliatus* disease. *Chinese Journal of Parasitic Disease Control* [English abstract] 9, 172.

Maclean, J.D., Arthur, J.R., Ward, B.J., Gyorkos, T.W., Curtis, M.A. and Kokoskin, E. (1996) Common-source outbreak of acute infection due to the North American liver fluke *Metorchis conjunctus. Lancet* 347, 8895, 154-158.

Malek, E.A. (1980) *Snail-transmitted Parasitic Diseases*. Vol. II. CRC Press: Boca Raton, Florida

Milleman, R.E. and Knapp, S.E. (1970) Biology of *Nanophyetus salmincola* and 'salmon poisoning' disease. *Advances in Parasitology* 8, 1-41.

Miyazaki, I. (1978) Two types of lung fluke which have been called *Paragonimus westermani* (Kerbert 1978). *Medical Bulletin of Fukuoka University* 5, 251-263.

Mohamed, A.R.E. and Mummery, V. (1990) Human dicrocoeliasis, report on 208 cases from Saudi Arabia. *Tropical and Geographical Medicine* 42, 1-7.

Muller, R. (1975) *Worms and Disease: a Manual of Medical Helminthology*. Heinemann Medical, London.

Murrell, K.D. (1995) Food borne parasites. *International Journal of Environmental Health Research* 5, 63-85.

Nasr, M. (1941) The occurrence of *Prohemistomum vivax* (Sonsino, 1892) Azim 1933 infection in man, with a redescription of the parasite. *Laboratory Medical Progress* 2, 135-149.

Niemi, D.R. and Macy, R.W. (1974) The life cycle and infectivity to man of *Apophallus donicus* (Skrjabin and Lindtrop, 1919) (Trematoda: Heterophyidae) in Oregon. *Proceedings of the Helminthological Society of Washington* 41, 223-229.

Nishida, H. (1989) Paragonimiasis in Japan, with special reference to species and their symptoms. *Saishin Igaku* [Eng. summary] 44, 843-850.

Pearson, J.C. (1956) Studies on the life cycles and morphology of the larval stages of *Alaria orisaemoides* Augustine and Uribe, 1927 and *Alaria canis* La Rue and Fallis. *Canadian Journal of Zoology* 34, 295-387.

Pearson, J.C. and Johnson, A.D. (1988) The taxonomic status of *Alaria marcianae* (Trematoda: Diplostomidae). *Proceedings of the Helminthological Society of Washington* 55, 102-103.

Petithory, J.C. and Ardoin, F. (1990) Prevalence en France et en Italy de *Toxocara canis* et autres helminthes chez le chien en 1987-1989. *Bulletin de la Societé Francaise de Parasitologie* 8, 257-266.

Radomyos, P., Charoenlarp, P. and Radomyos, B. (1991) Human *Episthmium caninum* (Digenea, Echinostomatidae) infection: report of two more cases. *Journal of Tropical Medicine and Parasitology* 14, 48-50.

Radomyos, P., Radomyos, B. and Tungtrongchitr, A. (1994) Multi-infection with helminths in adults from northeast Thailand as determined by post-treatment fecal examination of adult worms. *Medicine and Parasitology* 45, 133-135.

Rausch, R.L., Scott, M. and Rausch, V.R. (1967) Helminths in Eskimos in western Alaska, with particular reference to *Diphyllobothrium* infection and anaemia. *Transactions of the Royal Society of Tropical Medicine and Hygiene* 61, 351-357.

Rollinson, D. and Simpson, A.J.G. (1987) *The Biology of Schistosomes: From Genes to Latrines*. Academic Press, London.

Ryang, Y.S., Ahn, Y.K., Kim, W.T., Shin, K.C., Lee, K.W. and Kim, T.S. (1986) Two cases of human infection by *Echinostoma cinetorchis*. *Korean Journal of Parasitology* 24, 71-76.

Sachs, R. and Cumberlidge, N. (1990) The dog as natural reservoir host for *Paragonimus uterobilateralis* in Liberia, West Africa. *Annals of Tropical Medicine and Parasitology* 84, 101-102.

Savioli, L., Renganatham, E., Montresor, A., Davis, A. and Behbehani, K. (1997) Control of schistosomiasis - a global picture. *Parasitology Today* 13, 444-448.

Schultz, M.G. (ed.) (1982) *CRC Handbook Series in Zoonoses. Section C, Parasitic Zoonoses III.* CRC Press, Boca Raton, Florida.

Semenova, N.N. and Ivanov, V.M. (1990) Current situation of opisthorchiasis of animals in the Volta Delta, USSR. *Vetererinarya, Moskva* [Eng. summary] 1, 45-46.

Shalaby, S.I. and Trenti, F. (1994) Trematode parasites transmitted to man and fish eating mammals through *Tilapia nilotica*. First records in Egypt. *18th World Buiatrics Congress, Bologna* 1, 901-904.

Shalaby, S.I., Easa, M.E.S. and Trenti, F. (1994) Trematode parasites transmitted to man and fish eating mammals through *Tilapia nilotica*. 2. New trematodes. *18th World Buiatrics Congress, Bologna* 2, 1577-1580.

Shoop, W.L. (1989) Vertical transmission in the Trematoda. *Journal of the Helminthological Society of Washington* 61, 153-161.

Shoop, W.L. (1990) Transmammary transmission in primates with *Alaria marcianae* (Trematoda). *Bulletin de la Societé Francaise de Parasitologie* 8 (suppl. 2), 695.

Shoop, W.L. (1994) Vertical transmission in the Trematoda. *Journal of the Helminthological Society of Washington* 61, 153-161.

Shoop, W.L. and Corkum, K.C. (1983a) Transmammary infection of paratenic and definitive host with *Alaria marcianae* (Trematoda) mesocercariae. *Journal of Parasitology* 69, 731-735.

Shoop, W.L. and Corkum, K.C. (1983b) Migration of *Alaria marcianae* in domestic cats. *Journal of Parasitology* 69, 912-917.

Shoop, W.L., Salazar, M.A., Vega, C.S., Font, W.F. and Infante, F. (1989) *Alaria nasuae* (Trematoda: Diplosomidae) from domestic dogs. *Journal of Parasitology* 75, 325-327.

Smales, L.R., Miller, A.K. and Obendorf, D.L. (1990) Parasites of the water rat, *Hydromys chrysogaster,* from Victoria and South Australia. *Australian Journal of Zoology* 37, 657-663.

Smyth, J.D. (1995) Rare, new and emerging helminth zoonoses. *Advances in Parasitology* 36, 1-47.

Sugano, H., Yogo, S., Fukase, T., Chinone, S. and Itagaki, H. (1989) Canine paragonimiasis in Ehime Prefecture, Japan. *Journal of the Japanese Veterinary Medical Association* [Eng. summary] 42, 495-498.

Tadros, G. and El-Mokaddem, E.E.A. (1983) Observations on heterophyids affecting man in Egypt. *Bulletin of the Zoological Society of Egypt* 33, 107-111.

Tani, S. (1976) Studies on *Echinostoma hortense*. I. and II. *Japanese Journal of Parasitology* 25, 461 and 262.

Thrasher, S.P. (1964) Canine schistosomiasis. *Journal of the American Veterinary Medical Association* 144, 1119.

Toscano, C., Hai, Y.S., Nunn, P., Mott, K.E. and Yu, S.H. (1995) Paragonimiasis and tuberculosis - diagnostic confusion: a review of the literature. *Tropical Diseases Bulletin* 92, R1-R27.

Wang, X., Liu, Y., Wang, Q., Zhan, Q., Yu, M. and Yu, D. (1985) Clinical analysis of 119 cases of *Paragonimus szchuanensis*. *Journal of Parasitology and Parasitic Diseases* 3, 5-8.

WHO (1995) *Control of Foodborne Trematode Infections*. WHO Technical Report Series 849. WHO, Geneva.

Xiao, X., Lu, D.B., Wang, T.P., Gao, J.F., Wu, W.D., Peng, H.C., Zhang, B.J., Xu, M.R. and An, J.S. (1994) Epidemiological studies on *Echinochasmus liliputanus* infection. I. Parasite infection and distribution in final hosts. *Chinese Journal of Parasitic Disease Control* [Eng. abstract] 7, 285-287.

Yokogawa, M. (1965) *Paragonimus* and paragonimiasis. *Advances in Parasitology* 3, 99-158.

Yokogawa, M. (1969) *Paragonimus* and paragonimiasis. *Advances in Parasitology* 7, 375-388.

Yu, S.-H. and Mott, K.E. (1994) Epidemiology and morbidity of food-borne intestinal trematode infections. *WHO/SCHISTO* 94, pp. 108.

Chapter Seven

Dogs and Cestode Zoonoses

Calum N.L. Macpherson and Philip S. Craig

The domestication of the dog some 12,000 to 14,000 years ago has undoubtedly been of great benefit to humans. From a Darwinian perspective wolves that started to cohabit with humans made a smart choice given the nearly ubiquitous distribution of dogs around the world today and the patchy and limited distribution of wolves. The human:dog relationship may be as close as pampered and cosseted lap dogs to strays and feral dogs which live a precarious existence on the fringes of human society. The diversity of breeds of dogs and uses to which we put them may lead to their exposure to infectious organisms and their unwitting participation in the transmission of over 60 zoonotic infections (see Chapters 3-10; Hubbert *et al.*, 1975; Baxter and Leck, 1984). Undoubtedly human behavior plays a pivotal role in the perpetuation of parasitic zoonoses, including with the tapeworms or cestodes, many of which are important food and/or water borne zoonoses (Macpherson *et al.*, 2000). This chapter reviews the role of dogs in the life cycles of the main cestode zoonoses with a focus on *Echinococcus granulosus* and *Echinococcus multilocularis,* the two most important species from a public health point of view.

Echinococcus spp.

The genus *Echinococcus* comprises a complex of species and sub-species (see Thompson *et al.*, 1995 for review). Two species, *E. granulosus* the causative organism of cystic echinococcosis (CE) in humans and livestock and *E. multilocularis,* which causes human alveolar echinococcosis (AE) are of major public health importance. The dog is the major definitive host of *E. granulosus* and dogs are becoming increasingly recognized as a source of human infection with *E. multilocularis.* Two other species of *Echinococcus, Echinococcus vogeli* and *Echinococcus oligarthrus*, are geographically limited to Mesoamerica and South America and rarely cause disease in humans. Dogs play an increasingly recognized role in the transmission of *E. vogeli* to humans. Felids are the main definitive hosts of *E. oligarthrus* and dogs play no part in the transmission of this species, which will not be considered further.

Echinococcus granulosus (Batsch, 1786)

Dogs as definitive hosts of *Echinococcus granulosus*

Although susceptibility between and even within different breeds occurs, globally dogs are definitive hosts *par excellence* for *E. granulosus*. Dogs and other suitable carnivores become infected when they ingest protoscoleces found in hydatid cysts. These are most commonly found in the liver or lungs, and to a lesser extent in any other internal organ, of an enormous range of domestic and wild mammalian intermediate host species. The protoscoleces evaginate in the small intestine and the rostellum of the scolex attaches to the base of the crypt of Lieberkühn and the suckers attach to the base of the intestinal villi. The adults grow to a length of between 2 and 11 mm, are hermaphrodites and the prepatent period varies between 34 and 58 days (Thompson, 1995).

Worm burden

The mean worm burden in dogs varies considerably between endemic localities but in most endemic regions in developed countries (Europe, New Zealand, North America) worm burdens of around 200 are usually found (Gemmell *et al.*, 1987). Much heavier worm burdens have been reported in dogs living in many of the drier parts of the world, which must increase the biotic potential of the parasite and would be useful for the survival of the parasite in areas where the climatic conditions are inimical to the survival of the eggs (Wachira *et al.*, 1991). For example, one infected wild dog (domestic dog and dingo hybrid) in Australia was found to harbor over 300,000 worms (Jenkins and Morris, 1991) and wild dogs in general tend to have heavy worm burdens (Jenkins *et al.*, 2000). Heavy infections have also been reported in Kenya where of 274 infected dogs examined in the Turkana District, 122 (44.5%), 54 (19.7%) and 98 (35.8%) had light (1-200) medium (201-1000) and heavy (> 1000) worm burdens, respectively. Many of the heavily infected dogs had over 50,000 adults which completely carpeted the entire length of the small intestine (Macpherson *et al.*, 1985). Fertility of hydatid cysts in Turkana is high both in humans (Macpherson, 1983) and livestock (Macpherson, 1981) which would facilitate heavy worm burdens in dogs. Heavy worm burdens have been reported in the Levant country of Jordan where the heaviest worm load was 16,467 in a single dog fed offal by a slaughterhouse worker (Abdel-Hafez and Kamhawi, 1997). In Iraq, the mean worm burden in 57 infected dogs was 1,844 with 61.4% of the dogs having worm burdens of > 1000 worms (Molan and

Baban, 1992). The heaviest infected dog in this study harbored 15,182 worms. Heavy worm burdens have not been reported from all dry endemic regions and have not been reported from dogs in north Africa or from the Middle East (Dar and Alkarmi, 1997; Ibrahem and Gusbi, 1997; Ouhelli *et al.*, 1997; Eslami and Hosseini, 1998). In Morocco the average number of worms in 34 infected dogs was 219 (Ouhelli *et al.*, 1997).

Egg production, dispersal and survival

Egg production may be synchronous or asynchronous with proglottids being produced roughly every 2 weeks. Egg production may reach over a million a day. Expulsion of eggs has been shown to be continuous for at least 80 days (Heath and Lawrence, 1991).

The routes for the transfer of eggs from the definitive host to intermediate hosts and their successful establishment in the intermediate host remain arcane. This process must involve a complex mixture of environmental and parasite factors (particularly intraspecific strain variation), host assemblages, host genetics, nutritional status and immunity, animal husbandry and slaughter practices and socio-cultural and behavioral factors. One study, which documented the movements of 31 dogs for 24,541 observation-minutes, in areas of high, medium and low human CE prevalence, found that the amount of time dogs spent in their houses was significantly correlated with an increased prevalence of CE (Spearman's rank correlation coefficient (rs) = +0.986, $P < 0.01$). A significantly positive correlation was also found for homesteads which allowed dogs to defecate in the home area, clean children and to lick eating utensils (Watson-Jones and Macpherson, 1988). Other studies have shown eggs in water holes and in the home area, locations which probably required no dispersal mechanisms (Craig *et al.*, 1988; Macpherson *et al.*, 1989a; Macpherson and Craig, 1991). In these studies *E. granulosus* eggs were differentiated from the morphologically identical taeniid eggs by immunological means (Craig *et al.*, 1986).

The mechanisms for the dispersal of eggs are unclear but are likely to be a combination of a number of factors. These range from the movements of the proglottids away from the fecal mass to dispersal by water, wind, flies (especially blowflies) and other insects and birds. Most eggs remain within a 180 m of their deposition but under certain circumstances eggs appear to be able to disperse over considerable distances. For example, eggs of *Taenia hydatigena* have been shown to move over 60 km upwind by the activities of birds and insects (Torgerson *et al.*, 1992, 1995).

Egg survival is dependent on temperature and relative humidity. At 7 and 21°C eggs survive for over 200 and 50 days, respectively (Gemmell, 1977). At temperatures of over 40°C survival is only a few hours but is prolonged if the eggs are in water (Wachira *et al.*, 1991). In the hot, arid regions of the world transfer of eggs from dogs to intermediate hosts must be rapid to be successful. Mathematical models have been generated that predict that the biotic potential per infected dog would be 28 viable cysts. This is based on the assumption that an infected dog produces 8470 eggs a day and that 0.0033 of these eggs develop into viable cysts (Gemmell *et al.*, 1987). The longevity of the adult worm in dogs is unknown but is possibly 1-2 years.

Diagnosis of *Echinococcus granulosus* in dogs

Identification of infected dogs may be important for diagnostic, epidemiologic or control/surveillance reasons. Almost all hydatid control programs necessitate consideration of quantification of canine echinococcosis (Gemmell, 1990). Diagnosis is most effective by autopsy and examination of the small intestine, which is also the only accurate method of recording worm burdens. Anti-mortem diagnosis has been carried out for many years using arecoline purgation, however, although this method is highly specific it has many drawbacks including poor sensitivity, it is biohazardous and logistically problematic with up to 20% of dogs failing to purge (Wachira *et al.*, 1990; Craig *et al.*, 1995; Craig, 1997). The development of *Echinococcus* spp. coproantigen ELISA tests has dramatically improved the capability of sensitive and highly specific ante-mortem diagnosis of *E. granulosus* in dogs (Allan *et al.*, 1992; Deplazes *et al.*, 1992). Specificity is around 96% and sensitivity > 80% when worm burdens are greater than 50. Pre-patent infections are detectable by coproantigen ELISA and antigen levels return to normal within 5 days post-treatment. Coproantigens remain stable in formol saline preserved samples and also in fecal samples left in the "open" for up to 6 days (Jenkins *et al.*, 2000). To date coproantigen ELISA for *E. granulosus* has been used to screen sheep farm dogs in Wales, Uruguay, Australia and Peru (Palmer *et al.*, 1996; Cohen *et al.*, 1998; Moro *et al.*, 1997, 1999; Jenkins *et al.*, 2000) nomadic community dogs in Northwest China (Wang *et al.*, 2000), stray dogs in Spain, Jordan and Nepal (Deplazes *et al.*, 1992; Baronet *et al.*, 1994; El-Shehabi *et al.*, 2000) and feral dogs and dingoes in Australia (Jenkins *et al.*, 2000). Coproantigen positive rates ranged from < 5.0 to 46%. Currently differentiation between *E. granulosus* and *E. multilocularis* is not possible by coproantigen detection as the tests are genus-specific. Presently a PCR-based DNA detection assay has not been developed for *E. granulosus* in contrast to *E. multilocularis* (Deplazes and Eckert, 1996; Dinkel *et al.*, 1998).

Treatment of *Echinococcus granulosus* in dogs

Since the 1970s the treatment of choice is praziquantel, given in a single oral dose of around 5 mg per kg body weight. The drug is well tolerated by dogs. To date no drug resistance has been reported. The drug is metabolized within 1 hour and consequently reinfection may occur not long after treatment.

Epidemiology and public health importance

Infections with *E. granulosus* occur world-wide. A so-called European form, primarily involving synanthropic hosts in its cycle, has a nearly cosmopolitan distribution (Rausch, 1995). This form is a major public health and economic problem in many rural areas of the world. The Northern form is prevalent in northern parts of the North American continent and Eurasia and is probably the archetypal form (Rausch, 1995). Globally, little data exist on the overall prevalence and economic importance of CE (Craig *et al.*, 1996). Regions with good documentation where a relatively high prevalence in defined geographical areas has been reported include the whole Mediterranean area including Southern Europe, Egypt, Libya, Tunisia and Morocco (Rausch, 1995; Schantz *et al.*, 1995). Another focus occurs in Africa south of the Sahara in the semi-arid areas of East Africa, including Kenya, Uganda, Sudan, Ethiopia and Tanzania and in the rural areas of Nigeria and South Africa (reviewed by Macpherson and Wachira, 1997). Large foci are also known to occur in the sheep rearing countries of South America, including Uruguay (Carmona *et al.*, 1998), Argentina (in the Patagonian Provinces of Rio Negro, Chebut, Santa Cruz and Tierra del Fuego) (Frider *et al.*, 1988; Perdomo *et al.*, 1997, 1999), Brazil (Rio Grande do Sol), and the high sierra areas of Chile, Peru and Bolivia (Williams *et al.*, 1971; Ramirez, 1979; Schantz *et al.*, 1995) and Eastern Europe (Bulgaria, Romania, Poland) Russia, Central Asian Republics (Kazakhstan, Uzbekistan, Kyrgystan, Mongolia), (Schantz *et al.*, 1995; Shaikenov *et al.*, 1999) and parts of China (Craig *et al.*, 1991, 1992; Wen and Yang, 1997).

Africa and the Middle East

There are three broad categories of dogs in this region of the world, viz: feral or stray dogs, which usually comprise the largest population, working sheepdogs, used particularly in north Africa and in the Middle East to herd sheep, and pet dogs which are kept mostly for guarding property and in rural areas to protect against wild animals (see Chapter 2). Very few dogs are considered as household pets with no other function. Stray dogs usually are not very visible during the day but emerge at night to scavenge from rubbish dumps and around human settlements. In many north African, Levant and Middle Eastern countries owned pet dogs are not restricted to the home area and are allowed to roam freely with stray dogs and many authorities consider these dogs, together with strays, as the main sources of infection for livestock and humans, due to their free roaming, scavenging lifestyle (Moch *et al.*, 1974; Kilani *et al.*, 1986; Gusbi *et al.*, 1990; Kamhawi and Abdel-Hafez, 1995; Abdel-Hafez and Kamhawi, 1997; Ouhelli *et al.*, 1997). The generally high prevalence of *E. granulosus* in dogs in north Africa and the Middle East is thought to be also due to a lack of appreciation of the life cycle of the parasite by abattoir workers, butchers, meat inspectors and dog owners and the lack of infrastructure and the enforcement of regulations governing infected offal disposal. Home slaughter, particularly for religious and special ceremonial events occurs throughout the region and at such times meat inspection is not enforced. In Morocco, feeding of infected offal to dogs was found to occur in all areas and since between 70-90% of owned dogs are allowed to roam free there exists ample opportunities for exposure to infection (Ouhelli *et al.*, 1997). Muslims, whose religious teachings advise that dogs are impure ("If a dog licks from the utensils of anyone of you it is essential to wash it seven times"..."Angels do not enter a house where there is a dog" "The Prophet has ordered the killing of dogs, except for a hunting dog, or a sheep or cattle dog" – sayings of the Prophet Muhammad, related by Muslim, Ahmed, Abu Dawood, Al-Bukhari and Al-Behaqi) still find that dogs are useful or even essential to guard the home or livestock and so are kept in large numbers: over 3 million dogs are thought to occur in Morocco (National Laboratory for Epidemiology and Zoonoses, 1993) which has a human population of just over 26 million. Children throughout the Middle East and in North Africa regularly have contact with dogs and CE has a relatively high prevalence in children less than 15 years of age in this region. Responsibility for feeding and looking after dogs in Morocco, and in the region in general, is usually left to women and this increased contact may be partly responsible for the higher incidence of CE amongst women compared to men (Shambesh *et al.*, 1992, 1999; Abdel-Hafez and Kamhawi, 1997; Ouhelli, *et al.*, 1997).

A history of dog ownership has been shown to be important in some areas. For example, CE patients in Beirut were 21 times more likely to have had a history of dog ownership than other Beirutis (Abou Daoud and Schwabe, 1964). The use of dogs for hunting wild pigs by Christians and Druze people and feeding the offal to the dogs is thought to be a risk factor increasing the incidence of CE amongst these groups compared to Arabs in Israel (Yarrow *et al.*, 1991).

In sub-Saharan Africa, in addition to domestic dogs, there are a number of wild carnivores which serve as definitive hosts, but it is unlikely that any of these wild species plays an important role in human infection (Macpherson and Wachira, 1997). A number of prevalence studies have been conducted in different countries and these are presented in Table 7.1. As in North Africa and the Middle East there are large numbers of stray dogs and most owned dogs are free to roam and scavenge. Dogs are maintained for guarding from intruders and wild animals but are usually not used for herding. Dogs spend most of their day in their home area but are rarely trained or shown affection. There have been few attempts to control their numbers in any of the sub-Saharan countries and dog populations are therefore restricted by food, water and shelter availability (see Chapter 2). In urban areas dogs living close to abattoirs are often infected with *E. granulosus* (Wachira *et al.*, 1993). In the hyperendemic focus amongst the nomadic pastoralists of East Africa (Figure 7.1), there are usually no veterinary and scarce medical and educational facilities, no abattoirs, little knowledge about the parasite and food for dogs is scarce, so infected offal is invariably fed to dogs. In such areas droughts are common and it is thought that animals that die in huge numbers during drought years are very important for creating ideal conditions for the rapid

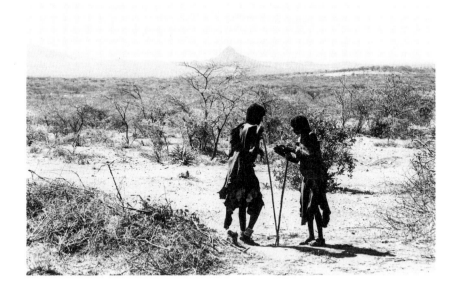

Figure 7.1. Two Hamar women who live a nomadic lifestyle in southern Ethiopia. Educational, medical, veterinary, communication facilities, and safe water supplies are virtually non-existent in this area: a situation which stretches across the contiguous arid areas of southern Sudan, northern Kenya and Uganda.

expansion of the infected dog population (Wachira *et al.*, 1990; Macpherson, 1994).

A lack of hygiene, the use of water holes for drinking water which dogs have access to (Figure 7.2) and where *E. granulosus* eggs survive longer (Wachira *et al.*, 1991) may be important sources of human infection. Additionally, the preparation of food where dogs lick up the remnants (Figure 7.3) and a close association of dogs with women in particular (Watson-Jones and Macpherson, 1988) allows almost ideal conditions for the continuous transmission of the parasite in this region. It is not surprising that there is a continuous exposure to infection and the prevalence of CE increases with age (Macpherson *et al.*, 1987, 1989b).

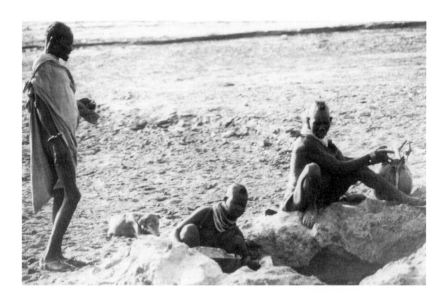

Figure 7.2. Turkana obtaining their drinking water from a hole dug in a dry river bed. Dogs are often observed lying in these cool water holes during the day.

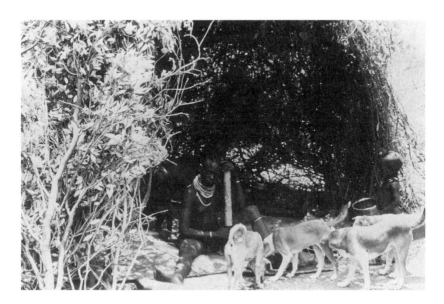

Figure 7.3. A large number of dogs scavenging scraps of food during its preparation. Dogs are allowed to lick clean cooking and eating utensils.

Table 7.1. Reported prevalence of *Echinococcus granulosus* in dogs in Africa.

Country - location	Dogs exam.	% dogs infected	Reference
North Africa			
Algeria	172	9.9	Senevet, 1951
Egypt	570	3.9	Moch *et al.*, 1974
	510	1.6	Hegazi *et al.*, 1986
Libya	243	29.6	*Ibrahem and Gusbi, 1997
Morocco (1920-1949)	331	1-70	*Ouhelli *et al.*, 1997
(1979-1985)	103	48.3	*Ouhelli *et al.*, 1997
1995	282	33.3	*Ouhelli *et al.*, 1997
Tunisia	348	22.7	Kilani *et al.*, 1986
		1.2	Bernard *et al.*, 1967
Sub-Saharan Africa			
Chad - Central	117	3.4	Troncy and Graber, 1969
-Fort-Lamy	-	2	Provost, 1971
Kenya -Turkana	695	13-63.5	Macpherson *et al.*, 1985
-Maasailand	92	37	Nguzi, 1986
-Nairobi	156	10	Wachira *et al.*, 1993
Mozambique - Maputo	643	0.5	Ferreira Pirez, 1980
Nigeria - (in general)	549	1.2-6.2	Dada, 1979, 1980; Dada *et al.*, 1979
Somalia	-	23	Macchioni *et al.*, 1985
South Africa - Pretoria	1063	0.9	Verster, 1979
Sudan - Khartoum	33	3	El-Badawi *et al.*, 1979
-Central	25	51	Saad and Magzoub, 1986
-South	76	52.6	Eisa *et al.*, 1962
Tanzania - Maasailand	10	60	Macpherson *et al.*, 1989a

*Review, summarizing data from numerous sources

Asia

From China (including Tibet), through Mongolia, Siberia, Kazakhstan, the central Asian Republics, Nepal, Bhutan, Pakistan, India to Iran, the dog is the principal definitive host of *E. granulosus* (Schantz *et al.*, 1995; Shaikenov *et al.*, 1999). Over this huge area of grazing steppe and montane pastures dogs have traditionally and continue to be associated with nomadic, semi-nomadic and settled pastoral communities.

In China, six provinces or autonomous regions, including Xinjiang, Gansu, Ningxia, Inner Mongolia, Qinghai and Tibet have the highest reported prevalences of CE (Craig *et al.*, 1991). Dogs are used as guards, particularly in the towns and cities and as shepherd dogs in the vast sheep rearing areas (Liu, 1993). Autopsy surveys of dogs revealed high rates of infection in Xinjiang, 7-71%; Gansu, 27%; Ningxia, 56%; Quinghai, 11-47% (Zhang, 1983; Yan, 1983;

Yang, 1992). In the Xinjiang Uygur Autonomous Region between 1957-1991, 8.1% of 27,186 dogs were found to harbor *E. granulosus* infections, as determined by either autopsy or arecoline purgation (Liu, 1993). In this region home slaughter was an important risk factor and infection rates in dogs was higher in pastoral than agricultural areas. Kazak, Mongolian and Kergez peoples who are mostly pastoralists have correspondingly higher infections in their dogs compared to Han, Hui or Uygur ethnic groups.

In Kathmandu, Nepal a coproantigen study revealed a prevalence of 5.7% (5/88) in domestic dogs living near the area of the city where livestock was slaughtered, and 1.8% (3/171) domestic dogs from all areas of the city (Baronet *et al.*, 1994). As is the case elsewhere in Asia there were a large number of street dogs (some of which were "owned" by the community), each apparently with its own "territory" and domestic and street dogs were allowed to roam freely and had access to livestock viscera.

Australia

A number of studies involving only a few animals have been undertaken on the role of domestic dogs in the transmission of *E. granulosus* in Australia (Baldock *et al.*, 1985; Thompson *et al.*, 1988; Gasser *et al.*, 1990; Jenkins and Andrew, 1993; Grainger and Jenkins, 1996). The limited data available suggest that in some rural and urban areas up to 10.2% of domestic dogs are infected. This is likely to be an underestimation of the true prevalence level, as the studies relied upon arecoline purgation and detection of serum antibodies to determine parasite presence. Dogs are infected by ingestion of raw offal from sheep, wild pigs or macropod marsupials. Classes of dogs found infected include those belonging to recreational pig hunters, suburban residents of Perth and Aboriginal communities in New South Wales (Thompson *et al.,* 1988; Jenkins and Andrew, 1993; Thompson *et al.*, 1993; Jenkins *et al.*, 1996). Domestic dogs are rarely treated for intestinal worms.

Between 48-93% of wild dogs, consisting of dingoes and dingo/domestic dog hybrids, have been found infected with very heavy *E. granulosus* worm burdens in Queensland (Baldock *et al.*, 1985), Victoria (Granger and Jenkins, 1996) and New South Wales (Jenkins and Morris, 1991). In addition to a wildlife cycle wild dogs may also be responsible for sheep and human infection.

New Zealand

Fifty years ago approximately 10% of sheepdogs in the rural areas and over 56% of dogs owned by professional rabbit hunters were infected with *E. granulosus* (Sweatman and Williams, 1962). A national control program eradicated the parasite and the country now is in a "maintenance of eradication" phase (see Chapter 12).

North America

The cervid strain is mainly maintained in a wildlife cycle involving wolves as definitive hosts and moose (*Alces alces*) as intermediate hosts. Dogs fed offal from wild ungulates are the most important source of infection for humans. Wolves recently translocated from British Columbia and Alberta to Yellowstone National Park were coproantigen tested prior to movement and found to have high rates of *Echinococcus* antigen positivity 75.6% (62/82), most likely the cervid strain (S. Storandt and P.S. Craig, unpublished).

   E. granulosus (sheep strain) was probably introduced to Utah by sheepdogs imported from Australia in 1938 (Crellin *et al.*, 1982). Infection then spread in the western states by movement of infected sheep. Transmission occurs between sheep and the large numbers of dogs used to herd them, which are maintained in a transhumant system employed by the Basque Americans living in the Central Valley of California and in native Americans in Utah. (Araujo *et al.*, 1975; Andersen *et al.*, 1983). CE is also found amongst native Americans who practice home slaughter in Arizona and New Mexico (Schantz, 1977).

South and Central America

In Florida, Uruguay, dogs are used for herding sheep, home slaughter is frequent and in one study in a rural area 13.2% of dogs were found infected. Reinfection 2-4 months after treatment was high (Cabrera *et al.*, 1996). Mean worm burden (by arecoline purgation) in Durazno Department (Uruguay) was 67 (range 1-1020) where the prevalence was 20% (Cohen *et al.*, 1998). Feeding of offal to dogs was significantly correlated with *E. granulosus* infections in dogs and CE infection in humans (Carmona *et al.*, 1998).

   The prevalence of infection of dogs in Peru is high in the central and southern highlands, ranging from a prevalence rate of 8-46% in Junin and 32-37% in Puno. In urban areas, prevalence rates range from 3.42% in Lima to 48.2% in Arequipa (Moro *et al.*, 1997).

   CE is prevalent throughout Chile (Arambulo, 1997), but is especially common in the south of the country where active control programs have been in place for many years (see Chapter 12). CE is also common in the high sierra of Bolivia and in the Rio Grande do Sol in Brazil (Schantz *et al.*, 1995).

   CE infection in Central America is rare and most probably maintained in a pig-dog cycle. In many countries poor abattoir conditions exist with dogs gaining access to discarded offal (Schwabe, 1984).

Diet

The diet available to dogs obviously plays a pivotal role in their becoming infected with *E. granulosus*. In most nomadic or transhumant populations dogs are fed scraps and scavenge from around the temporary encampments. In many instances human feces comprises an important part of the dog's diet and dogs are welcomed for the sanitary role that they play (Watson-Jones and Macpherson, 1988). Food availability varies considerably, even within regions where socio-cultural and socioeconomic conditions are similar. For example, in Turkana 63.5% of 263 dogs were found infected in the northwest of the district whilst only a few hundred miles east none of 80 dogs owned by Turkana's living along the shores of Lake Turkana were infected (Macpherson *et al.*, 1985). The lake shore dogs fed almost exclusively on fish scraps whilst the dogs in the west had fed on livestock that had died during the 1978-1981 drought. In Turkana dogs may scavenge from human cadavers increasing the role of humans in the life cycle of the parasite there (Macpherson, 1983). There are no abattoirs outside the major towns of Lodwar, Kakuma, Lokitaung and Lokichoggio, so offal from infected animals that are slaughtered at the temporary nomadic homes are also sources of infection for dogs.

In developing countries conditions at abattoirs are not always appropriate for control of *E. granulosus* infection in dogs and dogs are allowed to scavenge from carcasses or from offal that is discarded (Figure 7.4) (Moch *et al.*, 1974; Schwabe, 1984; Irshadullah *et al.*, 1989; Wachira *et al.*, 1993; Ibrahem and Gusbi, 1997; Ouhelli *et al.*, 1997).

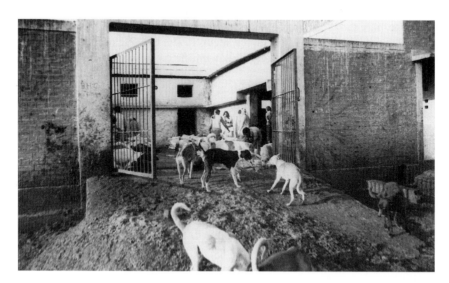

Figure 7.4. Dogs exiting an abattoir for water buffaloes in Aligarh, Uttah Pradesh, India. Dogs not only have access to offal but hydatid cysts are often thrown to them by the abattoir workers.

Thus in some countries, such as in India and North and sub-Saharan Africa urban cycles of *E. granulosus* occur. In Egypt, Moch *et al.* (1974) found that dogs had a higher prevalence of *E. granulosus* in areas where there were abattoirs that in areas that did not.

Dogs used for herding in many continents are at risk from infection when they scavenge from dead livestock, particularly sheep (Schwabe, 1984). Ample opportunities for this occur, particularly in nomadic or transhumant situations where livestock are moved over vast distances. These scavenging opportunities increase the risk for human CE amongst such peoples (Arajou *et al.*, 1975; Macpherson, 1995).

In a number of countries in West Africa and Asia some people eat dogs which would be hazardous to the people preparing them as well as the consumers (Simoons, 1961; Schwabe, 1991). In Turkana, jackals and hyenas were consumed during periods of drought but the people denied ever eating dogs (Macpherson *et al.*, 1983).

Socioeconomic factors

A number of socioeconomic factors operating at the individual, community and national levels, which vary in different parts of the world, contribute to the transmission of *E. granulosus* including:

- Education, specifically a lack of knowledge about the life cycle of *E. granulosus*, is an important factor affecting the public health importance of CE in endemic communities. In endemic countries information about the transmission of the parasite and its prevention is rarely taught, outside of specific control activities.
- Lack of veterinary and medical facilities including abattoirs.
- Lack of diagnostic centers where a diagnosis of CE may be made in humans and livestock and *E. granulosus* infections in dogs.
- Lack of trained personnel.
- Lack of baseline information on the public health and veterinary importance of CE.
- Lack of separate or integrated veterinary and healthcare policies regarding the control of the disease.
- Lack of a safe piped water supply. Hygiene in such areas is naturally compromised if water has to be carried over long distances to the home.
- Inability to pay for treatment of owned dogs and for treatment of individuals with CE.
- Pastoralists are at greater risk of CE than agriculturists or urban dwellers.
- Transhumant or nomadic pastoralists who live in many parts of the world appear to consistently have the greatest risk of CE.
- Abattoir workers are a high risk group for CE, particularly those who work in developing countries.

A greater understanding of these factors and also particular socio-cultural factors is essential to the successful implementation of control programs.

Control and surveillance

There have been a number of island and continental control programs for *E. granulosus*: these are covered in Chapter 12 and only a brief overview of control measures that are applied to dogs will be considered here. Many control programs have been implemented and several have been very successful in reducing the annual incidence of CE in humans and sheep and *E. granulosus* infections in dogs. One country, Iceland, has succeeded in eradicating the disease.

A number of options are available for control (Chapter 12) but most programs have had similar strategies to control *E. granulosus* in dogs, which include:

- Education of the local population (Figure 7.5). An important aspect with any educational program is compliance with the control approach, for example, complying with dog registration and treatment schedules, not feeding cysts to dogs, etc.
- Dog registration.
- Elimination of stray and unwanted dogs.
- Population management of wanted dog populations (spaying programs: see Chapter 11).
- Prevention of access of dogs to infected offal. This may be achieved through strict rules of disposal of infected offal in abattoirs and preventing dogs from gaining access to such facilities. In the absence of such facilities, such as occurs in nomadic and transhumant communities, and in places where animals are slaughtered on farms and at home for religious or ceremonial occasions, education of those who carry out home slaughter and meat inspection should be implemented.
- Regular dosing of dogs with praziquantel. Some programs implement an intense dosing schedule every 6 weeks whereas others examine epidemiological factors and dosing is timed to prevent transmission when the intensity is likely to be highest and the greatest cost:benefit value is obtained. Regular dosing of dogs is thought to comprise a very important method of reducing the basic reproductive rate of *E. granulosus* (R_o) below unity thus achieving control (Ming *et al.*, 1992).

Surveillance in dogs may be carried out through arecoline surveys. This is a hazardous procedure and is not very sensitive in detecting *E. granulosus* infections, particularly light infections (< 200 worms). This method will most likely be replaced by coproantigen tests which are less hazardous, have a greater sensitivity and can detect prepatent infections. Field tests with this technique are currently under investigation in a number of countries.

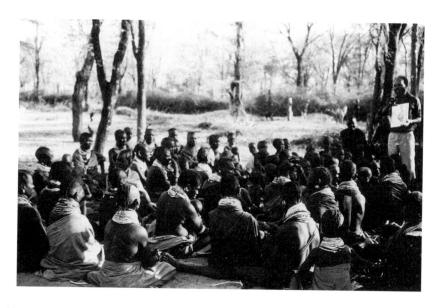

Figure 7.5. In Turkana, northwestern Kenya, the educational part of the control program focused on women who had almost three times the incidence of CE. Particular attention was paid to stressing that dogs should not be fed cysts. In this area the educational methods relied on songs, role plays and routine purgation of dogs in the presence of their owners.

Echinococcus multilocularis (Leuckart, 1863)

The small (1.2-4.5 mm) adult tapeworms live in the small intestines of wild canids. Throughout most of the parasite's range the red fox (*Vulpes vulpes*) is the main definitive host. In the northern tundra zone of North America and in northern Russia the arctic fox (*Alopex lagopus*) is an important definitive host. In central north America between 6 and 35% of coyotes (*Canis latrans*) have been found infected (Eckert, 1998, for review). Other relatively important wild definitive hosts include wolves (*Canis lupis*) and sand fox (*Vulpes corsac*) which may be commonly infected in Eurasia. Domestic dogs and cats also serve as definitive hosts (see below). Small mammals including microtine and arvicolid rodents, and occasionally other groups such as ochotonidae, are intermediate hosts for *E. multilocularis*. In these hosts the parasite develops rapidly, in contrast to the much slower developing metacestode of *E. granulosus*.

Distribution

E. multilocularis is predominantly maintained in predator:prey wildlife cycles and in most endemic areas humans, with their domestic animals, are ecologically separated. The parasite is found over an extensive area of the northern hemisphere extending from the tundra zone of North America, through northern and central Europe and Eurasia to China and the northern islands of Japan. Its southernmost limits in Asia are northern India, Iran and eastern Turkey (Rausch, 1995; Eckert, 1998). *E. multilocularis* eggs have become adapted to cold climates and can survive temperatures of -50°C. Eggs can thus overwinter and be viable when the intermediate hosts emerge after the winter (Schiller, 1955).

Dogs as definitive hosts of *Echinococcus multilocularis*

Dogs appear to be relatively susceptible to *E. multilocularis* and infection occurs when dogs ingest infected intermediate hosts. Huge worm burdens may result in both dogs and foxes. On St Lawrence Island mean infection rates in Arctic foxes was 7400-54,000 (range 1-84,000) (Rausch *et al.*, 1990). In the red fox in urban areas of Zurich infections of over 10,000 individuals was found in 8% of the 133 infected foxes (Hoffer *et al.*, 2000). The prepatent period is slightly shorter than for *E. granulosus* at about 28 days and proglottids contain only between 200 and 300 eggs. The adult parasites probably live for between 2-5 months (Ishige *et al.*, 1990) with maximum egg excretion 8-13 weeks after infection. More than 100,000 eggs per gram of feces may occur. The suitability of cats as definitive hosts is somewhat equivocal with some authors reporting retarded development and lower worm burdens than dogs (Thompson and Eckert, 1983) whilst other, more recent studies (Deplazes *et al.*, 1999), have suggested that development rates are only slightly slower to that found in dogs.

　　In China dogs have been found to be infected in Gansu (6 out of 58) and Sichuan Provences (Craig *et al.*, 1992). In south Gansu dog ownership *per se* was not a risk factor for human AE, rather, number of dogs and period of dog ownership and dog-carer were risk factors (Craig *et al.*, 2000). In this montane agricultural region a semi-domestic cycle between dogs and microtine rodent species is likely to occur during periods of high population density for susceptible rodent species.

　　Within Tibetan communities on the Qinghai-Tibet plateau (includes west Sichuan province), domestic dogs are also probably involved in semi-domestic transmission of *E. multilocularis* involving the common lagomorph species in this biotype, *Ochotona curzonae*. In both Gansu and Sichuan higher AE rates in women may be related to closer contact of females with dogs as has been shown in nomadic people in East and North Africa.

　　In Japan stray dogs have been found infected on Reubun Island (1.6% of 3224) (Yamashita, 1973) and in 2% of dogs on the island of Hokkaido (Iida, 1969). In both areas the red fox is perceived as the main definitive host.

In North America *E. multilocularis* is currently an important public health problem only amongst the Yupik Eskimos in the northern tundra zone of Alaska, despite the parasite's wide distribution, including as far south as Canada (Rausch, 1995; Schantz *et al.*, 1995). The parasite has been found on a number of the subarctic islands, including St Lawrence Island, where in the 1950s 12% of dogs autopsied were infected (Rausch *et al.*, 1990). Dog ownership and tethering dogs near houses was an important risk factor for patients found to have AE (Stehr-Green *et al.*, 1988).

It has been speculated that dogs may have been the route through which the parasite was spread from the northern tundra zone to southern Canada and to central areas of the northern USA, especially North Dakota and northern Manitoba (Rausch, 1967). The parasite has spread from these areas and has now been reported in 11 contiguous states in the USA and in three Canadian provinces (Schantz *et al.*, 1995). So far the parasite in this area has not been found in domestic dogs and only two human AE cases have been confirmed in the last 50 years (Schantz *et al.*, 1995).

In Europe, little is known about the importance of dogs in the transmission of *E. multilocularis* to humans as there are few stray dogs and, until recently, the only means of diagnosis was necropsy. Studies which were carried out generally involved small numbers of dogs and salient risk factor assessment was lacking (Romig *et al.*, 1999). The recent development of *ante mortem* diagnostic tests (see below) has facilitated much larger studies. A recent ELISA coproantigen study with confirmation by PCR of 660 dogs in Switzerland found a prevalence of 0.3% (Deplazes *et al.*, 1999). In Austria, cat ownership and hunting in the forest were found to be important risk factors whereas dog ownership was not (Kreidl *et al.*, 1998). In Austria, as elsewhere in Europe, dogs are mostly pets and not used for hunting.

In an attempt to estimate the relative capacities of foxes, dogs and cats to contaminate the environment with *E. multilocularis* eggs, a model calculation was carried out for the Canton of Zurich, Switzerland (Eckert and Deplazes, 1999). The population size and prevalence of *E. multilocularis* in the three definitive host species was calculated (Table 7.2). Foxes were the largest group of *E. multilocularis* carriers whereas the numbers of infected dogs and cats were much smaller and represented only 7% and 16% of the number of infected definitive hosts, respectively. Apparently, in this epidemiological situation foxes were the main contaminators of the environment with *E. multilocularis* eggs. Such calculations can provide a few suggestions of the importance of the various definitive hosts but they are woefully incomplete as many other factors play a role. For example, although the prevalence rate in dogs and cats was small they have a closer contact with humans than foxes providing greater opportunities for being the source of human infection. On the other hand it has been recently noted that fox populations are increasing in the cities in Europe and in Zurich, Switzerland it has been estimated that there are between 300-400 foxes within the city limits with 47% being infected with *E. multilocularis* (Hoffer *et al.*, 2000). It is known that such foxes visit public parks and swimming pools (Deplazes *et al.*, 1999) and infection with *E. multilocularis* in urban areas from foxes may become more important in the future.

Table 7.2. Relative significance of foxes, dogs and cats as definitive hosts for *Echinococcus multilocularis*: model calculation for the Canton of Zurich, Switzerland (modified from Eckert and Deplazes, 1999).

Host Species	Estimated populated size (1992)	Infected with *E. multilocularis* Per cent of definitive hosts		
		%	Number	Population
Fox	4,700	33.0	1,551	77
Dog	48,400	0.3	145	7
Cat	145,200	0.2	319	16

The prevalence rates in cats in Europe varies between 0 and 5.5% (Eckert, 1998) and they must therefore pose a source of infection to humans. The introduction of new diagnostic tests may not only be used for *ante mortem* diagnosis of dogs and cats but also potentially be able to detect *E. multilocularis* infections in fecal samples collected in the field. This will facilitate studies to examine the relative contribution of dogs and cats compared to that made by foxes to environmental contamination and enable studies to be carried out to examine potential routes of infection for humans.

Diagnosis of *Echinococcus multilocularis* in dogs

Until recently the only means of accurately diagnosing *E. multilocularis* infections in dogs was by autopsy and the subsequent morphological identification of the adult worms. The development of ELISA and PCR tests for screening feces for coproantigens or worm DNA has revolutionized diagnosis of not only patent but also prepatent infections in definitive hosts (Dinkel *et al.*, 1998; Deplazes *et al.*, 1999). The coproantigen test has a sensitivity of 80% and a specificity of 95 to 99.5%. Confirmation of infection may be made using the PCR to detect *E. multilocularis* DNA which increases the sensitivity to 94% and has a specificity of 100% (Deplazes and Eckert, 1996; Dinkel *et al.*, 1998).

Treatment of *Echinococcus multilocularis* in dogs

The treatment of choice is praziquantel. As with *E. granulosus* no resistance to the drug has yet been reported and the drug is effective in a single dose.

Epidemiology and public health importance

Foxes contaminated with *E. multilocularis* eggs have traditionally been considered to be an important health hazard to fox hunters, however there is no direct evidence for this. When hunters in the USA and Japan were screened by serological tests no increased risk of seropositivity was observed (see Schantz *et al.*, 1995).

Indirect contact with fox feces contaminated environment, e.g. wild fruits and/or herbs, has been considered an important mode of infection - though detailed studies are lacking. Dog (or cat) ownership over a reasonable period (years) within endemic areas is possibly a greater risk factor for human AE (see above), together with an agricultural occupation or background and households close to landscape/biotype capable of sustaining susceptible intermediate host populations (Bresson-Hadni *et al.*, 1994; Craig *et al.*, 2000).

Control and surveillance

The only example of eradication of *E. multilocularis* occurred on Reuben Island (Japan) 30 years after the parasite had been introduced inadvertently with translocated red foxes (in 1924-1926). Approximately 1% of the population (129 AE cases) was infected, 19% of red foxes and 1.6% of dogs. A 5 year fox and dog culling control program appeared to eliminate the parasite by 1995 (Yamashita, 1973; Craig *et al.*, 1996).

There has been a single trial to treat dogs as part of a control program for *E. multilocularis*. This took place in St Lawrence Island where dogs were treated monthly with praziquantel over a 10 year period. This reduced the infection in the rodent intermediate hosts from 29% to 5%. The prevalence rate in the intermediate hosts, however, rebounded to the original rates soon after dosing of dogs was discontinued (Schantz *et al.*, 1995).

In southern Germany a trial to reduce the prevalence of *E. multilocularis* in wild foxes (*V. vulpes*) demonstrated that after six treatments the prevalence of the parasite in these definitive hosts fell from 32% to 4% (Schelling *et al.*, 1997). it has been proposed that only those dogs and cats at risk of infection through eating wild-caught intermediate hosts should be treated regularly with praziquantel (Eckert and Deplazes, 1999). The possibility of introducing a dog screening program with ELISA tests to detect coproantigens provides an exciting new approach to *E. multilocularis* epidemiology and surveillance.

Echinococcus vogeli (Rausch and Bernstein, 1972)

E. vogeli has a restricted global distribution and has only been reported within the range of its wild definitive and intermediate hosts in Central and South America: in Costa Rica, Panama, Colombia, Ecuador, Venezuela, Brazil and Bolivia (Rausch, 1995 for review). The disease in humans who serve as accidental intermediate hosts is known as polycystic echinococcosis (PE) or hydatid disease. The adult parasites were first described from specimens recovered from the small intestine of the bush dog, *Speothos venaticus* (Rausch and Bernstein, 1972) which is the only known wild definitive host species of this parasite. The animal had been captured in its natural habitat in Esmeraldas Province, Ecuador and kept in the Los Angeles Zoo. The bush dog was responsible for infecting five different species of non-human primates housed in nearby cages and most of them subsequently died of PE (Howard and Gendron, 1980). There were no human cases but this incidence does highlight how infective the eggs are for non-human primates.

The paca, *Cuniculus paca* serves as the main intermediate host. Agoutis (*Dasyprocta* spp.) and spiny rats (*Proechimys* spp.) have also been found to harbour *E. vogeli* protoscoleces (Rausch *et al.*, 1981). Domestic dogs can also serve as definitive hosts and experimental infections of dogs with cysts from an agouti were confirmed as being *E. vogeli* (Rausch *et al.*, 1984). In its natural habitat *E. vogeli* is maintained in a predator:prey cycle. As *Speothos* spp. hunt in packs many bush dogs may be infected from a single paca kill. The risk of human infection from wild definitive hosts would be rare since bush dogs are secretive and very wary of humans and move further into the forest when humans encroach on their territory. Contact rarely occurs. In endemic areas, dogs are used to hunt and are commonly fed viscera from pacas so that human infections are probably acquired from the feces of infected dogs. Feeding dogs paca offal is an important risk factor and in Colombia a hunter's dog has been found to have the adult parasites (D'Alessandro *et al.*, 1979, 1981). In Brazil, Meneghelli *et al.* (1990) found that seven patients with polycystic hydatid disease had all had contact with dogs that had been fed offal from pacas.

The disease in humans on radiological examination gives the appearance of multiple cysts of *E. granulosus* (Meneghelli *et al.*, 1992a). Cysts are usually located in the liver but also infect the lungs, spleen, pancreas, peritoneal cavity and mesentery (Meneghelli *et al.*, 1992b). Differentiation between *E. vogeli* and *E. granulosus* is possible using protoscolex hook morphology, PCR and ELISA. Human infections have been reported in most countries within its known range in neotropical America (D'Alessandro *et al.*, 1979, 1981; Meneghelli *et al.*, 1992a; Nunez *et al.*, 1993; Rausch, 1995). In Ecuador at least 12 human cases have been diagnosed coming from diverse geographic regions, including the coastal plain, Amazon basin and Andean plateau (Nunez *et al.*, 1993). In Brazil, most cases have been reported from the Amazon region but a few from the state of Sao Paulo (Meneghelli *et al.*, 1992b).

Albendazole given over a period of several months successfully treated four of six patients (Meneghelli *et al.*, 1986, 1992a). The remaining two patients had some remission of the disease. It would be impossible to control the parasite in its natural habitat but making hunters aware of the dangers of feeding offal from pacas to their dogs would help decrease human exposure in endemic regions. Regular treatment with praziquantel of dogs who are fed such offal would also be advisable.

Diphyllobothriosis

Within the group of tapeworms belonging to the genus *Diphyllobothrium*, *Diphyllobothrium latum* is the predominant species with regard to numbers of human infections which amount to approximately 20 million. *D. latum*, known as the "broad" tapeworm, as the proglottids are usually wider than they are long, is the largest tapeworm of humans, growing to a length of 3-25 m and a width of 1-2 cm. The parasite is especially prevalent in countries where fish is a major source of protein and is often eaten raw or only partially cooked (i.e. smoked). Offal from the fish is often available to domestic animals and cats, pigs and especially dogs may serve as definitive hosts. In some areas infection levels in dogs reach 34-47% and they likely serve as the main definitive hosts (Witenburg, 1964). Major foci occur in European freshwater lakes, in areas of the former Soviet Union, Finland, Scandinavia, the alpine zone, Asia and in America where eating undercooked salmon, sushimi, is becoming increasingly popular (Ruttenber *et al.*, 1984). Marine diphyllobothriasis occurs in marine mammals, e.g. seals, and occasionally humans who eat raw or undercooked fish. Human infections have been recorded in Peru, Chile and Japan, however, susceptibility of dogs is unknown (Miyazaki, 1991).

The life cycle of *Diphyllobothrium* spp. includes copepods as first intermediate hosts (proceercoid stage) and freshwater fish as second intermediate hosts (plerocercoid stage) (Rahkonen and Valtonen, 1997). Following ingestion by definitive hosts, such as humans and a range of other fish-eating carnivores, and in particular domestic animals such as dogs, cats and pigs (see above) the plerocercoid larvae mature to adult tapeworms that may contain up to 3000 proglottids. Experimental infections in dogs have shown that egg production starts about 21 days after infection (Wardle and Green, 1941).

Intestinal infection with *D. latum* is usually asymptomatic. In some cases, mild gastrointestinal obstruction, rarely diarrhea and abdominal pain, and occasionally leukocytosis with eosinophilia are present. Perhaps the most serious clinical manifestation is the onset of pernicious anemia which occurs in approximately 2% of the patients as shown in studies performed in Finland. This is caused by the extensive absorption of vitamin B_{12} by the adult tapeworm (von Bonsdorff, 1977).

Prevention and control measures include appropriate cooking of fish and treatment of infected individuals and domestic animals, particularly dogs, with praziquantel. Regular treatment with praziquantel of domestic carnivores, especially those being fed raw fish, can dramatically reduce environmental contamination of natural water resources with parasite eggs and thus reduce transmission. Preventing access of wild carnivores to aquaculture facilities, by appropriate fencing, also helps control the parasite in such areas.

Cestode species of minor zoonotic importance

Dipylidium caninum

Dipylidium caninum is one of the commonest tapeworms of dogs and cats in most parts of the world (Boreham and Boreham, 1990). It is especially common in neglected dog populations which have large ectoparasite populations. Children under 10 years of age also serve as definitive hosts and adults only rarely (Moore, 1962); this is probably due to increased opportunities for children to become infected. The adult parasite lives in the small intestine and rarely exceeds 50 cm in length. Proglottids migrate out of the anus or are shed in feces and are easily identifiable as they resemble a large rice grain and are either passed singly or as a short ribbon of up to 10 proglattids. A hand-lens inspection of freshly passed proglottids reveals the lateral genital pores and egg packets, which can be used to differentiate this parasite from the taeniids. Each *D. caninum* proglottid contains up to 20 egg packets each containing 6-12 infective eggs. Fleas (*Ctenocephalides felis* and *Ctenocephalides canis*) and the dog louse (*Trichodectes canis*) serve as intermediate hosts. Biting lice can ingest oncospheres at any stage in their life cycle as all stages have chewing mouthparts, but fleas are only infected in the larval stage as the adults have piercing mouthparts. Development in the obligate ectoparasite, the louse, takes up to 30 days whilst in the flea larvae in the environment may take up to a couple of months, depending on the ambient temperature. The cysticercoid in the louse or flea is ingested by the definitive hosts and the prepatent period is about 3 weeks.

The adults, which may number several hundred, are not pathogenic. Proglottids passing out of the anus may cause mild puritis.

Treatment of children, dogs and cats is with praziquantel, niclosamide or nitroscanate. Control of the ectoparasite intermediate hosts should be carried out simultaneously (see Chapter 9). Special attention should be paid to the sleeping area of domestic dogs and cats.

Taenia spp.

There are at least 3 taeniid species, *Taenia multiceps*, *Taenia serialis* and *Taenia brauni* which have dogs and other canids as definitive hosts and a few humans have been identified to be infected with the larval stage. In addition, *Taenia silium* cysticercosis has been recorded in dogs.

Taenia multiceps (Syn. *Multiceps multiceps*)

The parasite is regarded as being common in dogs in Australia, Europe, South America and Africa but has disappeared from New Zealand and the US. A prevalence of 26.6% of dogs in Wales has been reported (Hackett and Walters, 1980). The prepatent period in dogs is between 38 and 43 days (Willis and Herbert, 1987), adult worms grow up to about 100 cm and proglottids are shed in the feces. Intermediate host species include wild ruminants, chamois, cattle, goats and most importantly sheep. Ingested eggs hatch in the small intestine and the oncosphere penetrates the gut and lodges primarily in the central nervous system, especially the brain. Here over a period of about 8 months it develops into a coenurus (*Cysticercus cerebralis*), giving rise to many hundreds of daughter protoscoleces hence multiple worm infections are common in dogs. Clinical manifestations depend on the location of the cyst(s) and may include circling, paraplegia, peculiarities in gait known as "gid". Only a dozen or so human cases have been reported (Smyth, 1994).

Taenia serialis and *Taenia brauni*

Intermediate hosts include lagomorphs and rarely rodents. Cysts are usually located intramuscularly or subcutaneously. Protoscoleces align in rows or series in such cysts, hence the name *T. serialis*. Differential diagnosis with *T. multiceps* may be difficult in both adult and cystic stages (for human infections). Intermediate hosts of *T. brauni* are rodents. Most human infections are subcutaneous or intraocular and most have been reported from Africa (Lloyd, 1998).

Spirometra spp.

Adult *Spirometra* spp. are found in dogs, cats and a range of wild carnivores in many parts of the world particularly eastern Asia, but also in Africa, North and South America and Australia. The life cycle of these tapeworms is similar to that of *D. latum* and two intermediate hosts are normally required. The procercoids are found in crustaceans and the plerocercoids in a range of intermediate host species including amphibians, birds, snakes, mammals and humans (Smyth and Heath, 1970). Humans can be infected in three different ways, viz: by ingesting procercoids in crustaceans (*Cyclops* spp.) in drinking water, through ingesting plerocercoids in undercooked amphibia, snakes, birds and mammals such as pigs, or by applying poultices (such as split frogs) to skin wounds and especially to the eyes. In the latter case plerocercoids migrate from the poultice into the local tissue. This mode of transmission is most commonly found in China and Southeast Asia. Plerocercoids can grow up to 30-40 cm. The disease is known as sparganosis (*Sparganum* was the old name for the plerocercoid stage). Ingested procercoids or plerocercoids penetrate the intestinal mucosa, wander through tissues and may end up in subcutaneous sites where they may encyst. They may cause edema and inflammation of the periorbital area, the predilection site of the plerocercoids.

There are many different species of *Spirometra* but the dog is the known definitive host of *Spirometra mansoni*, the dominant species in Asia and South America; snakes serve as intermediate hosts for this species. In lions examined in the Serengeti National Park (Tanzania) *Spirometra* was the commonest intestinal helminth recorded (Muller-Graf *et al.*, 1999).

Rarely the parasite proliferates producing a large number of plerocercoids, which may be fatal (Mueller, 1974). Diagnosis is by finding the plerocercoid, often incidentally when a biopsy of a lump is made. Treatment is by surgically removing the plerocercoid and occasionally praziquantel may be used, especially in heavy or cerebral infections.

Mesocestoides lineatus

Dogs can serve as both secondary intermediate as well as definitive hosts for *Mesocestoides lineatus*. The parasite has a wide distribution in Asia, Europe and Africa. Adult worms have been recorded in humans in Japan, China and Korea (Miyazaki, 1991; Lloyd, 1998). Mites serve as the first intermediate hosts and have the cysticercoid stage. Dogs, other carnivores, amphibia, reptiles and birds serve as secondary intermediate hosts with the tetrathyridia stage. The tetrathyridia can multiply asexually in the peritoneum or may develop into adults. The scolex has no hooks. Clinical symptoms include severe diarrhea, abdominal pain, hunger and dizziness. In Japan, human infection probably occurs as a result of eating/taking uncooked blood or organs of snakes and turtles as tonics (Miyazaki, 1991).

References

Abdel-Hafez, S.K. and Kamhawi, S.A. (1997) Cystic echinococcosis in Levant countries (Jordan, Palastinian Autonomy, Israel, Syria and Lebanon). In: Andersen, F.L., Ouhelli, H. and Kachani, M. (eds), *Compendium on Cystic Echinococcosis in Africa and in Middle Eastern Countries With Special Reference to Morocco*. Brigham Young University, Provo, Utah, pp. 292-316.

Abou Daoud, K. and Schwabe, C.W. (1964) Epidemiology and echinococcosis in the Middle East. III. A study of hydatid disease patients from the city of Beirut. *American Journal of Tropical Medicine* 13, 681-685.

Allan, J.C., Craig, P.S., Garcia Noval, J., Liu, D., Wang, Y., Wen, H., Zhou, P., Stringer, R., Rogan, M. and Zeyhle, E. (1992) Coproantigen detection for immunodiagnosis of echinococcosis and taeniasis in dogs and humans. *Parasitology* 104, 347-355.

Andersen, F.L., Crellin, J.R., Nichols, C.R. and Schantz, P.M. (1983) Evaluation of a program to control hydatid disease in Central Utah. *Great Basin Naturalist* 43, 65-72.

Arambulo III, P. (1997) Public health importance of cystic echinococcosis in Latin America. *Acta Tropica* 67, 113-124.

Araujo, F.P., Schwabe, C.W., Sawyer, J.C. and Davis, W.G. (1975) Hydatid disease transmission in California: a study of the Basque connection. *American Journal of Epidemiology* 102, 291-302.

Baldock, F.C., Arthur, R.J. and Lawrence, A.R. (1985) A meatworks survey of bovine hydatidosis in southern Queensland. *Australian Veterinary Journal* 62, 238-243.

Baronet, D., Waltner-Toews, D., Craig, P.S. and Joshi, D.D. (1994) *Echinococcus granulosus* in the dogs of Kathmandu, Nepal. *Annals of Tropical Medicine and Parasitology* 88, 485-492.

Baxter, D.N. and Leck, I. (1984) The deleterious effects of dogs on human health: 2. Canine zoonoses. *Community Medicine* 6, 185-197.

Bernard, J., Osman, F.B. and Juminer, B. (1967) Enquetas sur les helminthes parasites du chien a Tunis. *Archives de Institut Pasteur, Tunis* 44.

Boreham, R.E. and Boreham, P.F.L. (1990) *Dipylidium caninum*, life cycle epizootiology and control. *Compendium of Continuing Education for the Practising Veterinarian* 12, 667-674.

Bresson-Hadni, S., Laplante, J.J., Lenys, D., Rohmer, P., Gottstein, B., Jacquier, P., Mercet, P., Meyer, J.P., Miguet, J.P. and Vuitton, D.A. (1994) Seroepidemiologic screening of *Echinococcus multilocularis* infection in a European area endemic for alveolar echinococcosis. *American Journal of Tropical Medicine and Hygiene* 51, 837-846.

Cabrera, P.A., Parietti, S., Harian, G., Benavidez, U., Lloyd, S., Perera, G., Valledor, S., Gemmell, M.A. and Botto, T. (1996) Rates of reinfection with *Echinococcus granulosus*, *Taenia hydatigena*, *Taenia ovis* and other cestodes in a rural dog population in Uruguay. *International Journal of Parasitology* 26, 79-83.

Carmona, C., Perdomo, R., Carbo, A., Alvarez, C., Monti, J., Grauert, R., Stern, D., Perera, G., Lloyd, S., Bazini, R., Gemmel, M.A. and Yarzabal, L. (1998) Risk factors associated with human cystic echinococcosis in Florida, Uruguay: results of a mass screening study using ultrasound and serology. *American Journal of Tropical Medicine and Hygiene* 58, 599-605.

Cohen, H., Paolillo, E., Bonifacino, R., Botta, B., Parada, P., Snowden, K., Gasser, R., Tessier, R., Dibarboure, L., Wen, H., Allan, J.C., Soto de Al Faro, H., Rogan, M.T. and Craig, P.S. (1998) Human cystic echinococcosis in a Uruguayan community: a sonographic, serologic and epidemiologic study. *American Journal of Tropical Medicine and Hygiene* 59, 620-627.

Craig, P.S. (1997) Immunodiagnosis of *Echinococcus granulosus* and a comparison of techniques for diagnosis of canine echinococcosis. In: Andersen, F.L., Ouhelli, H. and Kachani, M. (eds) *Compendium on Cystic Echinococcosis in Africa and in Middle Eastern Countries With Special Reference to Morocco.* Brigham Young University, Provo, Utah, USA, pp. 85-118.

Craig, P.S., Macpherson, C.N.L. and Nelson, G.S. (1986) The identification of eggs of *Echinococcus* by immunofluorescence using a specific monoclonal antibody. *American Journal of Tropical Medicine and Hygiene* 35, 152-158.

Craig, P.S., Macpherson, C.N.L., Watson-Jones, D. and Nelson, G.S. (1988) Immunodetection of *Echinococcus* eggs from naturally infected dogs and from environmental contamination sites in settlements in Turkana, Kenya. *Transactions of the Royal Society of Tropical Medicine and Hygiene* 82, 268-274.

Craig, P.S., Liu, D. and Ding, Z.X. (1991) Hydatid disease in China. *Parasitology Today* 7, 46-51.

Craig, P.S., Deshan, L., Macpherson, C.N.L., Shi Dazhong, Reynolds, D., Barnish, G., Gottstein, B. and Zhirong, W. (1992) A large focus of alveolar echinococcosis in central China. *Lancet* 340, 326-331.

Craig, P.S., Gasser, R.B., Parada, L., Cabrera, P., Parietti, S., Borgues, C., Acuttis, A., Agulla, J., Snowden, K. and Paolillo, E. (1995) Diagnosis of canine echinococcosis: comparison of coproantigen and serum antibody tests with arecoline purgation in Uruguay. *Veterinary Parasitology* 56, 293-301.

Craig, P.S., Rogan, M.T. and Allan, J.C. (1996) Detection, screening and community epidemiology of Taeniid cestode zoonoses: Cystic Echinococcosis, Alveolar Echinococcosis and Neurocysticercosis. *Advances in Parasitology* 38, 169-250.

Craig, P.S., Giraudoux, P., Shi, D., Bartholomot, B., Barnish, G., Delattre, P., Quere, J.P., Harraga, S., Bao, G., Wang, Y., Lu, F., Ito, A. and Vuitton, D.A. (2000) An epidemiological and ecological study of human alveolar echinococcosis transmission in south Gansu, China. *Acta Tropica*. In press.

Crellin, J.R., Andersen, F.L., Schantz, P.M. and Condie, S.J. (1982) Possible factors influencing distribution and prevalence of *Echinococcus granulosus* in Utah. *American Journal of Epidemiology* 116, 463-474.

Dada, B.J.O. (1979) Helminth parasites of stray dogs in Kaduna State and their public health significance. *Nigerian Medical Journal* 9, 693-694.

Dada, B.J.O. (1980) Taeniasis, cysticercosis and echinococcosis/hydatidosis in Nigeria, IV. Prevalence of *Echinococcus granulosus* infection in stray dogs. *Journal of Helminthology* 54, 299-301.

Dada, B.J.O., Adegboye, D.S. and Mohammed, A.N. (1979) A survey of gastro-intestinal helminth parasites of stray dogs in Zaria, Nigeria. *Veterinary Record* 104, 145-146.

D'Alessandro, A., Rausch, R.L., Cuello, C. and Aristizabal, N. (1979) *Echinococcus vogeli* in man, with a review of polycystic hydatid disease in Columbia and neighbouring countries. *American Journal of Tropical Medicine and Hygiene* 28, 303-317.

D'Alessandro, A., Rausch, R.L., Morales, G.A., Collet, S. and Angel, D. (1981) *Echinococcus* infections in Columbian animals. *American Journal of Tropical Medicine and Hygiene* 30, 1263-1276.

Dar, F.K. and Alkarmi, T. (1997) Cystic echinococcosis in the Gulf Littoral States. In: Andersen, F.L., Ouhelli, H. and Kachani, M. (eds) *Compendium on Cystic*

Echinococcosis in Africa and in Middle Eastern Countries With Special Reference to Morocco. Brigham Young University, Provo, Utah, pp. 281-291.

Deplazes, P. and Eckert, J. (1996) Diagnosis of *Echinococcus multilocularis* infection in final hosts. *Applied Parasitology* 37, 245-252.

Deplazes, P., Gottstein, B., Eckert, J., Jenkins, D.J., Ewald, D. and Jimenez Palacios, S. (1992) Detection of *Echinococcus* coproantigens by enzyme-linked immunosorbent assay in dogs, dingoes and foxes. *Parasitology Research* 78, 303-308.

Deplazes, P., Alther, P., Tanner, I., Thompson, R.C.A. and Eckert, J. (1999) *Echinococcus multilocularis* coproantigen detection by enzyme-linked immunosorbent assay in fox, dog, and cat populations. *Journal of Parasitology* 85, 115-121.

Dinkel, A., Nickisch-Rosenegk, M., Bilger, B., Merli, M., Lucius, R. and Romig, T. (1998) Detection of *Echinococcus multilocularis* in the definitive host: Coprodiagnosis by PCR as an alternative to necropsy. *Journal of Clinical Microbiology* 36, 1871-1876.

Eckert, J. (1998) Alveolar echinococcosis (*Echinococcus multilocularis*) and other forms of echinococcosis (*Echinococcus vogeli* and *Echinococcus oligarthrus*). In: Palmer, S.R., Lord Soulsby and Simpson, D.I.H. (eds) *Zoonoses.* Oxford University Press, pp. 689-716.

Eckert, J. and Deplazes, P. (1999) Alveolar Echinococcosis in humans: The current situation in Central Europe and the need for countermeasures. *Parasitology Today* 15, 315-319.

Eisa, A.M., Mustafa, A.A. and Soliman, K.N. (1962) Preliminary report on cysticercosis and hydatidosis in southern Sudan. *Sudan Journal of Veterinary Science* 3, 97-108.

El-Badawi, E.S., Eisa, A.M., Slepenev, N.K. and Saad, M.B.A. (1979) Hydatidosis of domestic animals in the central region of the Sudan. *Bulletin of Animal Health Production in Africa* 27, 249-251.

El-Shehabi, F.S., Kamhawi, K., Schantz, P.M., Craig, P.S. and Abdel-Hafez, S.K. (2000) Diagnosis of canine echinococcosis: comparison of coproantigen detection with necropsy in stray dogs and red foxes from northern Jordan. *Journal of Parasitology* (in press).

Eslami, A. and Hosseini, S.H. (1998) *Echinococcus granulosus* infection of farm dogs of Iran. *Parasitology Research* 84, 205-207.

Ferreira Pirez, M.L. (1980) Occurrence of the multivesicular form of hydatidosis in cattle in Mozambique. *Bulletin of Animal Health and Animal Production* 28, 54-58.

Frider, B., Losada, C.A., Larrieu, E. and de Zavaleta, O. (1988) Asymptomatic abdominal hydatidosis detected by ultrasonography. *Acta Radiologica* 29, 431-434.

Frider, B., Larrieu, E. and Odriozola, M. (1999) Long-term outcome of asymptomatic liver hydatidosis. *Journal of Hepatology* 30, 228-231.

Gasser, R.B., Lightowlers, D.L. and Rickard, M.D. (1990) A recombinant antigen with potential for serodiagnosis of *Echinococcus granulosus* infection in dogs. *International Journal for Parasitology* 20, 943-950.

Gemmell, M.A. (1977) Taeniidae: Modification to the life span of the egg and the regulation of tapeworm infections. *Experimental Parasitology* 41, 314-328.

Gemmell, M.A. (1990) Australian contributions to understanding of the epidemiology and control of hydatid disease caused by *Echinococcus granulosus* - past, present and future. *International Journal of Parasitology* 20, 431-456.

Gemmell, M.A., Lawson, J.R. and Roberts, M.G. (1987) Population dynamics in echinococcosis and cysticercosis: evaluation of the biological parameters of *Taenia hydatigena* and *T. ovis* and comparison with those of *Echinococcus granulosus* in dogs and sheep. *Parasitology* 94, 161-180.

Grainger, H.J. and Jenkins, D.J. (1996) Transmission of hydatid disease from wild dogs to sheep in Victoria, Australia. *International Journal of Parasitology* 26, 1268-1270.

Gusbi, A.M., Awan, M.A.Q. and Beesley, W.N. (1990) Echinococcosis in Libya. IV. Prevalence of hydatidosis (*Echinococcus granulosus*) in goats, cattle and camels. *Annals of Tropical Medicine and Parasitology* 84, 477-482.

Hackett, F. and Walters, T.M.H. (1980) The prevalence of cestodes in farm dogs in mid-Wales. *Veterinary Parasitology* 7, 95-101.

Heath, D.D. and Lawrence, S.B. (1991) Daily egg-production of dogs infected with *Echinococcus granulosus*. *Archives de la Hidatidosis* 30, 321-328.

Hegazi, M.M., Abdel-Magied, S.A., Abdel-Wahab, F.M. and Atia, R.A. (1986) Epidemiological study of echinococcosis in Dakahlia Governorate, Egypt. *Journal of the Egyptian Society of Parasitology* 16, 541-548.

Hoffer, S., Gloor, S., Muller, U., Mathis, A., Hegglin, D. and Deplazes, P. (2000) High prevalence of *Echinococcus multilocularis* in urban red foxes (*Vulpes vulpes*) and voles (*Arivicola terrestris*) in the city of Zurich, Switzerland. *Parasitology* 120, 135-142.

Howard, E.B. and Gendron, A.P. (1980) *Echinococcus vogeli* infection in higher primates at the Los Angeles Zoo. In: Montali, R.J. and Migaki, G. (eds) *The Comparative Pathology of Zoo Animals.* Smithsonian Institution Press, Washington DC, pp. 379-382.

Hubbert, W.T., McCulloch, W.F. and Schnurrenberger, P.R. (1975) *Diseases Transmitted From Animals to Man*, 6th edn. Charles C. Thomas, Springfield, Illinois, USA.

Ibrahem, M.M. and Gusbi, A.M. (1997) Cystic echinococcosis in North Africa (excluding Morocco): Veterinary aspects. In: Andersen, F.L., Ouhelli, H. and Kachani, M. (eds) *Compendium on Cystic Echinococcosis in Africa and in Middle Eastern Countries With Special Reference to Morocco.* Brighman Young University, Provo, Utah, USA, pp. 207-222.

Iida, H. (1969) Epidemiology of *Multilocular echinococcosis* in Hokkaido, Japan. *Hokkaido Institute of Public Health,* Sapporo, Hokkaido, pp. 7-15.

Irshadullah, M., Nizami, W.A. and Macpherson, C.N.L. (1989) Observations on the suitability and importance of the domestic intermediate hosts of *Echinococcus granulosus* in Uttah Pradesh, India. *Journal of Helminthology* 63, 39-45.

Ishige, M., Yagi, K. and Itoh, T. (1990) Egg production and life span of *Echinococcus multilocularis* in dogs, Hokkaido, Japan. International Workshop on Alveolar Hydatid Disease, 7-8 June 1990, Anchorage, Alaska. *Abstracts*, pp. 14-15.

Jenkins, D.J. and Andrew, P.L. (1993) Intestinal parasites in dogs from an Aboriginal community in New South Wales. *Australian Veterinary Journal* 70, 115-116.

Jenkins, D.J. and Morris, B. (1991) Unusually heavy infections of *Echinococcus granulosus* in wild dogs in south-eastern Australia. *Australian Veterinary Journal* 68, 36-37.

Jenkins, D.J., Meek, P., Ardler, A. Hawksby, R. (1996) Aboriginal community dogs: worms, control and human health. In: *Dog Health in Indigenous Communities. Proceedings of a Conference Held as Part of the Western Pacific Veterinary Conference, Darwin, 1993,* edited and published by Shield I, Queensland Department of Primary Industries.

Jenkins, D.J., Fraser, A., Bradshaw, H. and Craig, P.S. (2000) Detection of *Echinococcus granulosus* coproantigens in Australian canids with natural or experimental infection. *Journal of Parasitology* 86, 140-145.

Kamhawi, S. and Abdel-Hafez, S.K. (1995) Cystic echinococcosis as a major public health problem in Jordan. XVII International Congress of Hydatidology, Limassol, Cyprus. *Abstract* A17.

Kilani, A., Dargouth, M.A., Lahmar, S., Jaoua, H. and Jemli, M.H. (1986) Dogs' role in the epidemiology of the hydatid cyst in Tunisia. *La Tunisie Medical* 64, 333-337.

Kreidl, P., Allerberger, F., Judmaier, G., Auer, H., Aspock, H. and Hall, A.J. (1998) Domestic pets as risk factors for alveolar hydatid disease in Austria. *American Journal of Epidemiology* 147, 978-981.

Liu, F.J. (1993) Prevalence of *Echinococcus granulosus* in dogs in the Xinjiang Uygur Autonomous Region, PRC. In: Andersen, F.L., Chai, J.J. and Liu, F.J. (eds) *Compendium on Cystic Echinococcosis.* Brigham Young University, Utah, pp. 168-176.

Lloyd, S. (1998) Other cestode infections hymenolepiosis, diphyllobothriosis, coenurosis, and other adult and larval cestodes. In: Palmer, S.R., Lord Soulsby, and Simpson, D.I.H. (eds) *Zoonoses.* Oxford University Press, pp. 651-663.

Macchioni, P.G.M., Lanfranchi, M.A., Abdallatif, and Testi, F. (1985) Echinococcosis and hydatidosis in Somalia. *Bulletin of Science Faculty of Zoology and Veterinary Medicine* 5, 179-189.

Macpherson, C.N.L. (1981) Epidemiology and strain differentiation of *Echinococcus granulosus* in Kenya. PhD thesis, University of London.

Macpherson, C.N.L. (1983) An active intermediate host role for man in the life cycle of *Echinococcus granulosus* in Turkana, Kenya. *American Journal of Tropical Medicine and Hygiene* 32, 397-404.

Macpherson, C.N.L. (1994) Epidemiology and control of parasites in nomadic situations. *Veterinary Parasitology* 37, 87-102.

Macpherson, C.N.L. (1995) The effect of transhumance on the epidemiology of animal diseases. *Preventive Veterinary Medicine* 25, 213-224.

Macpherson, C.N.L. and Craig, P.S. (1991) Echinococcosis - a plague on pastoralists. In: Macpherson, C.N.L. and Craig, P.S. (eds) *Parasitic Helminths and Zoonoses in Africa*. Unwin Hyman, London, pp. 25-53.

Macpherson, C.N.L. and Wachira, T.W.M. (1997) Cystic echinococcosis in Africa south of the Sahara. In: Andersen, F.L., Ouhelli, H. and Kachani, M. (eds) *Compendium on Cystic Echinococcosis in Africa and in Middle Eastern Countries With Special Reference to Morocco*. Brigham Young University, Provo, Utah, pp. 245-277.

Macpherson, C.N.L., Karstad, L., Stevenson, P. and Arundel, J.H. (1983) Hydatid disease in the Turkana District of Kenya iii. The significance of wild animals in the transmission of *Echinococcus granulosus,* with particular reference to Turkana and Masailand. *Annals of Tropical Medicine and Parasitology* 77, 61-73.

Macpherson, C.N.L., French, C.M., Stevenson, P., Karstad, L. and Arundel, J.H. (1985) Hydatid disease in the Turkana District of Kenya iv. The prevalence of *Echinococcus granulosus* infections in dogs and observations on the role of the dog in the lifestyle of the Turkana. *Annals of Tropical Medicine and Parasitology* 79, 51-61.

Macpherson, C.N.L., Romig, T., Zeyhle, E., Rees, P.H. and Were, J.B.O. (1987) Portable ultrasound scanner verses serology in screening for hydatid cysts in a nomadic population. *Lancet* i, 259-261.

Macpherson, C.N.L., Craig, P.S., Romig, T., Zeyhle, E. and Watschinger, H. (1989a) Observations on human echinococcosis/hydatidosis and evaluation of transmission factors in the Maasai of northern Tanzania. *Annals of Tropical Medicine and Parasitology* 83, 489-497.

Macpherson, C.N.L., Spoerry, A., Zeyhle, E., Romig, T. and Gorfe, M. (1989b) Pastoralists and hydatid disease: an ultrasound scanning prevalence survey in East Africa. *Transactions of the Royal Society of Tropical Medicine and Hygiene* 84, 243-247.

Macpherson, C.N.L., Gottstein, B. and Geerts, S. (2000) Parasitic food-borne and water-borne zoonoses. In: Pastoret, P.-P. (Coordinator), *An Update on Zoonoses. Revue Scientifique et Technique Office International des Epizooties* 19, 240-258.

Meneghelli, U.G., Barbo, M.L.P., Magro, J.E., Bullucci, A.D. and Llorach Velludo, M.A.S. (1986) Polycystic hydatid disease (*Echinococcus vogeli*) clinical and radiological manifestations and treatment with albendazole of a patient from the Brazilian Amazon region. *Arquivos de Gastroenterologia, Sao Paulo* 23, 177-183.

Meneghelli, U.G., Martinelli, A.L.C. and Llorach Velludo, M.A.S. (1990) Cistos de Echinococcus vogeli em figado de paca (*Cuniculus paca*) originaria do Estado do Acre, Brasil. *Revista da Sociedade Brasileira de Medicina Tropica* 23, 153-155.

Meneghelli, U.G., Martinelli, A.L., Bellucci, A.D., Villanova, M.G., Belludo, M.A. and Magro, J.E. (1992a) Polycystic hydatid disease (*Echinococcus vogeli*). Treatment with albendazole. *Annals of Tropical Medicine and Parasitology* 86, 151-156.

Meneghelli, U.G., Martinelli, A.L., Llorach Velludo, M.A., Belluci, A.D., Margro, J.E. and Barbo, M.L. (1992b) Polycystic hydatid disease (*Echinococcus vogeli*). Clinical, laboratory and morphological findings in nine Brazillian patients. *Journal of Hepatology* 14, 203-210.

Ming, R., Tolley, H.D., Andersen, F.L., Chai, J. and Chang, Q. (1992) Frequency distribution of *Echinococcus granulosus* in dog populations in the Xinjiang Uygur Autonomous Region, China. *Veterinary Parasitology* 43, 233-241.

Miyazaki, I. (1991) *Helminthic Zoonoses*. International Medical Foundation of Japan, Tokyo.

Moch, R.W., Fairchild, D.G., Botros, B.A.M. and Barsoum, I.S. (1974) Echinococcosis in Egypt. Prevalence of canine infection in Cairo area. *Journal of Tropical Medicine and Hygiene* 77, 163.

Molan, A.L. and Baban, M.R. (1992) The prevalence of *Echinococcus granulosus* in stray dogs in Iraq. *Journal of Tropical Medicine and Hygiene* 95, 146-148.

Moore, D.V. (1962) A review of human infections with the common dog tapeworm, *Dipylidium caninum*, in the United States. *Southwestern Veterinarian* 15, 283-288.

Moro, P.L., McDonald, J., Gilman, R.H., Silva, B., Verastegui, M., Malqui, V., Lescano, Falcon, N., Montes, G. and Bazalar, H. (1997) Epidemiology of *Echinococcus granulosus* infection in the central Peruvian Andes. *Bulletin of the World Health Organisation* 75, 553-561.

Moro, P.L., Bonifacio, N., Gilman, R.H., Lopera, L., Silva, B., Takvmoto, R., Verastegui, M. and Cabera, L. (1999) Field diagnosis of *Echinococcus granulosus* infection among intermediate and definitive hosts in an endemic focus of human cystic echinococcosis. *Transactions of the Royal Society of Tropical Medicine and Hygiene* 93, 611-615.

Muller-Graf, C.D.M., Woolhouse, M.E.J. and Packer, C. (1999) Epidemiology of the intestinal parasite *Spirometra* spp. in two populations of African lions. *Parasitology* 118, 407-415.

Mueller, J.F. (1974) The biology of *Spirometra*. *Journal of Parasitology* 60, 3-14.

National Laboratory for Epidemiology and Zoonoses (1993) Enquete rage/hydatidose (rapport partiel). Rapport du Laboratoire National d'Epidemiologique et des Zoonoses. Direction de l'Elevage. Ministere de l'Agriculture et de la Reforme Agraire.

Ngunzi, M.M. (1986) The effect of prolonged drought on infection of domestic dogs with *Echinococcus granulosus* in Maasailand, Kenya. In: Tukei, P.N., Koech, D.K. and Kimoti, S.N. (eds) *Recent Advances in the Management and*

Control of Infectious Diseases in Eastern Africa. English Press, Nairobi, pp. 231-239.

Nunez, G., Calvopina, M., Torres, A., Sarsoxa, M., Guderian, R. and Carrasco, E. (1993) IV. Hidatidosis poliquistica humana en paciente embarazada. Reporte del duodecima caso en Ecuador. *Revista de Medicina de la Hospital Vozandes* 6, 55-61.

Ouhelli, H., Kadiri, A., El Hasnaoui, M. and Kachani, M. (1997) Prevalence of *Echinococcus granulosus* in dogs in Morocco and potential role of dogs in transmission of cystic echinococcosis. In: Andersen, F.L., Ouhelli, H. and Kachani, M. (eds) *Compendium on Cystic Echinococcosis in Africa and in Middle Eastern Countries With Special Reference to Morocco*. Brighman Young University, Provo, Utah, pp. 145-155.

Palmer, S.R., Biffin, A.H., Craig, P.S. and Walters, T.M.H. (1996) The control of hydatid disease in Wales. *British Medical Journal* 312, 674-675.

Perdomo, R., Alvarez, C., Monti, J., Ferreira, C., Chiesa, A., Carbo, A., Alvez, R., Grauert, D., Stern, D., Carmona, C. and Yarzabal, L. (1997) Principles of the surgical approach in human liver cystic echinococcosis. *Acta Tropica* 64, 109-122.

Provost, A. (1971) Region de recherches veterinaires et zootechniques d'Afrique Centrale. Rapport annuel 1970. Laboratoire de Farcha. II. Institut d' Elevage Medecine Veterinaire Pays Tropicaux, 10 rue Pierre Curie, 94-Maisons-Alfort, France, 430.

Rahkonen, R. and Valtonen, E.T. (1997) Infection of brown trout with *Diphyllobothrium dendriticum* procercoids. *International Journal of Parasitology* 27, 1315-1318.

Ramirez, R. (1979) Epidemiology of human hydatid disease in Chile (1969-78). *Boletin Chileno de Parasitolgia* 34, 59-62.

Rausch, R.L. (1967) On the ecology and distribution of *Echinococcus* spp. (Cestoda: Taeniidae) and characteristics of their development in the intermediate host. *Annales de Parasitologie Humaine et Comparée* 42, 16-93.

Rausch, R.L. (1995) Life cycle patterns and geographic distribution of *Echinococcus* species: In: Thompson, R.C.A. and Lymbery, A.J. (eds) Echinococcus *and Hydatid Disease*. CAB International, Wallingford, UK, pp. 89-134.

Rausch, R.L. and Bernstein, J.J. (1972) *Echinococcus vogeli* sp. n. (Cestoda: Taeniidae) from the bush dog, *Speothos venaticus* (Lund). *Zeitschrift fur Tropenmedizin und Parasitologie* 23, 25-34.

Rausch, R.L., D'Alessandro, A. and Rausch, V.R. (1981) Characteristics of the larval *Echinococcus vogeli* Rausch and Bernstein, 1972 in the natural intermediate host, the paca, *Cuniculus paca* L. (Rodentia: Dasyproctidae). *American Journal of Tropical Medicine and Hygiene* 30, 1043-1052.

Rausch, R.L., D'Alessandro, A. and Ohbayashi, M. (1984) The taxonomic status of *Echinococcus cruzi* Brumpt and Joyeux, 1924 (Cestoda: Taeniidae) from an agouti (Rodentia: Dasyproctidae) in Brazil. *Journal of Parasitology* 70, 295-302.

Rausch, R.L., Fay, F.H. and Williamson, F.S. (1990) The ecology of *Echinococcus multilocularis* (Cestoda: Taeniidae) on St. Lawrence island, Alaska. II. Helminth populations in the definitive host. *Annals de Parasitologie Humaine et Comparee* 65, 131-140.

Romig, T., Bilger, B., Dinkel, A., Merli, M. and Mackenstedt, U. (1999) *Echinococcus multilocularis* in animal hosts: new data from western Europe. *Helminthologia* 36, 185-191.

Ruttenber, A.J., Weniger, F., Sorvillo, R., Murray, R.A. and Ford, S.L. (1984) Diphyllobothriasis associated with salmon consumption in Pacific coast states. *American Journal of Tropical Medicine and Hygiene* 33, 455-459.

Saad, M.B. and Magzoub, M. (1986) *Echinococcus granulosus* infections in dogs in Tambool, Sudan. *Journal of Helminthology* 60, 299-300.

Schantz, P.M. (1977) Echinococcosis in American Indians living in Arizona and New Mexico. A review of recent studies. *American Journal of Epidemiology* 106, 370-379.

Schantz, P.M., Junje, C., Craig, P.S., Eckert, J., Jenkins, D.J., Macpherson, C.N.L. and Thakur, A. (1995) Epidemiology and control of hydatid disease. In: Thompson, R.C.A. and Lymbery, A.J. (eds) Echinococcus *and Hydatid Disease.* CAB International, Wallingford, UK, pp. 233-331.

Schelling, U., Frank, W., Will, R., Romig, T. and Lucius, R. (1997) Chemotherapy with praziquantel has the potential to reduce the prevalence of *Echinococcus multilocularis* in wild foxes (*Vulpes vulpes*). *Annals of Tropical Medicine and Parasitology* 91, 179-186.

Schiller, E. (1955) Studies on the helminth fauna of Alaska XXVI. Some observations on the cold-resistance of eggs of *Echinococcus sibiricensis* Rausch and Schiller, 1954. *Journal of Parasitology* 41, 578-582.

Schwabe, C.W. (1984) *Veterinary Medicine and Human Health*, 2nd edn. Williams and Wilkins, Baltimore\London.

Schwabe, C.W. (1991) Helminth zoonoses in African perspective. In: Macpherson, C.N.L. and Craig, P.S. (eds) *Parasitic Helminths and Zoonoses in Africa.* Unwin Hyman, London, pp.1-24.

Senevet, G. (1951) Epidemiologie du kyste hydatique en Afrique du Nord. *Archivos Internationales Hydatidologie* 12, 113-120.

Shaikenov, B.S., Vaganov, T.F. and Torgerson, P.R. (1999) Cystic echinococcosis in Kazakhstan: An emerging disease since independence from the Soviet Union. *Parasitology Today* 15, 172-174.

Shambesh, M.K., Craig, P.S., Macpherson, C.N.L., Rogan, M., Gusby, A.M. and Echtuich, E.F. (1999) An extensive ultrasound and serologic study to investigate the prevalence of cystic echinococcosis in northern Libya. *American Journal of Tropical Medicine and Hygiene* 60, 462-468.

Shambesh, M.K., Macpherson, C.N.L., Beesley, W.N., Gusby, A. and Elsonosi, T. (1992) Prevalence of human hydatid disease in northwestern Libya: a crossectional ultrasound study. *Annals of Tropical Medicine and Parasitology* 86, 381-386.

Simoons, F. (1961) Eat not this flesh: food avoidance in the old world. University of Wisconsin Press, Madison.

Smyth, J.D. (1994) *Introduction to Animal Parasitology*, 3rd edn. Cambridge University Press.

Smyth, J.D. and Heath, D.D. (1970) Pathology of larval cestodes in mammals. *Helminthological Abstracts* 39, 1-23.

Stehr-Green, J.A., Stehr-Green, P.A., Schantz, P.M., Wilson, J.F. and Lanier, A. (1988) Risk factors for infection with *Echinococcus multilocularis* in Alaska. *American Journal of Tropical Medicine and Hygiene* 38, 380-385.

Sweatman, G.K. and Williams, R.J. (1962) Wild animals in New Zealand as hosts of *Echinococcus granulosus* and other taeniid tapeworms. *Transactions of the Royal Society of New Zealand* 2, 221-250.

Thompson, R.C.A. (1995) Biology and systematics of *Echinococcus*. In: Thompson, R.C.A. and Lymbery, A.J. (eds) Echinococcus *and Hydatid Disease*. CAB International, Wallingford, UK, pp. 1-50.

Thompson, R.C.A. and Eckert, J. (1983) Observations on *Echinococcus multilocularis* in the definitive host. *Zeitschrift fur Parasitenkunde* 69, 335-345.

Thompson, R.C.A., Lymbery, A.J., Hobbs, R.P. and Elliot, A.D. (1988) Hydatid disease in urban areas of Western Australia: an unusual cycle involving western grey kangaroos (*Macropus fuliginosus*), feral pigs and domestic dogs. *Australian Veterinary Journal* 65,188-190.

Thompson, R.C.A., Robertson, I.D., Gasser, R.B. and Constantine, C.C. (1993) Hydatid disease in Western Australia: a novel approach to education and surveillance. *Parasitology Today* 9, 431-433.

Thompson, R.C.A., Lymbery, A.J. and Constantine, C.C. (1995) Variation in *Echinococcus*: towards a taxonomic revision of the genus. *Advances in Parasitology* 35, 145-176.

Torgerson, P.R., Gulland, F.M.D. and Gemmell, M.A. (1992) Observations on the epidemiology of *Taenia hydatigena* on St Kilda. *Veterinary Record* 131, 218-219.

Torgerson, P.R., Pilkington, J., Gulland, F.M.D. and Gemmell, M.A. (1995) Further evidence for long distance dispersal of taeniid eggs. *International Journal for Parasitology* 25, 265-267.

Troncy, P. and Graber, M. (1969) L'echinococcose-hydatidose en Afrique Centrale. III. Taeniasis des carnivores a *Echinococcus granulosus* (Batsch, 1786-Rudolphi, 1801). *Revue d'Elevage Medecine Veterinaire Pays Tropicaux* 22, 75-84.

Verster, A. (1979) Gastro-intestinal helminths of domestic dogs in the Republic of South Africa. *Onderstepoort Journal of Veterinary Research* 46, 79-82.

von Bonsdorff, B. (1977) *Diphyllobothriasis in man*. Academic Press, London.

Wachira, T.M., Macpherson, C.N.L. and Gathuma, J.M. (1990) Hydatid disease in the Turkana District of Kenya V11: analysis of the infection pressure between definitive and intermediate hosts of *Echinococcus granulosus*, 1979-1988. *Annals of Tropical Medicine and Parasitology* 84, 361-368.

Wachira, T.M., Macpherson, C.N.L. and Gathuma, J.M. (1991) Release and survival of *Echinococcus* eggs in different environments in Turkana and their possible impact on the incidence of hydatidosis in man and livestock. *Journal of Helminthology* 65, 55-61.

Wachira, T.M., Sattran, M., Zeyhle, E. and Njenga, M.K. (1993) Intestinal helminths of public health importance in dogs in Nairobi. *East African Medical Journal* 70, 617-619.

Wang, Y.H., Rogan, M.T., Vuitton, D.A., Wen, H., Bartholomot, B., Macpherson, C.N.L., Zou, P.F., Ding, Z.X., Zhou, H.X., Zhang, X.F., Luo, J., Xiong, H.B., Fu, Y., McVie, A., Giraudoux, P., Yang, W.G. and Craig, P.S. (2000) Cystic echinococcosis in semi-nomadic pastoral communities in northwest China. *Transactions of the Royal Society of Tropical Medicine and Hygiene.* In press.

Wardle, R.A. and Green, N.K. (1941) The rate of growth of the tapeworm *Diphyllobothriasis latum. Canadian Journal of Research* 19, 245-257.

Watson-Jones, D.L. and Macpherson, C.N.L. (1988) Hydatid disease in the Turkana district of Kenya VI. Man:dog contact and its role in the transmission and control of hydatidosis amongst the Turkana. *Annals of Tropical Medicine and Parasitology* 82, 343-356.

Wen, H. and Yang, W.G. (1997) Public health importance of cystic echinococcosis in China. *Acta Tropica* 67, 133-145.

Williams, J.F., Lopez Adaros, H. and Trejos, A. (1971) Current prevalence and distribution of hydatidosis with specific reference to the Americas. *American Journal of Tropical Medicine and Hygiene* 20, 224-236.

Willis, J.M. and Herbert, I.V. (1987) A method for estimating the age of coenuri of *Taenia multiceps* recovered from the brains of sheep. *Veterinary Record* 121, 216-218.

Witenburg, G.G. (1964) Cestodiases. In: van der Haeden, J. (ed.) *Zooparasitic Diseases.* Elsevier, Amsterdam, pp. 648-707.

Yamashita, J. (1973) *Echinococcus* and echinococcosis. *Progress of Medical Parasitology in Japan 5*, 65-123. Meguro Parasitological Museum, Tokyo.

Yan, Q. (1983) An investigation of *Echinococcus granulosus* infection in sheep and cattle in Huangnan Prefecture of Qinghai Province. *Qinghai Journal of Zootechnics and Veterinary Science* 4, pp. 34.

Yang, F. (1992) Investigations on hydatid infection in animals and its hazard in Qinghai Province. *Bulletin of Hydatid Disease Control and Research*, No. 3. National Hydatid Disease Center of China, Urumqi.

Yarrow, A., Slater, P.E., Gross, E.M. and Costin, C. (1991) The epidemiology of echinococcosis in Israel. *Journal of Tropical Medicine and Hygiene* 94, 261-267.

Zhang, J. (1983) A preliminary survey of *Echinococcus* infection in man and animals in Ningxia Hui Autonomous Region. *Abstracts of Papers Presented at Scientific Conference on Parasitic Diseases*, 234 pp.

Chapter Eight

Dogs and Nematode Zoonoses

Paul A.M. Overgaauw and Frans van Knapen

Dogs and humans have lived together in close association for more than ten thousand years (see Chapter 1). Worms in dogs have always been apparent and are often assumed to be similar to worms in man or at least capable of producing infection in man. Medical and veterinary professionals still have difficulty recognizing specifically human or dog parasites from zoonoses, which involve both hosts in their life cycles. Parasitic infections of man caused by dog nematodes are widely publicised. The presence of similar parasites in both man and dogs does not necessarily mean a zoonotic infection. The definition of a zoonosis is that a natural transmission from dogs to man should occur (direct or indirect, via the environment or vectors). In some dog-human zoonoses, dogs play a major role in the infection (e.g. *Toxocara*, *Gnathostoma*) but in others the parasites would persist in humans whether dogs were present or not (e.g. *Brugia*, *Dioctophyma*).

The ubiquitous problem of stray dogs in urban areas (see Chapter 2) emphasizes the need to diagnose, treat and prevent zoonoses including parasitic nematodes. Regional differences in the epidemiology of zoonoses, such as rabies and hydatidoses, may overshadow the relative importance of dog nematode zoonoses. In many developed countries, considered as free from serious infectious diseases in man, dogs still harbor prevalent nematode infections, causing mostly chronic sub-clinical infections. This chapter reviews all presently known dog: human nematode zoonoses.

Toxocarosis

Toxocara canis, a roundworm of the dog, is probably the most common gastro-intestinal helminth of domestic canids world-wide. Infection is reported in domestic and wild Canidae. Adult *T. canis* generally inhibit the small intestine. Adults do not attach to the mucosa and live on intestinal contents. The reported infection rates in domestic dog populations vary from 3.5% (adults) to 79% (pups) and in foxes up to 80%. Widespread environmental contamination with *Toxocara* eggs facilitates human infection. *Toxocara* infection is the (covert) infection following ingestion of *Toxocara* eggs, or ingestion of larvae that can lead to (overt) clinical disease, toxocarosis.

Mode of transmission

The life cycle of *T. canis* is complex (Parsons, 1987; Overgaauw, 1997a). Adult worms in the intestinal tract of infected dogs shed large numbers of eggs via the feces into the environment where they are ingested by natural hosts and paratenic hosts. *Toxocara* eggs are unembryonated and not infectious when passed into the environment. Within a period of between 3-6 weeks to several months, depending on soil type and climatic conditions, such as temperature and humidity, eggs will develop to an infectious stage that can survive under optimal circumstances for at least 1 year.

Several studies from all over the world demonstrated high rates (10-30%) of soil contamination with *Toxocara* eggs in parks, playgrounds, sandpits and other public places. In the intestine the larvae hatch and migrate via blood vessels all over the body. This is called visceral larva migrans (VLM). In young animals a tracheal migration occurs via the lungs and trachea and, after swallowing, the larvae mature in the intestinal tract. In paratenic hosts and most adult dogs that have some degree of acquired immunity, the larvae undergo somatic migration to remain as somatic larvae in the tissues. After predation of *Toxocara*-infected paratenic hosts by dogs, larvae will be released and develop in most cases directly to adult worms in the intestinal tract.

In the pregnant bitch, "dormant" tissue larvae are reactivated and migrate across the placenta to infect the fetuses. Newborn puppies also acquire infection through ingestion of larvae via the milk.

Toxocarosis is a public health problem (Schantz, 1989; Overgaauw, 1997b; Lloyd, 1998a). Man acts as an unnatural host in which *Toxocara* larvae will not develop but migrate and survive for a long time.

The mode of transmission to humans is by oral ingestion of infective *Toxocara* eggs from contaminated soil (sapro-zoonosis), from unwashed hands or consumption of raw vegetables. Some infections may occur from ingestion of larvae in under-cooked organ and muscle tissue of infected paratenic hosts such as chickens, cattle and sheep (Glickman and Schantz, 1981; Stürchler *et al.*, 1990). Vertical transplacental transmission in pregnant women as a result of activated somatic larvae, similar to the situation in the dog, does not occur (Taylor, 1993).

Direct contact with infected dogs is not considered as a potential risk because embryonation of *Toxocara* ova to the stage of infectivity requires a minimum of 3 weeks. *T. canis* infections are therefore more likely to be a hazard for people exposed to contaminated environments.

Disease in animals

Clinical symptoms

The clinical symptoms depend on the age of the animal and on the number, location and stage of development of the worms (Parsons, 1987). After birth, puppies can suffer from pneumonia associated with the tracheal migration and die within 2 to 3 days. At an age of 2 to 3 weeks, puppies can show emaciation and digestive disturbances, caused by mature worms in the stomach and intestine. Diarrhea, constipation, vomiting, coughing and nasal discharge can be found at clinical examination. Distension of the abdomen ("potbelly") can occur, probably as the result of gas formation caused by dysbacteriosis. Although rare, mortality is possible due to obstruction of the gall bladder, bile duct, pancreatic duct and rupture of the intestine.

The prevalence of patent *T. canis* infections in adult dogs is low and clinical symptoms are rare. During somatic larval migration, dogs seldom manifest signs of clinical disease. Larval migration to the eyes (Ocular Larval Migrans) by *T. canis* larvae is described.

Diagnosis

Patent *Toxocara* infection in dogs and cats can be tentatively diagnosed from the medical history, particularly the lack of an appropriate anthelmintic schedule, and the clinical symptoms. Confirmation of the diagnosis can be obtained by finding dark brown colored eggs with thick-pitted shells in fecal samples after flotation (Lindsay and Blagburn, 1995).

The ELISA test, using TES antigens, is described as a sensitive technique for determining whether or not a bitch is carrying somatic larvae (Scheuer, 1987).

Methods of control

There are two reasons for *Toxocara* control; to prevent human infection and to reduce the risk of infection to pets. *Toxocara* eggs are very resistant to adverse environmental conditions and may remain infective for years. Since no practical methods exist for reducing environmental egg burdens, prevention of initial contamination of the environment is the most important tool. This can be achieved by taking measures such as eliminating patent infections in dogs and cats, preventing defecation by pets in public areas, hygiene, and education of the public.

A decrease in contamination can be achieved by methods including: restriction of uncontrolled dogs and cats, cleaning up feces from soil and on pavements by dog owners, preventing access of dogs and cats to public places (especially children's playgrounds) and by strategic anthelmintic treatment of dogs and cats with emphasis on puppies and nursing bitches (Schantz, 1981). *Toxocara* eggs are not destroyed by composting and can survive sewage treatment. Infective eggs can therefore be present in potty soil. A complicating factor in the prevention of environmental contamination is the presence of infected wild and stray canines.

The most serious and concentrated source of infection is the bitch nursing a litter and puppies aged between 3 weeks and 6 months (Jacobs *et al.*, 1977). A major aim of long-term prophylactic anthelmintic programs is to suppress *T. canis* egg-output throughout the whole of puppyhood using a multidose schedule. Anthelmintic treatment should be started before the age of 3 weeks. Because milk transmission occurs continuously for at least 5 weeks post partum, repeated treatments are necessary. Larvae that reach the intestine need at least 2 weeks to mature and start passing eggs, therefore the treatment should be repeated every 14 days. Re-infection can occur throughout the suckling period and treatment should at least be continued until the time when the last larvae arrive through the milk to the puppies' intestine at 7 weeks of age. Bitches should always be included in the treatment at the same time as the puppies (Jacobs, 1987).

Control in older dogs can be achieved by periodic treatments with anthelmintics whose efficacy can be limited to the intestinal stages, or by treatments prescribed based on the results of periodic diagnostic fecal examinations.

Elimination of the larvae from the tissues and therefore prevention of vertical intra-uterine and transmammary transmission would have a significant effect on the parasite population (Kassai, 1995). Deworming of bitches during pregnancy is sometimes advised in anthelmintic schedules, but this advice is questionable. Efficacy of nearly all licensed anthelmintics with various dosages and treatment periods, against somatic larvae in experimental animals and bitches, has been intensively investigated (Bosse and Stoye, 1981; Burke and Roberson, 1983; Lloyd and Soulsby, 1983; Schnieder *et al.*, 1996; Fok and Kassai, 1998). In general it can be concluded that anthelmintics at the recommended doses are not effective against inhibited somatic larvae (Epe *et al.*, 1996) and treatment of bitches before mating and 2 weeks before the anticipated whelping date has no useful effect on prenatal transmission (Fisher *et al.*, 1994). Prenatal infection can be substantially reduced by daily treatments with fenbendazole (25mg per kg) given to the bitch from the 40th day of pregnancy to two days post-partum, but this treatment regime is too expensive for general use (Bartiga, 1988).

Hygiene can be achieved by removing feces and by thorough cleaning of kennels. Expelled worms have to be destroyed. Dog owners can help to avoid contamination of the environment with *Toxocara* eggs and the exposure of other persons to unnecessary risks of *Toxocara* infections. Proper information about this zoonosis and the social concept of responsible pet ownership is required. Pet owners should be advised about deworming schemes, effective anthelmintics and the need to prevent their animals from defecating on children's playgrounds.

Veterinarians should be the most appropriate source of information for their clients regarding the dangers and the control of toxocarosis (Harvey *et al.*, 1991; Overgaauw, 1996).

Toxocara worms should be removed by treatment with an effective and larvicidal anthelmintic with a low toxicity. For this purpose benzimidazoles and newer generation avermectins (e.g. selamectin) are recommended.

Disease in man

Children are reported to be more frequently infected than adults. VLM with severe clinical symptoms is mainly found in children 1-3 years of age. Risk factors include the behavior of young children who often play in potentially contaminated soil in yards and sandpits. Children may also put their fingers into their mouth and sometimes eat dirt. The tendency of some children to eat dirt (geophagic pica) is a major risk factor (Schantz, 1981). The compulsion to eat dirt as a behavior disorder may affect 2 to 10% of children between the ages of 1 to 6 years. Around 40% of patients with ocular involvement showed a history of pica. There is no need to deny the opportunity for young children to play with puppies if good hygiene is practiced.

In contrast with the existence of clinical toxocarosis mainly in young children, anti-*Toxocara* titers are more frequently found in older people (van Knapen *et al.*, 1983). This is due to *Toxocara* titers that last for many years and an increasing prevalence with age simply reflects continuous exposure over time.

Clinical symptoms

Asymptomatic toxocarosis

In most cases, positive toxocaral antibody titers and/or eosinophilia can occur in the absence of symptoms or signs following infection by small numbers of larvae in the recent or more distant past. After ingestion of infective *Toxocara* eggs by humans, *Toxocara* larvae hatch in the stomach and migrate into the mucosa of the upper small intestine. There they penetrate via blood and lymphatic vessels and can be transported in the blood throughout the body, resulting in somatic larvae in many types of tissues (Glickman and Shofer, 1987). The liver is an important site for controlling the migration of *Toxocara* larvae (liver entrapment). Dissemination occurs via the bloodborne route, through tissues and body cavities.

Most of the larvae of *T. canis* seem to be distributed to the brain. *T. canis* second- or third-stage larvae have a particular affinity for nervous tissue and may therefore be responsible for neurological disease in man. Larvae do not migrate continuously, but tend to rest periodically before continuing their migration. During such periods of reduced movement, the larvae induce an immunologically mediated inflammatory response. Larvae in the brain are not encapsulated and do not induce immunological reaction by the host.

Visceral Larva Migrans

When a large number of *T. canis* larvae migrate to the tissues, a more marked, inflammatory, immune response ensues called Visceral Larva Migrans syndrome or VLM (Gillespie, 1993). This multisystem invasion can be associated with varied, non-specific clinical symptoms as a result of the host's immune response. VLM is mainly diagnosed in children between 1 to 7 years of age (mean age 2 years) and is characterized by persistent eosinophilia, leukocytosis, elevated glutamate transaminase level and hypergamma-globulinemia. Eosinophilia is seen more often in children than in adults and this may be one of the reasons why toxocarosis is often overlooked in adults (Ljungström and van Knapen, 1989). Clinical symptoms often include general malaise, fever, abdominal complaints (vague upper abdominal discomfort attributed to hepatomegaly), wheezing or coughing. Larvae that remain in the liver can be associated with an eosinophilic granulomatous hepatitis. *Toxocara* infection should be considered in the differential diagnosis of any child with a persistent and unexplained eosinophilia or recurrent abdominal pain. Toxocarosis can be considered as common, especially in children, and is associated with clinical features that are generally regarded as non-specific but together form a recognizable complex of symptoms. An allergy-like reaction, characterized by chronic "idiopathic" urticaria in adults and children, is found strongly associated with the presence of antibodies to *Toxocara* and may be caused by liberation of larval ES-antigens. If subsequent exposure to *Toxocara* eggs is avoided, the disease is usually self-limiting. Severe clinical symptoms are reported including life-threatening pneumonia after massive infection and eosinophilic meningo-encephalitis in children. Fatal cases as result of an exaggerated immunological response or extensive larval migration through the myocardium or central nervous system are rare.

Toxocara larvae have the ability to avoid the host's immune responses and can survive in tissues for at least 10 years. The immune evasion is caused by the extraordinarily rapid turnover and shedding of the whole length of the outer surfaces of the larvae ("dynamic larval surface"). The inflammatory response is formed round shed surface components shed during larval migration. As a result, the granulomas that form do not frequently contain histologically identifiable larval fragments ("verminous tracks").

Ocular Larva Migrans

Migrating *Toxocara* larva(e) can induce granulomatous retinal lesions, which are characterized by complaints of loss of visual acuity, squint and "seeing lights". This is called Ocular Larva Migrans syndrome (OLM) (Girdwood, 1986). In a minority of cases, total blindness of one or both eyes can result. A commonly found clinical syndrome in OLM is a posterior pole granuloma mimicking a retinoblastoma. If not recognized, this can finally lead to enucleatio bulbi.

The mean age of patients with OLM is 8 years, but it is diagnosed in adults as well (Ljungström and van Knapen, 1989). The relative number of eye disorders may increase with age as well as the percentage of seropositive cases in a normal (subclinical) population without particular association. Low numbers of larvae could escape the host immunity if provoked and finally reach the eye. Even low ELISA antibody titers may be indicative for OLM. The reported higher mean age of patients with OLM can be explained by a longer incubation period, because larvae can persist in the body for more than 10 years and periodically resume migration. Another explanation for the difference can be the difficulty of recognizing visual impairment in young children (Glickman and Schantz, 1981). OLM is usually caused by no more than a single larva. It is apparent that patients with VLM indeed have higher *Toxocara* titers than OLM patients. The highest titres were found in the few cases in which OLM was associated with VLM.

Covert toxocarosis

A milder form of toxocarosis called "covert toxocarosis" (CT), was described in patients with a variety of non-specific clinical symptoms that do not fall within the categories of VLM or OLM but which are nevertheless associated with a positive toxocaral antibody and/or eosinophilia (Taylor *et al.*, 1987). Symptoms such as hepatomegaly, cough, sleep disturbances, abdominal pain, headaches and behavioral changes have been associated with raised *Toxocara* antibodies. In older children beyond the toddler stage, the combination of abdominal pain, headache and cough was more significantly associated with a high *Toxocara* ELISA titer than were individual clinical features. The diagnosis "Idiopathic Abdominal Pain of Childhood" is usually made in children. The diagnosis of toxocarosis should be considered in children with cough and wheeze and having an additional history of headache and abdominal pain. It was postulated that patients with covert toxocarosis are less able to develop a protective immune response, permitting unlimited larval migration, so that even a small number of larvae induce severe immunopathology (Smith, 1993).

Concurrent diseases

Besides the complex of clinical symptoms discussed, there are other important arguments that support the requirement for an optimal prevention of *Toxocara* infection.

A relationship between *Toxocara* seroprevalence and the incidence of asthma, elevation of serum IgE concentration, the presence of allergen-specific IgE and eosinophilia was established. Occurrence of asthma or recurrent bronchitis and hospitalization due to asthma was significantly related to seroprevalence, while eczema tended to be more frequent. It was concluded that allergic phenomena in children who are predisposed to asthma, are more frequently manifested after *Toxocara* infection (Buijs *et al.*, 1997; Obwaller *et al.*, 1998).

Toxocara larvae that enter the central nervous system may cause neurological disorders such as subtle neurological deficits or behavioral disorders in children. In one study, infected children performed worse on neuropsychological tests of motor and cognitive function than did uninfected controls (Marmor *et al.*, 1987).

Diagnosis

Direct diagnosis of *Toxocara* infection is not easy, because patients do not excrete parasite material such as eggs or larvae, and migrating larvae are not easily found in biopsy material.

Accurate histopathological diagnosis of larval toxocarosis in biopsy material is possible and may show patterns of antigen deposition in acute infections and in granulomas, empty or centered around larvae. Identification of ascaridoid larvae in human tissue is possible with a recently developed PCR-method (Jacobs *et al.*, 1997).

Serodiagnostic techniques, such as the *Toxocara* ELISA, are reliable tools to detect antibodies and circulating antigens (Knapen and Buijs, 1993). The Western-blotting procedure (testing specific IgG) for the immunodiagnosis of human toxocarosis is used with high sensitivity and specificity, avoiding problems of cross-reactivity with sera infected with other helminth diseases (Magnaval *et al.*, 1991).

In experimentally infected animals antibody responses to TES antigens become detectable 4 days to 4 weeks after infection and can persist for months to years. As few as five infective eggs can produce symptoms and seroconversion in mice.

Finding a positive serum titer is not always proof of a causative relationship between *Toxocara* infection and the patient's current illness. In many cases it reflects the prevalence of asymptomatic toxocarosis. It should also be emphasized that serological prevalence is not synonymous with infection rate, because it depends on the sensitivity and specificity of the serological method used to quantify the antibody response.

The serological tests for OLM have a lower sensitivity, probably as result of low larval burden and/or the longer period between infection and testing. The mean period between onset of illness and serodiagnostic testing was less than 6 months for VLM and 2 years for OLM. In a small proportion of OLM patients, antibodies cannot be detected in serum. In rare cases, if larvae migrate through the ocular tissues, they can be visualized using ophthalmoscopy. Standardized echography has been used to identify *Toxocara* granulomas hidden by active inflammation in the eye. It was concluded that in combination with the history, clinical examination, and ELISA, standardized echography may be useful in establishing the diagnosis of ocular toxocarosis in cases of leukocoria in which nematode endophthalmitis is suspected (Wan *et al.*, 1991). Negative serological results and normal blood eosinophilia are due to a physiological barrier between blood and ocular fluids (immunological blood-eye barrier). A solution to provide a definitive diagnosis would be the demonstration of antibodies in the vitreous humor using the ELISA TES-test or the micro Ouchterlony test that requires only small amounts of ocular fluid (10-20 µl). Criteria for the diagnosis of OLM are formulated by Petithory *et al.* (1987) as positive immunological tests for nematode antigens and eosinophilia of vitreous or aqueous humors and the presence of ocular lesions.

Many people infected with *Toxocara* are undiagnosed because signs are absent or non-specific and serological tests are not requested for most patients. In different parts of the world seroprevalence studies for *Toxocara* have demonstrated a variation between 4.6 to 7.3% in children in the USA, 2.5% in Germany to 83% for children in the Caribbean. In tropical climates high ambient temperature and humidity probably favor transmission. Reviews of reported cases of toxocarosis (VLM and OLM) from all over the world revealed that more than half of the patients were less than 3 years old, one fifth were adults and 60% were males (Ehrhard and Kernbaumm, 1979). In a survey in Scotland, 16% of patients with unexplained eosinophilia and hepatomegaly, 15% of patients with ocular lesions and 14% in cases of hayfever, asthma or eczema tested positive for *Toxocara* (Girdwood *et al.*, 1978). In a recent study in Spain sera of a selected group of patients with clinical symptoms such as eosinophilia, splenomegaly and recurrent pain and asthma were assayed for *Toxocara* antibodies using the ELISA method. The results were that 23% of 30 adults, 33% of 332 children and 18% from 45 patients of unknown age tested positive (Fenoy *et al.*, 1997). In The Netherlands between 4% and 15% in people younger than 30 years and 30% in adults older than 45 years has been reported (Melker *et al.*, 1995). Titers fall gradually over a period of about 3 years, but should be considered as a balance between the fading memory of the immune system and its stimulation by continuing ingestion of viable ova or reactivation of dormant larvae.

Methods of control

Control is important from the point of view of welfare, for the quality of human life and also for the economic costs to society. These costs can be estimated depending on the incidence of clinical disease, estimated number of physician visits per patient, hospitalization rate and average length of stay in clinically significant disease, the costs of pharmaceuticals and income losses. Prevention of toxocarosis is possible by the institution of certain measures: appropriate health care for pets including regularly anthelmintic treatments, reducing the number of uncontrolled and stray pets, preventing contamination of the environment with feces and promoting responsible pet ownership (Stehr-Green and Schantz, 1987).

To increase awareness of pet owners about the potential zoonotic hazards, veterinary practitioners, general practitioners and public health agencies should provide sufficient information and advice in order that appropriate measures can be taken to minimize the risk of infection.

Treatment of patients

Patients with severe *Toxocara* infections, particularly if there is central nervous system involvement, can be treated with systemic acting and larvicidal anthelmintics. Effective results are reported with use of diethylcarbamazine, albendazole, oxfendazole, cambendazole, fenbendazole, mebendazole and levamisole. Most of these results are obtained from experiments on animals (mice) where administration of higher doses of anthelmintics started directly after inoculation with *Toxocara* larvae (mimicking acute infection) and continued for several days.

Clinicians should balance the risk of therapy with the severity of the disease, because treatment can lead to severe hypersensitivity reactions caused by dying larvae. Toxic reactions of the used anthelmintics can occur especially in OLM cases. The anthelmintic dose should be increased gradually over a period of days and covered by the concomitant administration of steroids. Good results and a low rate of adverse reactions in man is described for mebendazole at a daily dose of 20-25 mg per kg for 21 days (Magnaval, 1995).

Laser photocoagulation can be used if OLM lesions are located. Marked allergic reactions or an inflammatory reaction, for example in the eyes, can be suppressed with systemic or local corticosteroid therapy without the risk of enhancing the infection.

Ancylostomosis

Hookworms (Ancylostomatoidea) are, after the ascarids, the most commonly found nematodes in carnivores. They inhibit the small intestine and show a dorsal bend in the anterior body that enables "hooking" on to the intestinal mucosa, which explains their name. Dogs may harbor two genera of importance, *Ancylostoma* and *Uncinaria*. Their geographic distribution is the result of the capacity of the eggs to develop under high or low temperatures. The eggs of *Uncinaria stenocephala* can develop at temperatures below 15°C and the parasite is found in northern Europe and America, and in southern Australia. *Ancylostoma caninum, Ancylostoma braziliense* and *Ancylostoma ceylanicum* require temperatures higher than 20°C. *A. caninum* is found in most tropical and temperate zones of the northern and southern hemisphere. *A. braziliense* is more restricted geographically than the other hookworms of dogs and occurs in Africa, southern Asia, tropical Australia, South and Central America, and the Gulf states of the USA (Miller, 1971). *A. ceylanicum* is found in cats and wild felidae in Asia, including Indonesia and Japan, and parts of South America. The reported infection rates in domestic dog populations are low, but prevalence can be high in kennel dogs, hounds and foxes.

Only two zoonotic hookworms are known to use humans as definitive hosts, *A. ceylanicum* often successfully, and *A. caninum* only occasionally, and without developing to full maturity. *A. braziliense* is mainly responsible for the cutaneous larva migrans or "creeping eruption" in man, which is caused by percutaneous infection of L_3 larvae from the environment. It is questionable if *U. stenocephala* is zoonotic, because natural infections of humans have not been reported (Prociv, 1998).

Mode of transmission

Hookworm eggs are excreted in the feces of infected dogs. L_1 larvae develop that leave the egg. After two moults, hosts can ingest infectious L_3 larvae after licking or eating soil or grass or by skin penetration. Two subsequent molts occur before the worms mature in the intestine.

Penetration of the skin or buccal mucosa by the L_3 larvae is the principal route of infection for *A. caninum* with a pre-patent period of 2 to 3.5 weeks. *A. caninum* larvae enter dermal lymphatics or blood capillaries and use the systemic circulation for migration to the lungs. From here the larvae puncture alveoli to then reach the gut by tracheal migration or enter the systemic circulation to have a somatic migration to the intestinal wall and skeletal muscles. The arrested larvae in the tissues are a relatively inaccessible reservoir of infection. This reservoir "leaks" larvae directly or via the lungs to the intestinal lumen of the adult dog and infects the litter with the milk for up to 20 days after whelping. Continuous infection of young dogs result in gradually increased egg shedding up to 7 to 8 months of age, after which immunity develops. Adult worms live an average of 6 months (Miller, 1971). Infective *A. braziliense* larvae will follow the tracheo-esophageal route after skin penetration and the pre-patent period in puppies is 2 weeks. Transmission through paratenic hosts is described for both *A. caninum* and *A. braziliense. A. ceylanicum* can have a direct cycle after oral exposure or a tracheal migration after cutaneous infection. The pre-patent period is 2 weeks.

Disease in animals

The pathogenicity for *U. stenocephala* is low as a result of the nearly exclusive direct route of infection without migration in the body (Pearson *et al.*, 1982). Furthermore, this is not a hematophagous parasite. Clinical symptoms of uncinariosis are sometimes present as mild transitory diarrhea and mild anemia in young dogs with heavy infections. Percutaneous infections via interdigital skin are rare and only a few larvae will continue to migrate. Hypersensitivity reactions like transitory pruritus can be noticed in relation with the invasion of larvae through the skin.

    A. caninum is, in contrast to *U. stenocephala*, one of the most pathogenic parasites of the dog. Penetration of the skin of the feet by larvae cause pruritus, erythema, papulae, eczema, ulceration, and secondary bacterial infection resulting from scratching, especially on the paws. Via hair follicles and apocrine sweat glands, the larvae migrate to the dermis. Interdigital dermatitis with wet eczema and swelling of the foot can be noticed. In chronic cases, secondary bacterial infections can contaminate the wounds and ultimately result in claw deformations. Hemorrhagic pneumonia and respiratory symptoms is possible as result of migration of larvae through the lungs, also in combination with the anoxia as result of the anemia. Blood leukocytosis and eosinophilia will follow infection. Percutaneous invading larvae and migration in the lungs causes damage and hypersensitivity reactions. The pre-adult and adult intestinal stages are very harmful due to their damage to the mucosa in the jejunum and their habit of frequently changing their position. Mucosal damage includes destruction of blood capillaries, which result in hemorrhages, blood loss, hypochromic anemia and ulcers. The intestinal absorption is disturbed and, in combination with significant blood losses especially in puppies, the clinical signs are presented as dark colored diarrhea with mucus. After lactogenic infection, massive blood loss will start from day 8 and anemia and hypo-proteinemia will develop in the second week of life, before the infection is patent. In severe infection lethargy, epistaxis and death occur. In chronic infection, the animals are anorexic and wasted and the anemia is often accompanied by weight loss. The patent infection of *A. caninum* is relatively long, 6 to 18 months. Adult dogs show age resistance, even when contact with the parasite at a young age is limited.

    A. braziliense causes negligible blood loss and signs of infection are restricted to gastrointestinal disturbances, such as mild diarrhea or protein-loosing enteropathy *A. ceylanicum* infection may cause diarrhea with blood and mucus and induces blood eosinophilia (Miller, 1971).

Diagnosis

Dogs, mainly puppies of 1 to 2 weeks of age, with dark diarrhea in combination with clinical or hematologically determined anemia, but without fever, in (sub) tropical areas are very suspicious for ancylostomosis. The diagnosis can be confirmed coprologically by finding the typical strongylid eggs with thin shells. Clinical signs of acute disease may be apparent before the infection is patent. Specification requires adult worms or can be based on characteristics of larvae in feces older than 2 days.

Methods of control

It is nearly impossible to prevent environmental infection, because wild and stray animals play a role in the epidemiology of hookworms. Floors of kennels and dog runs should be kept as smooth and dry as possible, preferably in sunlight. A flame gun can be used to destroy nematode eggs in runs with concrete floors. The efficacy of the flame gun is higher than that of chemicals (Pegg, 1977). Dog owners should avoid non-hygienic places with their animals. Periodic anthelmintic treatments for dogs at risk at 1-3 month intervals and for dogs after returning from high-risk areas reduce shedding of eggs and therefore environmental contamination. Repeated administration of anthelmintics after 3 to 4 weeks are necessary to eliminate recently matured adults. For this purpose benzimidazoles, milbemycin oxime, nitroscanate and pyrantel pamoate can be used. Milbemycin has limited efficacy for uncinarosis (Bowman, 1991). Nursing litters should be treated weekly up to 6 weeks of age and at 2-week intervals from 6-12 weeks of age. Special attention is required to treat the lactating bitches simultaneously. A single subcutaneous injection of doramectin to the bitch at day 55 of gestation (Schnieder *et al.*, 1994) prevented lactogenic infections.

Hygiene can be achieved by removing the feces and thorough cleaning of kennels. Pet owners should be advised to prevent their animals from defecating in parks and on children's playgrounds.

Treatment of patients

Adult hookworms as well as the pre-adult intestinal stages can be removed by treatment with most presently used anthelmintics. Effective agents include benzimidazoles, pyrantel pamoate, milbemycin oxime and nitroscanate (Hendrix *et al.*, 1996). The extra-intestinal stages are more difficult to reach with anthelmintics. In practice, veterinarians frequently encounter dogs with hookworm infections that refuse to disappear even after repeated wormings with a variety of drugs over the course of many months. The "larval leak" phenomenon provides a plausible explanation for such refractory cases (Georgi and Georgi, 1990). In clinical cases, supportive iron and fluid therapy should treat the anemia. Blood transfusions are sometimes required in puppies. Bitches should be dosed at least once during pregnancy (Kalkoven, 1987).

Disease in man

Hookworm infection is most common in children and in adults in areas with warm, moist climate who are sunbathing, playing or going frequently barefoot in moist, sandy soil areas contaminated with larval hookworms. Professionals at risk are construction workers, such as plumbers, electricians, and technicians working in the crawl space beneath a house and gardeners tending flower beds and vegetable gardens (Hendrix *et al.*, 1996). Clinical manifestations in human zoonotic hookworm infection involve the skin, blood, and intestine. Infection is obtained from soil that is contaminated by dog and cat feces. The percutaneous invasion of the third-stage infectious larvae of *A. braziliense* and *A. caninum* will cause skin lesions. *A. caninum* has been reported to be able to develop to pre-adults in the human gut and to induce an eosinophilic enteritis. Infection with *A. ceylanicum* occurs mainly peroral and the parasite can complete its life cycle in humans causing abdominal symptoms and anemia.

Clinical symptoms

After cutaneous infection, usually via hair follicles, the larvae will not migrate to deeper skin areas but remain in the epidermis as a form of cutaneous larva migrans. *A. braziliense* can invade the skin directly or through damp clothing and cause only in humans the classical linear skin lesions or cutaneous larva migrans, also known as creeping eruption, dermal larval migrans, ground itch, plumber's itch and sandworms. One hour after infection papules and local itching develop. Multiple serpiginous, elevated, reddened, linear, tunnel-like, pruritic skin eruptions appear within 1 to 4 days, lasting up to 3 months or more. Within weeks to months after the initial infection, the larvae die and are reabsorbed by the host. Visceral migration is rare, but lung involvement with petechiae and leukocytic infiltration is described as reaction on migrating larvae or as systemic allergic response. Blood eosinophilia and transient radiological pulmonary opacities may accompany respiratory symptoms (Prociv, 1998).

    A. caninum larvae produce only transient small papules and pustules. The lesions are highly pruritic and some of these may be followed by short migratory tracks, which can recur at variable intervals and in widely separated sites for up to 7 months. An eosinophilic folliculitis can be found at histological examination with several larvae arrested in the hair follicles. Myositis caused by hypobiotic L_3 may be common, but would be difficult to diagnose (Little *et al.*, 1983; Miller *et al.*, 1991). Recent studies in Queensland, Australia indicate that enteric infection with *A. caninum* is a leading cause of human eosinophilic enteritis. This disorder is also described in relation with circulating antibodies to excretory-secretory antigens of adult *A. caninum* (Loukas *et al.*, 1992; Prociv and Croese, 1996). In some cases single adult, but not patent, hookworms could be identified in the intestine of patients. The eosinophilic inflammation represents an allergic response to the secreted antigens of developing L₃, L₄ or adult worms and may present as acute, mild, intermittent or chronic disease. Although the infections may be subclinical, the chief symptom is abdominal pain, which is frequently severe with sudden onset.

Experimental and natural infections with *A. ceylanicum* in humans cause occasionally cutaneous lesions or anemia. In most cases acute gastrointestinal symptoms occur 2 to 3 weeks after infection and 1 to 2 weeks before eggs appear in stools. Under natural conditions *A. ceylanicum* causes only light human intestinal infections with few eggs. The infection behaves as if in an unsuitable host (Carroll and Grove, 1986).

Diagnosis

Diagnosis of hookworm infection rests on the history, with special attention for travellers returning from the tropics and sub-tropics, and on clinical recognition of the characteristic lesions. Symptoms commence between 1 and 29 days after returning home (Davies *et al.*, 1993). Present serology is neither adequately sensitive nor specific. In cases of eosinophilic enteritis, the blood eosinophilia suggests the diagnosis.

Methods of control

A common misconception is that infection is acquired from direct contact with dogs. There is no increased risk of infection, because transmission is only by contact with the infective larvae. The source of human infection is damp, shady soil or grass that has been contaminated with animal feces some time previously (Prociv, 1998). Protection can be achieved by wearing shoes in such areas. Pet owners should not allow their pet's feces to accumulate at beaches and in the lawn or garden environment and children's sandboxes should remain covered when not in use. If free roaming dogs defecate in a public area, the feces should be promptly removed. Further measures are prohibition of dogs and cats on playgrounds and beaches and increasing the awareness among public health workers, veterinarians and pet owners.

Treatment of patients

Topical thiabendazole (10% suspension or 15% cream) or systemic therapy with 400 mg albendazole daily for 3 to 5 days are reported to be effective (Davies *et al.*, 1993) as well as a single dose of 12 mg oral dose ivermectin (Caumes *et al.*, 1993). Although pruritus ceased rapidly for patients after application of anthelmintic agents, it may be necessary to combine the first treatment with antipruritics (0.1% dexamethasone cream) for 3 days or sedatives. Antibiotics may be indicated to control secondary infection. Surgical treatment is unsuccessful, because the larvae cannot be localized and removed surgically. Freezing the lesion using carbon dioxide snow, ethyl chloride spray or liquid nitrogen is no longer recommended. It may cause blisters and chronic ulcerations, while the cutaneous larva migrans continues to spread (Jelinek *et al.*, 1994; Tan, 1997).

Filariosis

The filarial nematodes are characterized by their location in the deeper tissues of the body and their dependence upon blood-feeding anthropod vectors for transmission (Mims *et al.*, 1993). The most important zoonotic species can cause inflammatory responses in the lungs (*Dirofilaria immitis*), or subcutis (other *Dirofilaria* species), or lymphatics (*Brugia*).

Dirofilaria immitis

Dirofilaria immitis causes heartworm in domestic and wild canine and feline species in tropical, subtropical and temperate regions of the world. Humans, as well as several other mammals, serve as accidental hosts in which the life cycle is not completed.

The worms are found primarily in the pulmonary arteries in animals with low worm burdens. In severe infections, they may also be found in the right side of the heart and, occasionally, the vena cava. Female worms produce microfilariae into the bloodstream where they circulate for up to 2.5 years. When bloodsucking mosquitoes take up the microfilariae, they develop within 2 to 3 weeks into infective L_3 stages. These are inoculated into a new host during a bloodmeal. Within 70 to 110 days, the L_3 and L_4 stages mature in the subcutaneous tissue and muscles of the host before they migrate to the thorax and enter the vascular system via penetration of peripheral veins. In the pulmonary arteries, preferentially those within the caudal lung lobes, they mature within another 3 months. The adult worms copulate and the female subsequently produces microfilariae (Schrey, 1996). The prepatent period is 6 to 7 months and the mean life expectancy of the worms in dogs is approximately 5 years. Transplacental infection of puppies or via blood transfusion with microfilariae is known, but in that case they cannot develop into adult worms (Todd and Howland, 1983).

D. immitis is prevalent in North America, Latin America and the Caribbean, Africa, Asia, Australia and southern Europe. Imported cases of *D. immitis* infections of dogs have been reported from several north and middle European countries. It is found that, within the last 20 years, the worm has established itself in northeastern regions of the USA and Canada, northern Italy and northeastern France. There is no clear explanation for this migration to colder climate zones.

Disease in animals

The migrating larvae produce minimal tissue damage and clinical signs are absent during the prepatent period. Chronic heartworm disease results from progressive proliferative endarteritis and thromboembolism of the a. pulmonalis, caused by adult *D. immitis* worms and worm antigen. The progressive vascular changes lead to pulmonary hypertension, right ventricular hypertrophy or dilatation with decompensation and cor pulmonale. Worm burdens up to 30 adults can remain asymptomatic; while clinically affected dogs generally have more than 50 adult worms. The first symptoms of dogs with right heart failure include exercise intolerance and a sporadic cough, in a later stage followed by weight loss, lethargy, hepatomegaly, ascites, syncope and respiratory symptoms such as dyspnoea, tachypnoea, chronic cough and hemoptysis. Anemia is commonly present as a result of mechanical damage to erythrocytes produced by atrial turbulence and by hemolysis caused by platelet activation and fibrin formation in small vessels. The venous congestion is in the final stages responsible for chronic liver congestion with ascites. Immune mediated glomerulonephritis (immune-complex deposition) and amyloid nephrosis may develop in association with the heartworm infection.

Acute heartworm disease can occur in heavy infestations, when masses of adult *D. immitis* worms have a retrogade migration from pulmonary arteries into the right side of the heart and, rarely, to the vena cava. Sometimes it causes a disruption of the tricuspid apparatus. This so called vena caval syndrome is characterized by acute weakness, anorexia, dyspnoea, and shock as result of valvular insufficiency, heart failure and a haemolytic crisis caused by intravascular hemolysis and disseminated intravascular coagulation (DIC) (Strickland, 1998).

Allergic pneumonitis with chronic, severe cough, dyspnoea and cyanosis is another phenomenon that can develop in combination with anorexia and weight loss (Schrey, 1996).

Occasionally, adult worms may be found in the anterior chamber of the eye, (the skin or the central nervous system) as a result of aberrant somatic migration of juvenile larvae (ectopic *D. immitis* infection) (Quinn *et al.*, 1997).

Diagnosis

A suspicion of heartworm infection arises when the clinical history indicates travelling or residence in an endemic area with exposure to mosquitoes.

The symptoms and clinical signs are related to right heart disease and thoracic radiography shows right ventricular and atrial cardiomegaly, enlarged and tortuous pulmonary arteries, and patchy pulmonary interstitial or alveolar infiltrates. Diffuse pulmonary interstitial or alveolar infiltrates are present in cases with allergic pneumonitis.

Echocardiography may show enlargement of the right heart and ventricular wall hypertrophy. Sometimes worms can be visualized in the pulmonary arteries and the heart. Pericardial effusion and tricuspid valve insufficiency can also be found. A sinus arrhythmia (tachycardia), enlargement of the right ventriculum and atrium and conductive disturbances can be noticed on an electrocardiogram (ECG). Haematological findings include eosinophilia, basophilia and normocytic, hypochromic anemia. Proteinuria is present as result of glomerulonephritis.

High numbers of microfilaria can be detected with microscopic examination of direct blood smears or a microhematocrit blood sample taken close to the buffy coat layer. Reliable isolation methods are the Knott's concentration method or Millipore filter technique. There is no seasonal or daily variation to microfilarial numbers and microfilaria are able to persist in the circulation, even after adult worm death, for as long as 2.5 years.

Failure to detect circulating microfilariae does not rule out infection. This is because of the presence of occult infections, prepatent infections, microfilaricidal therapy, unisex and ectopic infections. Heartworm preventive medication is a common cause of occult infections in dogs, because it kills the microfilariae while the adult worms are not affected.

Isolated microfilariae can be differentiated using the acid phosphatase histochemical stain, which is a quick and reliable method (Chalifoux and Hunt, 1971). Species-specific staining patterns enable easy identification of the different filarial larvae. *D. immitis* is highly pathogenic and *Dirofilaria repens* is considered as mildly pathogenic. *Dipetalonema reconditum*, *Dipetalonema dracunculoides* and *Dipetalonema grassi* (extremely rare) are non-pathogenic.

There are several commercial, semiquantative, *D. immitis* ELISA tests with high sensitivity and specificity available, employing monoclonal antibody, for detecting circulating antigen of *D. immitis*. The ELISA tests are useful in pretreatment evaluation, treatment and in detection of occult infections. Male worms, non-gravid females, or single (ectopic) worm infections are difficult to detect.

In endemic areas *Angiostrongylus vasorum*, the lungworm, should be considered as a differential diagnosis (Schrey, 1996).

Methods of control

The most practical approach for preventing heartworm infection is to avoid travelling with dogs to areas where heartworm is present. In endemic areas, mosquito control and continuing chemoprophylaxis of dogs is required. For these purposes the oral administration of the following prophylactic drugs can be used monthly: ivermectin 6-12 μg per kg, moxidectin 3 μg per kg, and milbemycin 0.5-0.9 mg per kg. Finally, the spot-on formulation selamectin can be used at a dosage of 6 mg per kg. Diethylcarbamazine in a dosage of 6.6 mg per kg orally, once daily, can be used prophylactically but should not be used in dogs with patent infections because of the risk of circulatory collapse. Melarsomine (2.2 mg per kg) is also effective as a prophylactic drug when given by two intramuscular injections 3 hours apart 4 months after mosquito activity. The treatment should be repeated two months later and can be continued every 4 months in case of sustained mosquito activity.

Treatment of dogs starts with adulticidal drugs. This is hazardous because it may result in pulmonary thrombosis with fatal consequences. Melarsamine dihydrochloride, given as a deep intramuscular injection in the lumbar muscles at a dose of 2.5 mg per kg on two consecutive days (Rawlings and McCall, 1996) or 2.2 mg per kg twice 3 hours apart (McTier *et al.*, 1994), is currently the most effective treatment for patent infections in dogs. Sodium thiacetarsamide, another adulticidal drug, is less effective and has potentially more side effects. Dogs with cardiac or pulmonary failure are treated with a single injection of melarsomine, thereby reducing the risk of thrombosis, a potential complication of chemotherapy in heavy infections. The two-injection regimen is then used 2 months later to eliminate residual infection. Surgical extraction of the worms is recommended in dogs with evidence of vena caval syndrome (Quinn *et al.*, 1997).

Six weeks later, microfilaricidal therapy is recommended. A single oral administration of ivermectin (0.05 mg per kg in propylene glycol 1:9) or milbemycin oxime (0.1-0.5 mg per kg) is highly effective against microfilariae, third- and fourth-stage larvae. For breeds that are highly sensitive to ivermectin, such as collies and bobtails, the alternative microfilaricidal drug levamisol (10 mg per kg per day for 7 days), can be used. The liberated microfilarial antigen can induce an anaphylactic reaction, especially in smaller dogs (< 16 kg) with high numbers of microfilariae (> 10,000 per ml blood). In order to prevent such reactions, measurement of microfilarial density is advised before treatment. If necessary, dividing the dose over a period of several days is recommended. Another option is to initiate heartworm prophylaxis with low dose microfilaricidal drugs to eliminate the microfilariae slowly over a period of 6 months.

A pre-treatment therapy with heparin (50-100 IU per kg t.i.d. subcutaneous) can be used for heartworm patients with cardiopulmonary and thromboembolic disease. Platelet aggregation inhibition should start 1 to 2 weeks before the adulticidal therapy. This prevents subsequent thromboembolic complications when adulticidal treatment is given. Strict cage rest for at least 3 weeks is required and the use of oxygen, bronchodilators and antibiotics may be necessary depending on the clinical symptoms and condition of the patient.

In cases of allergic pneumonia, the use of corticosteroids is indicated together with antibiotics. Two weeks later the adulticidal drug therapy can be started.

The treatment should be evaluated by performing a microfilaria isolation test 3 weeks after microfilaricidal therapy or an ELISA 12 weeks after adulticidal therapy (Henry and Dillon, 1994; Schrey and Trautvetter, 1998).

Disease in man

Humans are not hosts to the full development of any *Dirofilaria* species, but act as accidental dead-end hosts for immature female worms. There are several reports of *Dirotilaria repens* subcutaneous infection of humans (see below), but *D. immitis* infections are very rare. Most infections are reported from the USA and Japan (Beaver *et al.*, 1984). In Europe, clinical disease is reported from Spain and Italy (Schrey, 1996). After infection, *D. immitis* larvae undergo a somatic migration to reach a smaller branch of the a. pulmonalis. Patients may become symptomatic (43%) with a fever, persistent cough and even hemoptysis (Robinson *et al.*, 1977; Glickman and Magnaval, 1993). Eosinophilia is an inconsistent finding. In the lungs a 1-4 cm solitary spherical granuloma or 'coin lesion' with partly calcificated worms in the center will be formed. This does not appear to cause any problem, but it is frequently mistaken as a neoplasia and has led to numerous, unnecessary, open chest surgical removals of the lump (Denham, 1998). *D. immitis* has also been found in subcutaneous lesions in several patients in the USA and Canada.

Diagnosis

The diagnosis of *D. immitis* infection is made with ELISA, in combination with radiographic findings and by histology of biopsy material or surgically removed granuloma.

Methods of control

Humans can only prevent *Dirofilaria* infections by avoiding being bitten by mosquitoes in endemic areas. The use of repellents, containing diethyltoluamide (DEET) is recommended (Denham, 1998).

    In humans the worms are usually dead and therapy is therefore not indicated. Lung masses in which pulmonary dirofilariasis is suspected can be surgically removed.

Other *Dirofilaria* species

Dirofilaria species other than *D. immitis* infect dogs and other carnivora in Europe, Asia and Africa with subcutaneously dwelling adult worms. Subcutaneous dirofilariasis in the dog is due to *D. repens* and various mosquitoes can sometimes transmit the parasite to the human. Zoonotic infection produces subconjunctival or subcutaneous swelling or nodules enclosing an immature adult *D. repens*. The ocular form was a long time suspected to be caused by *Dirofilaria conjunctivae*, but electrophoretic analysis proved that the patterns were identical to *D. repens* (Cancrini *et al.*, 1991). The subcutaneous locations described are skulls, cheek, breast, inguinal area, buttocks, arms and legs. The infective larvae can have a painful migration in the subcutaneous tissues before an erythematous nodule (1-6 cm of diameter) develops in the skin. The lesions are of little significance, and subcutaneous dirofilariosis is often misdiagnosed as a tumor or a foreign body granuloma. The infection can be diagnosed by histological examination of the nodule or by extraction and morphological study of the worm. Blood eosinophilia or microfilariae are extremely rare (Gardiner *et al.*, 1978; Marty, 1997).

Brugia malayi

Brugia malayi, found in Southeast Asia (Malaysia, Indonesia) is strongly zoonotic and restricted to the tropics. The main animal reservoir is a leaf-eating monkey (*Presbytis* spp.), but this filarial nematode has also been found in many other mammals such as dogs. The finding of the same parasite in man and animals in the same environment does not prove it is a zoonosis and it is probable that these are the victims of transmission from *Presbytis* or even infected people (Denham, 1998). *Mansonia* spp. mosquitoes transmit zoonotic brugian filariosis. The female mosquitoes pick up microfilariae from infected hosts during blood-feeding. After migration, the microfilariae will develop in the flight muscles into infective L_3 larvae. The L_3 migrate to the mouthparts and emerge from the proboscis while the mosquito is feeding. In the host, the L_3 penetrate the lymph nodes and lymphatics of the limbs and inguinal region where they mature. After 2 months the female filaria produces microfilariae that migrate into the bloodstream. Further development occurs only after ingestion by a mosquito (Denham and McGreevy, 1977).

Another Brugia species, *Brugia pahangi*, was able to infect man experimentally, but this parasite has not been recognized in natural human infections. Natural infections of *B. pahangi* have been found in many mammals, including dogs.

Disease in animals

No clinical symptoms are reported in dogs in endemic areas. Only after experimental infection under laboratory conditions, dogs develop lymphadenitis, lymphangitis, and soft lymphoedema (Denham, 1998).

Methods of control

Despite the fact that clinical disease does not occur, it is advised in endemic areas to treat dogs and cats on a regular base with a benzimidazole carbamate to kill adult worms and to give protection against infection for several weeks. A once-monthly regime of 6 mg per kg is recommended (Denham, 1998).

Disease in man

Brugian filariosis may show few clinical signs, or suffer acute manifestations such as fever, rashes, eosinophilia, orchitis, and lymphadenitis and lymphangitis of the limbs and scrotum. The fever persists for 2-7 days and will repeat 3-6 times per year occasionally, but later more frequently. Acute lymphangitis can be infected with bacteria and result in abscess formation. After break through of an abscess, a painful ulcer exists, especially on the inside of the thighs. Filariosis is a progressive disease as long infection continues. Dilated varicosis of the lymph trunks may follow recurrent lymphangitis and chronic lymphangitis develops with enlarged lymph nodes and blocking of the lymphatics. Hydrocoele, lymphoedema and gross enlargement of breasts, scrotum and limbs develop (elephantiasis) with pigmentation changes (mainly hyperpigmentation). Some patients develop pulmonary symptoms known as "tropical pulmonary eosinophilia" (Bartoloni *et al.*, 1997) and late-stage interstitial pulmonary fibrosis can lead to cardiac failure (Quah *et al.*, 1997). Secondary fungal infections are common and skin wounds are frequently seen, soon infected with bacteria (Denham, 1998).

Without treatment, filarial lymphoedema is a progressive disease in endemic areas where patients will be bitten daily by infected mosquitoes.

Diagnosis

The diagnosis of filarial infections is based on the clinical symptoms and largely depends upon detection of microfilariae in the blood. In many infected people with lymphatic filariae, microfilariae are not detectable in the blood. An ELISA test for antifilarial IgG antibodies is available but this is not specific for *Brugia*. Monoclonal antibodies have been developed that are specific for detection of circulating antigens in lymphatic filariasis and species-specific DNA probes have been developed for *B. malayi* (Chandrashekar, 1997). Identification of which species is present is only possible by examination of the spicules of adult male worms. These can only be obtained after feeding infected blood to laboratory mosquitoes and injecting the L_3 intra-abdominal in the Mongolian gerbil.

Methods of control

Vector control and prevention of biting can minimize transmission of filariasis. As the *Mansonia* mosquitoes bite nocturnally, the use of bed nets is a good prevention. Unfortunately it is very difficult to prevent biting during the evening. The use of diethyltoluamide (DEET) can be used because of its repellent effect. It is not possible to control the mosquitoes in the forests, which are the mass breeding sites. The main reservoir, *Presbytis* monkeys, cannot be removed nor treated, but dogs and cats in endemic areas eventually can be treated on a regular basis with a benzimidazole carbamate to kill adult worms and to give protection against infection for several weeks. The preventive use of DEC by a once-monthly regime of 6 mg per kg is recommended (Denham, 1998).

Treatment of patients

Since many years the treatment of choice for *B. malayi* infection is diethylcarbamazine (DEC). Treatment with DEC-fortified cooking salt with the food of patients, in a mean daily dosage of 21 mg, showed excellent results after one year (Shenoy *et al.*, 1998b).

A single injection with ivermectin (dosage 20-200 μg per kg) reduced the geometric mean microfilarial count to less than 10% at 2 weeks and maintained it below 25% of the initial level even at 6 months post-treatment (Mak *et al.*, 1993).

In one trial, asymptomatic but microfilaremic patients were therefore treated with oral doses of 400 μg per kg ivermectin and 6 mg per kg DEC as single treatment. The combination demonstrated a microfilaricidal effect superior to that of either drug used alone. Both in the initial rapid clearance of microfilariae (clearance 97-100% and 57% of the individuals were amicrofilaraemic at 12 hours post-treatment) and in sustaining the effect for 1 year (mean clearance 99.9% and 68% amicrofilaraemic) (Shenoy *et al.*, 1998a).

The first grades of lymphoedema are susceptible to this treatment and affected legs often return to normal state (Partono *et al.*, 1981). The death, however, of large numbers of microfilariae, causes violent allergic responses (Mazzotti reaction) as side-effects due to the release of much protein into a host with large amounts of antibody.

Toxascariosis

Adult *Toxascaris leonina* ascarids occur in the small intestine of the dog, cat, fox and wild Canidae and Felidae in most parts of the world. *T. leonina* infection in the definitive host is similar to *Toxascaris canis*, but the parasite is generally less pathogenic. The zoonotic potential of *T. leonina* is considered in the literature as being absent or very limited. Few studies on this aspect, however, have been conducted.

Disease in animals

T. leonina larvae in the definitive host do not undergo a visceral, prenatal, or transmammary migration, but penetrate only the intestinal wall where they mature (mucosal migration). Clinical signs are rarely observed and the parasite is therefore not very pathogenic and may provoke only a mild inflammatory response associated with the larval development in the intestine (Parsons, 1987). There appears to be no age resistance in dogs to infection with eggs of *T. leonina*. Larvae may persist in the intestinal wall for at least 7 weeks up to 1 year and may mature to the adult stage following expulsion of an existing adult burden. Occasionally, in very heavy infections, larvae may migrate into the abdominal cavity or to the mesenteric lymph nodes, pancreas, liver, lungs, and muscle, where they may moult once but undergo no further development (Sprent, 1959).

Rodents and birds can act as paratenic host for *T. leonina* with larvae penetrating the intestinal wall to remain for a variable period. In mice and guinea pigs they undergo a somatic migration to the musculature, the liver, genital organs and the lungs. Not a single larva of *T. leonina* has been found in the brain (Matoff and Komandarev, 1963; Okoshi and Osui, 1968b; Prokopic and Figallova, 1982). In the paratenic host, the larvae, unlike those of *T. canis*, undergo considerable growth. Lactogenic transmission occurs in experimentallly infected mice (Karbach and Stoye, 1982), but has not been demonstrated or reported in the definitive host. In infected chickens, only a few larvae undergo somatic migration and most remain in the intestinal wall (Okoshi and Osui, 1968b; Dubey, 1969).

When dogs eat infected paratenic hosts, the larvae develop to maturity within the wall and lumen of the intestine. The development is slower following ingestion of paratenic hosts than with egg infections (Okoshi and Usui, 1968a).

Diagnosis and control is similar to that of *T. canis* infection.

Disease in man

Humans in a contaminated environment can ingest *T. leonina* eggs in the same way as *T. canis* eggs are swallowed. Presumably, they will then act as paratenic host with at least mucosal penetration occuring, if not visceral migration as well, as demonstrated in several laboratory models.

To investigate the pathogenicity of *T. leonina* in man, an ELISA-method using larval excretory-secretory antigens should be used for screening and diagnosis in suspected patients. Cross-reactions with antibodies to *T. canis* with such an ELISA-test were not observed in a study and a specific test seems therefore possible (Cuellar *et al.*, 1995).

Until the risk for *T. leonina* infections in humans is thoroughly evaluated, the parasite should be assumed a potential zoonosis. A recently developed PCR-based method for detection and identification of ascaridoid larvae in human tissues (Jacobs *et al.*, 1997) may be helpful in the future to evaluate the relative significance of *T. leonina* as a zoonosis.

Capillariosis

Capillaria aerophila, a lungworm found in canids, is reported to be zoonotic. The parasite is found in the upper respiratory tract of, mainly wild, canids and felids in North and South America, Europe, Russia, Asia, North Africa, and Australia. The prevalence rates seem to be highest in foxes with those raised for fur on farms most at risk. Human capillariosis, although quite rare (11 cases), have been reported from Russia, Morocco, France and Iran (Banzon, 1977; Vilella *et al.*, 1986). In the USA 0.8-9.6% of dogs are reported to found infected (Cross, 1998), but most of these infections are the nasal capillarid, *Capillaria boehmi*, which is believed to be a distinct species (Jordan *et al.*, 1993; Quinn *et al.*, 1997).

Disease in animals

C. aerophila invades the respiratory mucosa of the trachea, bronchi, and bronchioles. The eggs are coughed up, swallowed and pass in the feces. After embryonation in the environment for at least 40 days, earthworms ingest the eggs and the infection is then acquired by an animal after eating the earthworm. Direct transmission is also possible by ingestion of embryonated eggs. The prepatent period is 25-40 days in the host.

Clinical signs are usually mild. Large numbers of parasites may cause irritation, increased secretion and constriction of the lumen, especially in young animals. The symptoms are weight loss, anorexia, coughing, sneezing, superficial respiration, weakness, and progressive emaciation among uncomplicated cases with tracheitis and bronchitis. Secondary bacterial infection may cause bronchopneumonia and death. There is no age resistance.

Diagnosis of *C. aerophila* infection consists of the symptoms and finding the eggs in sputum or feces. Ivermectin (0.2 mg per kg) may be useful for anthelmintic treatment (Evinger *et al.*, 1985). Prevention consists of avoiding contaminated soil contact and prevention of scavenging.

Disease in man

Humans are infected when they ingest embryonated *C. aerophila* eggs from soil. The parasite develops to patency in the respiratory tract. The incubation period is 3-4 weeks. Fever and acute bronchopulmonary symptoms, such as cough, mucoid or bloody expectoration, and dyspnoea characterize the infection. The laboratory findings are leukocytosis, eosinophilia, and globulinemia. Radiographs show diffuse lung infiltrates and biopsies reveal granulomatous lesions containing the parasite. Finding the characteristic eggs in sputum or feces confirms the diagnosis. Complete cure is possible with administration of thiabendazole orally at a daily dose of 500 mg for 10 days or 25 mg per kg per day for 3 days (Banzon, 1977). Prevention consists of strict personal hygiene by animal caretakers, avoiding the ingestion of soil, and preventing children from playing in high-risk areas.

Dioctophymosis

Dioctophyma renale, the giant kidney worm of mink and other fish-eating mammals, occasionally also infects dogs. Information about the prevalence of the infection is difficult because most reports deal with isolated findings or clinical cases. Infestations have been reported throughout the world. Fewer than 20 human cases are described, most in North America, but also in Russia, Iran, Asia, Australia, and Spain (Lloyd, 1998b).

Disease in animals

D. renale eggs pass out in the urine and develop within 1 to 7 months in water (temperature dependent) to form a first-stage larva. After ingestion of the embryonated larvated eggs by aquatic annelid worms (*Lumbricus variegatus*), they develop to infective-stage larvae in 100 days. Dogs are infected with *D. renale* by eating infected worms or paratenic hosts such as fish, crayfish and some species of frogs (Measures and Anderson, 1985), in which the larvae become encapsulated in the tissues. The larvae migrate from the dog's intestine via the liver through the abdominal cavity to mainly the right kidney (80% of cases) to mature. A study in 96 infected dogs showed that only 40% had parasites in the renal location while the remainder were found in the abdominal cavity (Osborne *et al.*, 1969). The prepatent period is 3-6 months and the infection can be patent for 1 to 3 years. The blood-red, large (1-45 cm long) worms in the kidney can destroy kidney parenchyma forming a fibrous sac filled with sanguinopurulent fluid and adult worms. The parasite can also be found in the bladder and urethra, or in the peritoneal cavity causing chronic peritonitis with adhesions, ascites and hemorrhage. Infestations are often asymptomatic or mild. Weight loss and signs of cystitis (hematuria, frequent miction) and evidence of abdominal pain are occasionally present. In severe cases, obstruction of the urinary passages can lead to hydronephrosis with retention of urine and the development of uremia. History of ingestion of raw fish in endemic areas and the presence of characteristic clinical symptoms are suggestive of dioctophymosis. Demonstration of the worm(s) radiologically or ultrasonically and/or finding the characteristic, ring-like structured eggs in the urine can make the diagnosis. As therapy, surgery of the kidney (removing worms or nephrectomy) or the abdomen (removing worms from the peritoneal cavity) is required. Preventing the ingestion of raw fish or frogs is necessary to avoid infection (Barriga, 1977; Quinn *et al.*, 1997).

Disease in man

Dioctophymosis in man is a rare condition. The pathology in the human seems to be similar to that described in animals and occurs after ingestion of undercooked or raw infected fish (Barriga, 1977). A thick-walled cyst containing hemorrhagic debris is found in or on the right kidney and has been confused with a tumor (Sun *et al.*, 1986). Normally only one worm is present. Some patients are asymptomatic but symptoms include loin pain, renal colic and dysfunction, hematuria, and worms can be expelled from the urethra (Fernando, 1983). Larvae are also found in subcutaneous nodules on the chest (Lloyd, 1998b). Diagnosis, treatment, and prevention are the same as described for the dog.

Dracunculosis

Dracunculus medinensis, the guinea worm, was until recently an important parasite of rural populations in parts of Asia, the Middle East and parts of Africa. The introduction of a global eradication program in the early 1980s resulted in a restricted distribution of the parasite to a handful of countries in Africa (Muller, 1999). Significant numbers of cases now occur only in Sudan, Nigeria, Ghana, Burkino Faso and Togo (CDC, 2000). WHO has designated dracunculosis as the next disease scheduled to be eradicated after smallpox. Man is the principal definitive host, but natural infections have been reported in a variety of animals including monkeys, herbivores, and domestic and wild Canidae and Felidae. Dogs are considered as the major non-human hosts but still probably play only a minor role in the epidemiology of this mainly human infection (Kale, 1977a; Hugh-Jones *et al.*, 1995). Natural infections in dogs have been reported from India (Subrahmanyam *et al.*, 1976; Joseph and Kandazamy, 1980; Lalitha and Anandan, 1980), Argentina and in the former Soviet Union (Ghenis, 1972; Velikanov, 1984).

The species reported to occur in animals is *Dracunculus insignis* and the validity of this species is still in question (Muller, 1991). The parasite is found in raccoons, mink and other carnivores in North America and occasionally seen in dogs (Panciera and Stockham, 1988). A few cases of human infections with this parasite have been reported in the eastern USA.

Disease in animals

Female *Dracunculus* worms protrude from skin ulcers of their hosts and microfilariae larvae are expelled into water. Susceptible definitive hosts acquire the infection by ingesting drinking water containing infected crustacean intermediate hosts (*Cyclops* species) (Eberhard and Brandt, 1995; Quinn *et al.*, 1997). It is the only parasitic disease transmitted only through drinking water. Ingested larvae migrate via the lymphatics to deep subcutaneous and retroperitoneal tissues of the inguinal and axillary regions, the abdominal and thoracic walls and the limbs. The males die within 3 to 6 months after copulation and the females migrate to the surface of the body, particularly the extremities, emerging from there between the 9th and 14th month after infection had been acquired (Kale, 1977a). The females are found in fluctuating subcutaneous nodules with central ulceration and when the infected host enters water, the worm releases hundred of thousands of larvae. The female worm dies or is spontaneously extruded from the body of the host soon after parturition.

Rising blood eosinophilia, fever, restlessness and the eruption of irritating blister characterize the prepatent period. Pressure on the affected part causes part of the worm to protrude. The incubation period in experimentally infected dogs and monkeys is about 1 year. Puppies are more susceptible than older animals and dogs are able to extract protruding worms from their bodies with their teeth.

Diagnosis can be confirmed by identification of larvae in smears or exudate from lesions. Nodules containing parasites should be excised surgically and systemic acting anthelmintics may be of supportive therapeutic value.

Disease in man

The clinical manifestations are similar to those in animals. Infected persons may develop a generalized urticaria immediately preceding the emergence of the adult worm from under the skin, which is sometimes accompanied by erythema, pruritus, fever, nausea, vomiting, and diarrhea (Kale, 1977b). This allergic reaction lasts only for a few hours and 1 to 8 days later the patient experiences skin irritation at the site where a blister of 2-7 cm later forms. Within a week the blister ruptures and some fluid is discharged and the protruding end of the worm or part of its uterus can be seen. The worm will emerge completely from the body within 3-6 weeks. Breakage of the worm leads to painful and severe inflammation. Worms that do not emerge, die, form abscesses and are absorbed or calcified. Sepsis after the blister rupture is common (tetanus may be severe). Most patients harbor less than three worms (Kale, 1977a). The majority (> 98%) of the worms are found to emerge from the lower limbs and from nearly 1000 patients, 21% were totally incapacitated, 20% were seriously disabled, and 44% suffered mild incapacity, while 16% were unaffected (Okoye *et al.*, 1995).

Diagnosis in endemic areas can be made on the clinical symptoms, such as the onset of hypersensitization reaction that precedes the eruption of the characteristic blister. The identification of the emerging adult worm or the recovery of fragments, or the demonstration of first-stage larvae in smears from aspirate from the blister or discharges confirms a diagnosis. It may be possible to detect infection at least 6 months before the emergence of worms in an individual by using an ELISA-test for specific serum antibodies (Bapna and Renapurkar, 1996; Bloch and Simonsen, 1998). Immunodiagnosis for *D. medinensis*-specific antigens with Western blotting and ELISA failed and suggested that such antigens do not occur in infected individuals (Bloch *et al.*, 1998).

Treatments with anthelmintic drugs (diethylcarbamazine, albendazole, ivermectin, metronidazole, thiabendazole) may hasten expulsion of worms but does not kill them (Kale *et al.*, 1983; Eberhard *et al.*, 1990; Issaka-Tinorgah *et al.*, 1994). An exposed worm can be slowly removed by winding the protruding worm around a small stick.

Dracunculosis can be eradicated by the provision of safe drinking water. This can be achieved either by boiling or filtering water. Contamination of drinking water by infected individuals should be avoided. Education of people about the transmission of the parasite and instruction to change behavior and attitudes will hasten the eradication of this disease.

Gnathostomosis

The genus *Gnathostoma* contains several species from which *Gnathostoma spinigerum* was believed to cause human gnathostomosis in endemic areas in Southeast Asia (China, Japan, Thailand, Pakistan), Australia and central and South America (Mexico and Equador). From the early 1980s new zoonotic gnathomiasis infections appeared in urban areas in Japan that were caused by *Gnathostoma hispidum*, *Gnathostoma nipponicum* and *G. doloresi* (Nawa, 1991). *G. spinigerum* is found in gastric nodules of wild and domestic Canidae and Felidae that shed the eggs in their feces (Hinz, 1980). Human infection follows ingestion of fish or poultry containing third-stage larvae.

Disease in animals

The dog and cat are considered the most significant or principal reservoirs of the worm in many countries. The eggs of *G. spinigerum* hatch in water after 4 days and the L_1 are ingested by various copepods. Subsequently these larvae develop into advanced third-stage larvae when ingested by freshwater fish (loach, trout) and aquatic snakes as the second intermediate host. In a study of swamp eels, purchased from markets in Thailand, up to 33% were found to be infected (Nuamtanong *et al.*, 1998). Amphibians (frogs), reptiles, small mammals (rodents, pigs), and fowl may act as paratenic hosts with encysted L_3 in their flesh (Ando *et al.*, 1992). Ingesting either a second intermediate or a paratenic host infects dogs and cats. The larvae will migrate through the abdominal cavity, where they can cause extensive destruction of the liver and other organs, and musculature of the host before reaching the stomach wall (Quinn *et al.*, 1997). In the stomach the worms are located in one or two smooth and rounded, slightly protruding, gastric tumours (up to 3 cm in diameter) that consist of thick-walled cysts containing worms. They communicate with the stomach lumen through a very small opening. Communication with the peritoneal cavity may also be possible resulting in peritonitis. Most patients are asymptomatic but occasionally they may exhibit vomiting, appetite disturbances, weight loss and polydipsia. In heavy infestations blood may be seen in the feces. Rupturing of cysts may result in acute abdominal signs.

Diagnosis of gnathostomosis is made by fecal examination to find the eggs. Anthelmintics should be given to kill the parasite and prevention consists of preventing the ingestion of intermediate or paratenic hosts.

Disease in man

Humans acquire *Gnathostoma* infection from eating raw or undercooked fish or meat from paratenic hosts (mainly chicken). Very rarely drinking water with free-living third-stage larvae separated from the infected second intermediate host is the source of human infection (Daengsvang, 1976). Skin penetration by L_3 and occasional prenatal infection are described (Chen and Lin, 1991). Man is an accidental host and the adult parasite does not produce stomach tumors or lay fertilized eggs. The infection may or may not give rise to the symptoms of disease. Larvae and young adults migrate primarily in the skin, subcutaneous tissue, and mucous membrane causing inflammation and mechanical damage. The clinical manifestation develops within 3 to 4 weeks to several months and is characterized by localized, intermittent, migratory swellings of 5 mm in the skin and subcutaneous tissues, often in association with localized pain, pruritus, and erythema lasting 1-2 weeks (Rusnak and Lucey, 1993). Occasionally an abscess develops. The general health condition of the patient is usually normal but there may be several attacks in 1 year and these signs can persist for 8-12 years (Lloyd, 1998b). The worm can also migrate to deeper tissues and other organs including the respiratory tract, muscles, genitourinary system, and eye. When the CNS is involved encephalitis, radiculitis, myelitis, subarachnoid hemorrhage, and significant mortality can occur when *G. spinigerum* is migrating intracranially (Boongird *et al.*, 1977; Schmutzhard *et al.*, 1988). Other nervous symptoms may be acute radicular nerve root pain from the spine to the extremities, often followed by paralysis or severe headache, neck stiffness, vomiting, impairment of senses, and convulsions. The cerebrospinal fluid is bloody or xanthochromic (Punyagupta *et al.*, 1990). The parasite may also be visible in the eye (Biswas *et al.*, 1994). In heavy infections, transient gastrointestinal symptoms such as nausea, vomiting, abdominal cramps and diarrhea, may occur within 24 hours that may be confused with appendicitis. Malaise, chest discomfort, coughs, myalgia, weakness, and cutaneous migratory swellings may follow this (Migasena *et al.*, 1991).

Human gnathostomosis can be positively diagnosed by identification of recovered worms or by a history of dietary preferences, residence or travel in an endemic area, intermittent migratory swellings, and eosinophilia (values exceeding often 50% of the total white blood count). Using an ELISA-test, antibodies against *G. spinigerum* adult antigen in sera can be detected (Nopparatana *et al.*, 1991; Maleewong *et al.*, 1992).

Spontaneous recovery of the parasite is not very common. The worm can be very difficult to remove from CNS or cutaneous lesions, because it is fast moving and the edema and inflammation indicates its previous location (Lloyd, 1998b). Treatment with albendazole at a dosage of 400 mg twice daily for 2 weeks showed a significant higher outward migration of *Gnathostoma* than a placebo group. In this way, the worms could be recovered by excisional biopsy or by picking with a needle. Treatment with ivermectin at a dosage of 0.2-2.0 mg per kg in experimentally infected rabbits reduced the worm load by 74% and 84%, respectively (Anantaphruti *et al.*, 1992).

The prevention of the infection in man can be achieved by not eating raw or half-cooked preparations in any form of food prepared from animal flesh or other organs of the second intermediate or paratenic hosts. Handling raw animal organs, flesh, or carcasses of these animals should only be done wearing hand-gloves or be followed with frequent hand washing to prevent skin infection. Untreated freshwater likely to be contaminated with larvae should not be drunk. Health education of the public on the above principles of personal prevention of the infection is required (Daengsvang, 1977).

Thelaziosis

Thelaziosis is an infection of the conjunctiva of domestic and wild dogs and cats with the spiruroid nematode parasites *Thelazia californiensis* in western USA, and *Thelazia callipaeda* in dogs in Asia (Weinmann, 1977) and Europe (Rossi and Bertaglia, 1989). In the hilly or mountainous areas in California deer and jackrabbits are probably the principal reservoir hosts (Weinmann *et al.*, 1974). The disease is also known as eyeworms. Various muscoid non-biting flies serve as arthropod intermediate hosts that transmit the parasite. Infection in the conjunctival sac of man is occasionally reported.

Disease in animals

Adult worms live in the conjunctival sac, especially beneath the nictitating membrane, on the surfaces of the eye. Females produce embryonated eggs and flies pick up L_1-larvae by lapping eye secretions of infected animals. In the fly, the L_3 develops within 2 to 4 weeks, migrates to the mouthparts and will be transmitted to the final host where they mature within 2 to 6 weeks. Adults can survive in the eye for many years and larvae can overwinter in the dipteran pupae (Weinmann, 1977). Infections are commonly asymptomatic or with mild lacrimation, conjunctivitis and photophobia. Heavy infestations may cause keratitis and cornea lesions.

The diagnosis can be made on the clinical signs and by finding adult parasites in the conjunctival sac or microscopic identification of larvae in the lacrimal secretions.

The parasite, measuring 0.5 mm to 1.5 cm, can be removed under (local) anaesthesia with fine forceps or moistened cotton applicators. Levamisole, applied topically as a 1% aqueous solution (Quinn *et al.*, 1997) and avermectins at 200 µg per kg are effective as treatment (Lloyd, 1998b).

Control can be achieved by preventing contacts with flies and by the use of insect repellents in endemic areas.

Disease in man

Humans, mainly young children and babies, are infected when infected flies are feeding around their eyes. The disease is mild with symptoms limited to (unilateral) pain, conjunctivitis, increased lacrimation, and the sensation of a foreign body in the eye (Weinmann, 1977). The symptoms resolve in most cases immediately after removal of the worm(s) (Doezie *et al.*, 1996; Cheung *et al.*, 1998). The diagnosis and control can be made as described in animal infections.

Strongyloidosis

Strongyloides stercoralis is an intestinal threadworm of dogs, primates and man and is distributed in humid tropical and subtropical regions and warm temperate zones. The parasite is found in the southern USA and in southern European countries such as Spain, Portugal, Romania, and Italy. Threadworms have both free-living and parasitic generations. The growing importance of human strongyloidosis depends upon the unique ability of *S. stercoralis* to replicate within its host and behave as a potentially fatal opportunistic pathogen in immunocompromised hosts (Nolan *et al.*, 1998). The parasite can be present in man many years after leaving an endemic area.

Mode of transmission

Adult parthenogenetic female *S. stercoralis* worms are situated in the intestinal mucosa where they produce embryonated eggs that hatch internally. The L_1 rhabditiform pre-infective larvae that appear in the feces within 1 to 2 weeks, can give rise to L_3 infective filariform larvae. These larvae can survive about 2 weeks in the soil and are killed by drying or by excessive moisture. They invade the host by active penetration of the skin (direct development). The L_1 larvae can also develop to free-living adult male and female worms that produce eggs which may develop into either L_3 infective larvae (indirect development) or into free-living adults (Nolan *et al.*, 1998). After percutaneous entry, usually of the feet or lower legs, the larvae penetrate the circulation and arrive via different pathways, among which pulmonary and tracheal migration, in the intestines (Schad *et al.*, 1989). Oral infection is of limited importance because of the acid stomach as barrier.

A third life history alternative is autoinfection when eggs laid in the host develop to infectivity and re-infect the same host by penetration of the perianal skin or the wall of the large intestine. A persistent infection for decades or life-long can occur because of this autoinfection phenomena. This process of autoinfection can lead to hyperinfection in which there is an extremely high parasite burden or severe clinical condition known as "disseminated strongyloidosis".

Disease in animals

Concentration of infective larvae may occur in the vicinity of kennels leading to sporadic outbreaks of disease (Quinn *et al.*, 1997). In young pups, hyperinfective strongyloidosis occurs spontaneously (Schad *et al.*, 1993). The disease is usually mild and self-limiting, but in some cases verminous interstitial bronchopneumonia caused by migrating larvae and watery or mucus diarrhea due to adult worm activity can be seen (Genta *et al.*, 1986). Penetration of the infective larvae into the skin may produce an intense local pruritis and erythema. Older dogs are rarely severely infected and the prognosis is good, except in dogs infected with the southeast Asian (Indochinese) strain of the parasite (Nolan *et al.*, 1998). Hyperinfection in immunosuppressed dogs is reported (Schad *et al.*, 1984).

Diagnosis

The diagnosis of *S. stercoralis* infection by direct fecal examination is complicated because there is intermittent larval shedding and larvae may be absent from the feces even in symptomatic cases. The Baermann technique can be used to collect larvae from fresh feces, while transtracheal washing may reveal migrating L_3 larvae. Infectious stools held at room temperature for 24 to 96 hours might contain a variety of stages, including free-living adults.

Methods of control

Clinical cases should be isolated. The free-living larval stages are sensitive to desiccation and therefore a clean, dry environment provides effective control (Nolan *et al.*, 1998).

Treatment of patients with anthelmintics will not kill the migrating autoinfective L_3 larvae in very young or immunosuppressed dogs, but will remove adult *S. stercoralis* worms from the intestine. A 3-day course of thiabendazole (50 mg per kg orally, twice daily), a 5-day course of fenbendazole (50 mg per kg orally, once daily) (Quinn *et al.*, 1997), or one dose ivermectin 200 µg per kg (Mansfield and Schad, 1992) are effective. Reduction in serum antibody isotype responses to *S. stercoralis* following treatment may be used to assess the effectiveness of ivermectin in treating endemic strongyloidosis (Lindo *et al.*, 1996). When hyperinfection is suspected, fenbendazole once daily for 7 to 14 days at 50 mg per kg, or ivermectin 200 µg per kg, once every 4 days for 3 or 4 doses, can be used to prevent new autoinfective larvae from being produced (Mansfield and Schad, 1992). Follow-up fecal examinations are advised as control of parasitological cure.

Disease in man

The majority of *S. stercoralis* infections in man are either asymptomatic or have mild, non-specific symptoms. The skin penetration may cause a form of pruritic exanthema known as "ground itch", and the following passage through the lungs can cause diffuse pneumonitis. Symptoms of coughing, dyspnoea, eosinophilia, and fever may be present. Moderate infections are characterized by gastrointestinal symptoms such as abdominal pain, episodes of, sometimes bloody, diarrhea alternating with constipation.

Patients suffering from diseases that suppress immune function or that are being treated with immunosuppressive drugs are susceptible to the development of disseminated strongyloidosis. More autoinfective larvae complete the cycle (hyperinfection) and the number of parasitic adult worms increases (Genta, 1992). Massive larval migration in lungs, meningeal spaces, brain, liver, stomach, pancreas, kidneys, lymph nodes, cutaneous and subcutaneous tissues causes mechanical damage, inflammatory responses, Gram-negative bacterial infections carried from fecal material, and may cause the patient's death. Fulminant intestinal parasitism with severe enteritis is responsible for persistent and profuse diarrhea that may be watery, mucoid or bloody as a result of malabsorption, exudation (protein loosing enteropathy), and altered intestinal motility. Bacterial enterocolitis, sepsis with abscesses in various organs, and finally paralytic ileus has been reported (Igra-Siegmann *et al.*, 1981). In the lungs pulmonary bleeding, diffuse bronchopneumonia and the development of abscesses (pulmonary strongyloidosis) can occur (Berk and Verghese, 1988). Bacterial meningitis, as a result of cerebrospinal strongyloidosis is the most frequent central nervous system manifestation (Igra-Siegmann *et al.*, 1981). In some cases cerebral and cerebellar abscesses containing *S. stercoralis* larvae may be found (Masdeu *et al.*, 1982). Patients with chronic strongyloidosis may demonstrate different cutaneous manifestations such as urticarial rashes, characteristic dermatitis caused by migrating filariform larvae, or generalized cutaneous purpura (Kuster and Genta, 1989). Other reported rare systemic manifestations are arthritis caused by immune complexes containing *S. stercoralis* antigens (Brocq *et al.*, 1996), cardiac problems caused by migrating larvae in the myocardium, and genital lesions after passage of larvae in the sperm (Nolan *et al.*, 1998).

Diagnosis

The diagnosis may be suggestive by the clinical signs and symptoms, supported by the presence of eosinophilia, radiographic findings of the gastrointestinal tract and in the presence of dissemination of the respiration tract.

The only certain method of diagnosis is by identifying larvae in the feces by direct examination of several specimens of the stool or the Baermann technique, preferably after a charcoal culture of the feces. It is advised to examine several consecutive stool specimens because of the intermittent larval shedding (Dreyer *et al.*, 1996). A more sensitive and easy detection method is the use of modified agar plates (Koga *et al.*, 1991; Kaminsky, 1993). After 3 days examination, 96%

among positive cases could be detected (Moustafa, 1997). Eosinophilia is the only hematological abnormality in chronic strongyloidosis, but considerable variation is possible. Therefore several blood examinations are sometimes required to confirm the finding. Patients with disseminated strongyloidosis usually have normal eosinophil counts (Nolan *et al.*, 1998). The indirect immunofluorescence test and ELISA can be used to detect parasite-specific IgG antibodies (Bianco, 1993).

Methods of control

Proper and sanitary disposal and treatment of excrements can prevent infection with *S. stercoralis*. Wearing of shoes helps to avoid contact with possibly contaminated soil.

It is also important that, before any patient known to have resided in the tropics, even many years previously, is given immunosuppressive therapy, examination for *Strongyloides* should be made. Hyperinfection with *Strongyloides* should be considered in any patient from the tropics before laparotomy is performed.

Thiabendazole, at a dosage of 25 mg per kg per day for 2 days, is recommended for treatment of chronic, uncomplicated strongyloidosis. The side effects include nausea, vomiting, and dizziness in a high percentage of patients. For immunocompromised patients a double dosage is advised during a longer period. Multiple courses of therapy may be necessary to eradicate the parasite completely (Nolan *et al.*, 1998). Ivermectin (150-200 µg per kg in a single oral dose or on 2 consecutive days) is reported to be used successfully as treatment (Datry *et al.*, 1994; Marty *et al.*, 1996). All infected persons must be considered at risk for fatal hyperinfective strongyloidosis and treated with the goal of achieving parasitological cure (Nolan *et al.*, 1998).

References

Anantaphruti, M.T., Nuamtanong, S. and Waikagul, J. (1992) Effect of ivermectin on experimental gnathostomiasis in rabbits. *Tropical Medicine and Parasitology* 43, 65-67.

Ando, K., Tokura, H., Matsuoka, H., Taylor, D. and Chinzei, Y. (1992) Life cycle of *Gnathostoma nipponicum* Yamagutti 1941. *Journal of Helminthology* 66, 53-61.

Banzon, T. (1977) Capillariasis. In: Steele, J.H. (ed.) *CRC Handbook Series in Zoonoses*, Vol II. CRC Press, Boca Raton, Florida, pp. 63-65.

Bapna, S. and Renapurkar, D.M. (1996) Immunodiagnosis of early dracunculiasis. *Journal for Communicable Diseases* 28, 33-37.

Barriga, O.O. (1977) Dioctophymiasis. In: Steele, J.H. (ed.) *CRC Handbook Series in Zoonoses*, Vol II. CRC Press, Boca Raton, Florida, pp. 83-92.

Barriga, O.O. (1988) A critical look at the importance, prevalence and control of toxocariasis and the possibilities of immunological control. *Veterinary Parasitology* 29, 195-234.

Bartoloni, A., Dini, F., Farese, A., Rosso, A., Tinacci, L. and Paradisi, F. (1997) Tropical pulmonary eosinophilia. Report of a case. *Annuelles Médicine Interne* 148, 321-322.

Beaver, P.C., Jung, R.C. and Cupp, E.W. (1984) *Clinical Parasitology*. Lea and Febiger, Philadelphia.

Berk, S.L. and Verghese, A. (1988) Parasitic pneumonia. *Seminars in Respiratory Infection* 3, 172-178.

Bianco, A.E. (1993) Immunodiagnosis of *Strongyloides stercoralis* infection: a method for increasing the specificity of the indirect ELISA. *Transactions of the Royal Society for Tropical Medicine and Hygiene* 87, 173-176.

Biswas, J., Gopal, L., Sharma, T. and Badrinath, S.S. (1994) Intraocular *Gnathostoma spinigerum*. Clinicopathologic study of two cases with review of literature. *Retina* 14, 438-444.

Bloch, P. and Simonsen, P.E. (1998) Studies on immunodiagnosis of dracunculiasis. I. Detection of specific serum antibodies. *Acta Tropica* 70, 73-86.

Bloch, P., Vennervald, B.J. and Simonsen, P.E. (1998) Studies on immunodiagnosis of dracunculiasis. II. Search for circulating antigens. *Acta Tropica* 70, 303-315.

Boongird, P., Phnapradit, P., Siridej, N., Chirachariyavej, T., Chuahirun, S. and Vejjajiva, A. (1977) Neurological manifestations of gnathostomiasis. *Journal of Neurological Science* 31, pp. 279.

Bosse, M. and Stoye, M. (1981) Zur Wirkung verschiedener Benzimidazolcarbamate auf somatische Larven von *Ancylostoma caninum* ERCOLANI 1859 (Ancylosomidae) und *Toxocara canis* WERNER 1782 (Anisakidae). 2. Untersuchungen an der graviden Hündin. *Zeitblatt Veterinär Medizin* 28, 265-279.

Bowman, D.D. (1991) Effects of milbemycin oxime on adult *Ancylostoma caninum* and *Uncinaria stenocephala* in dogs with experimentally induced infection. *American Journal of Veterinary Research* 52, 64-67.

Brocq, O., Breuil, V., Agopian, V., Grisot, C., Flory, P., Bernard-Pomier, G., Ziegler, G. and Euller-Ziegler, L. (1996) Reactive arthritis induced by *Strongyloides stercoralis*. *Reviews Rheumatology* (English Edition) 63, 217-219.

Buijs, J., Borsboom, G., Renting, M., Hilgersom, W.H.H., Wieringen, J.C. van, Jansen, G. and Neijens, J. (1997) Relationship between allergic manifestations and *Toxocara* seropositivity: a cross-sectional study among elementary school children. *European Respiratory Journal* 10, 1467-1475.

Burke, T.M. and Roberson, E.L. (1983) Fenbendazole treatment of pregnant bitches to reduce prenatal and lactogenic infections of *Toxocara canis* and *Ancylostoma caninum* in pups. *Journal of the American Veterinary Medical Association* 183, 987-990.

Cancrini, G., d'Amelio, S., Mattiucci, S. and Coluzzi, M. (1991) Identification of *Dirofilaria* in man by multilocus electrophoretic analysis. *Annals of Tropical Medicine and Parasitology* 85, 529-532.

Carroll, S.M. and Grove, D.I. (1986) Experimental infection of humans with *Ancylostoma ceylanicum*: clinical, parasitological, haematological and immunological findings. *Tropical Geographic Medicine* 38, 38-45.

Caumes, E., Carrière, J., Datry, A., Gaxotte, P., Danis, M. and Gentilini, M.A. (1993) Randomized trial of ivermectin versus albendazole for the treatment of cutaneous larva migrans. *American Journal of Tropical Medicine and Hygiene* 49, 641-644.

CDC (2000) *Guinea Worm Wrap Up*. 97, Centers for Disease Control and Prevention, Atlanta, Georgia, pp. 12.

Chalifoux, L. and Hunt, R.D. (1971) Histochemical differentiation of *Dirofilaria immitis* and *Dipetalonema reconditum*. *Journal of the American Veterinary Medical Association* 158, 601-605.

Chandrashekar, R. (1997) Recent advances in diagnosis of filarial infections. *Indian Journal of Experimental Biology* 35, 18-26.

Chen, Q.Q. and Lin, X.M. (1991) A survey of epidemiology of *Gnathostoma hispidum* and experimental studies of its larvae in animals. *Southeast Asian Journal of Tropical Medicine and Public Health* 22, 611-617.

Cheung, W.K., Lu, H.J., Liang, C.H., Peng, M.L. and Lee, H.H. (1998) Conjunctivitis caused by *Thelazia callipaeda* infestation in a woman. *Journal of the Formosa Medical Association* 97, 425-427.

Cross, J.H. (1998) Capillariosis. In: Palmer, S.R., Lord Soulsby and Simpson, D.I.H. (eds) *Zoonoses. Biology, Clinical Practice and Public Health Control.* Oxford University Press, pp. 759-772.

Cuellar, C., Fenoy, S. and Guilen, J.L. (1995) Cross-reactions of sera from *Toxascaris leonina* and *Ascaris suum* infected mice with *Toxocara canis*, *Toxascaris leonina* and *Ascaris suum* antigens. *International Journal of Parasitology* 25, 731-739.

Daengsvang, S. (1976) Contributions to natural sources and methods of transmission of *Gnathostoma spinigerum* in Thailand. *Southeast Asian Journal of Tropical Medicine and Public Health* 7, pp. 95.

Daengsvang, S. (1977) Gnathostomiasis. In: Steele, J.H. (ed.) *CRC Handbook Series in Zoonoses*, Vol II. CRC Press, Boca Raton, Florida, pp. 147-161.

Datry, A., Hilmarsdottir, I., Mayorga-Sagastume, R., Lyagoubi, M., Gaxotte, P., Biligui, S., Chodakewitz, J., Neu, D., Danis, M. and Gentilini, M. (1994) Treatment of *Strongyloides stercoralis* infection with ivermectin compared with albendazole: results of an open study of 60 cases. *Transactions of the Royal Society for Tropical Medicine and Hygiene* 88, 344-355.

Davies, H.D., Sakuls, P. and Keystone, J.S. (1993) Creeping eruption: a review of clinical presentation and management of 60 cases presenting to a tropical disease unit. *Archives of Dermatology* 129, 588-591.

Denham, D.A. (1998) Zoonotic infections with filarial nematodes. In: Palmer, S.R., Lord Soulsby and Simpson, D.I.H. (eds) *Zoonoses. Biology, Clinical Practice and Public Health Control.* Oxford University Press, pp. 783-788.

Denham, D.A. and McGreevy, P.B. (1977) Brugian filariasis: epidemiological and experimental studies. *Advances in Parasitology* 16, 243-309.

Doezie, A.M., Lucius, R.W., Aldeen, W., Hale, D.V., Smith, D.R. and Mamalis, N. (1996) *Thelazia californiensis* conjunctival infestation. *Ophthalmic Surgery Lasers* 27, 716-719.

Dreyer, G., Fernandes-Silva, E., Alves, S., Rocha, A., Albuquerque, R. and Addiss, D. (1996) Patterns of detection of *Strongyloides stercoralis* in stool specimens: implications for diagnosis and clinical trials. *Journal of Clinical Microbiology* 34, 2569-2571.

Dubey, J.P. (1969) Migration and development of *Toxascaris leonina* in mice. *Tropical Geographical Medicine* 21, 214-218.

Eberhard, M.L. and Brandt, F.H. (1995) The role of tadpoles and frogs as paratenic hosts in the life cycle of *Dracunculus insignis* (Nematoda: Dracunculoidea). *Journal of Parasitology* 81, 792-793.

Eberhard, M.L., Brandt, F.H., Ruiz-Tiben, E. and Hightower, A. (1990) Chemoprophylactic drug trials for treatment of dracunculiasis using the *Dracunculus insignis*-ferret model. *Journal of Helminthology* 64, 79-86.

Ehrhard, T. and Kernbaum, S. (1979) *Toxocara canis* et toxocarose humaine. *Bulletin de l'Institut Pasteur* 77, 225-287.

Epe, C., Schnieder, T. and Stoye, M. (1996) Möglichkeiten und Grenzen der chemotherapeutischen Bekämpfung vertikaler Infektionen mit *Toxocara canis* und *Ancylostoma caninum* beim Hund. *Praktische Tierarzt* pp. 483-490.

Evans, N.A., Bishop, B.F., Bruce, C.I., Goudie, A.C., Gration, K.A.F., Gibson, S.P., Pacey, M.S., Perry, D.A. and Witty, M.J. (1999) Discovery and biological spectrum of selamectin. *Proceedings Pfizer Symposium 17th International Conference of the WAAVP,* Copenhagen, Denmark, pp. 11-15.

Evinger, J.V., Kazacos, K.R. and Cantwell, H.D. (1985) Ivermectin for treatment of nasal capillariasis in a dog. *Journal of the American Veterinary Medical Association* 186, 174-175.

Fenoy, S., Cuéllar, C. and Guillén, J.L. (1997) Serological evidence of toxocariasis in patients from Spain with a clinical suspicion of visceral larva migrans. *Journal of Helminthology* 71, 9-12.

Fernando, S.S. (1983) The giant kidney worm (*Dioctophyma renale*) infection in man in Australia. *American Journal of Surgery and Pathology* 7, 281-284.

Fisher, M.A., Jacobs, D.E., Hutchinson, M.J. and Dick, I.G.C. (1994) Studies on the control of *Toxocara canis* in breeding kennels. *Veterinary Parasitology* 55, 87-92.

Fok, E. and Kassai, T. (1998) *Toxocara canis* infection in the paratenic host: a study on the chemosusceptibility of the somatic larvae in mice. *Veterinary Parasitology* 74, 243-259.

Gardiner, C.H., Oberdorfer, C.E., Reyes, J.E. and Pinkus, W.H. (1978) Infection of man by *Dirofilaria repens*. *American Journal of Tropical Medicine and Hygiene* 27, 1279-1281.

Genta, R.M. (1992) Dysregulation of strongyloidiasis: a new hypothesis. *Clinical Microbiological Reviews* 5, 345-355.

Genta, R.M., Schad, G.A. and Hellman, M.E. (1986) *Strongyloides stercoralis*: parasitological, immunological and pathological observations in immunosuppressed dogs. *Transactions of the Royal Society for Tropical Medicine and Hygiene* 80, 34-41.

Georgi, J.R. and Georgi, M.E. (1990) Hookworm disease of dogs. In: Georgi, J.R. and Georgi, M.E. (eds) *Parasitology for Veterinarians*, 5th edn. W.B. Saunders, Philadelphia, pp. 172-177.

Ghenis, D.E. (1972) New cases of *Dracunculus medinensis* L., 1758 detected in domestic cats and dogs in Kazakhstan. *Medicale Parazitology Bol* 41, pp. 365.

Gillespie, S.H. (1993) The clinical spectrum of human toxocariasis. In: Lewis, R.M. and Maizels, R.M. (eds) *Toxocara and Toxocariasis, Clinical, Epidemiological and Molecular Perspectives*. British Society for Parasitology and Institute of Biology, London, pp. 55-61.

Girdwood, R.W.A. (1986) Human toxocariasis. *Journal of Small Animal Practice* 27, 649-654.

Girdwood, R.W.A., Smith, H.V., Bruce, R.G. and Quinn, R. (1978) Human *Toxocara* infection in west of Scotland. *Lancet* June 17, pp. 1318.

Glickman, L.T. and Magnaval, J.F. (1993) Zoonotic roundworm infections. *Infectious Diseases of North America* 7, 717-732.

Glickman, L.T. and Schantz, P.M. (1981) Epidemiology and pathogenesis of zoonotic toxocariasis. *Epidemiologic Reviews* 3, 230-250.

Glickman, L.T. and Shofer, F.S. (1987) Zoonotic visceral and ocular larva migrans. *Veterinary Clinics of North America* 17, 39-53.

Harvey, J.B., Roberts, J.M. and Schantz, P.M. (1991) Survey of veterinarians recommendations for treatment and control of intestinal parasites in dogs: Public health implications. *Journal of the American Veterinary Medical Association* 199, 702-707.

Hendrix, C.M., Homer, B.S., Kellman, N.J., Harrelson, G. and Bruhn, B.F. (1996) Cutaneous larva migrans and enteric hookworm infections. *Journal of the American Veterinary Medical Association* 209, 1763-1767.

Henry, C.J. and Dillon, R. (1994) Heartworm disease in dogs. *Journal of the American Veterinary Medical Association* 204, 1148-1151.

Hinz, E. (1980) Intestinal helminths in Bangkok: stray dogs and their role in public health. *Zentralblatt Bakteriologische und Mikrobiologische Hygiene B* 171, 79-85.

Hugh-Jones, M.E., Hubbert, W.T. and Hagstad, H.V. (1995) Dracunculiasis. In: Hugh-Jones, M.E., Hubbert, W.T. and Hagstad, H.V. (eds) *Zoonoses, Recognition, Control, and Prevention*, 1st edn. Iowa State University Press.

Igra-Siegmann, Y., Kapila, R., Sen, P., Kaminski, Z.C. and Louria, D.B. (1981) Syndrome of hyperinfection with *Strongyloides stercoralis*. *Reviews of the Infectious Diseases* 3, 397-407.

Issaka-Tinorgah, A., Magnussen, P., Bloch, P. and Yakubu, A. (1994) Lack of effect of ivermectin on prepatent guinea-worm: a single-blind, placebo-controlled trial. *Transactions of the Royal Society of Tropical Medicine and Hygiene* 88, 346-348.

Jacobs, D.E., Pegg, E.J. and Stevenson, P. (1977) Helminths of British dogs: *Toxocara canis*, a veterinary perspective. *Journal of Small Animal Practice* 18, 79-92.

Jacobs, D.E. (1987) Control of *Toxocara canis* in puppies: a comparison of screening techniques and evaluation of a dosing programme. *Journal of Veterinary Pharmacology and Therapy* 10, 23-29.

Jacobs, D.E., Zhu, X., Gasser, R.B. and Chilton, N.B. (1997) PCR-based methods for identification of potentially zoonotic ascaridoid parasites of the dog, fox and cat. *Acta Tropica* 68, 191-200.

Jelinek, T., Maiwald, H., Nothdurft, H.D. and Loscher, T. (1994) Cutaneous larva migrans in travelers: synopsis of histories, symptoms, and treatment of 98 patients. *Clinical Infectious Diseases* 19, 1062-1066.

Jordan, H.E., Mullins, S.T. and Stebbins, M.E. (1993) Endoparasitism in dogs: 21,583 cases (1981-1990). *Journal of the American Veterinary Medical Association* 203, 547-549.

Joseph, S.A. and Kandazamy, S. (1980) On the occurrence of the guinea-worm, *Dracunculus medinensis* (Linnaeus, 1758) Gallaidant 1773 in an Alsatian dog. *Cherion* 9, 198-199.

Kale, O.O. (1977a) Dracontiasis. In: Steele, J.H. (ed.) *CRC Handbook Series in Zoonoses*, Vol II. CRC Press, Boca Raton, Florida, pp. 111-122.

Kale, O.O. (1977b) The clinico-epidemiological profile of guinea-worm in the Ibadan district of Nigeria. *American Journal of Tropical Medicine and Hygiene* 26, pp. 208.

Kale, O.O., Elemile, T. and Enahoro, F. (1983) Controlled comparative trial of thiabendazole and metronidazole in the treatment of dracontiasis. *Annals of Tropical Medicine and Parasitology* 77, 151-157.

Kalkoven, U.P. (1987) Hookworms of dogs and cats. *Veterinary Clinics of North America* 17, 1341-1354.

Kaminsky, R.G. de (1993) Evaluation of three methods for laboratory diagnosis of *Strongyloides stercoralis* infection. *Journal of Parasitology* 79, 277-280.

Karbach, G. and Stoye, M. (1982) Occurence of prenatal and lactogenic infections caused by *Toxascaris leonina* Leiper 1907 (Ascaridae) in the mouse. *Zentralblatt Veterinärmedizin Reihe B* 29, 219-230.

Kassai, T. (1995) Chemotherapy of larval toxocarosis: progress and problems. Overview from veterinary aspects. *Helminthologia* 32, 133-141.

Knapen, F. van and Buijs, J. (1993) Diagnosis of *Toxocara* infection. In: Lewis, R.M. and Maizels, R.M. (eds) *Toxocara and Toxocariasis, Clinical, Epidemiological and Molecular Perspectives*. British Society for Parasitology and Institute of Biology, London, pp. 49-53.

Knapen, F. van., Leusden, J. van., Polderman, A.M. and Franchimont, J.H. (1983) Visceral Larva Migrans: examinations by means of enzyme-linked immunosorbent assay of human sera for antibodies to excretory-secretory antigens of the second-stage larvae of *Toxocara canis*. *Zeitschrift für Parasitenkunde* 69, 113-118.

Koga, K., Kasuya, S., Khamboonruang, C., Sukhavat, K., Ieda, M., Takatsuka, N., Kita, K. and Ohtomo, H. (1991) A modified agar plate method for detection of *Strongyloides stercoralis*. *American Journal of Tropical Medicine and Hygiene* 45, 518-521.

Kuster, L. von. and Genta, R.M. (1989) Cutaneous manifestations of strongyloidiasis. *Archives of Dermatology* 124, 1826-1830.

Lalitha, C.M. and Anandan, R. (1980) Guinea worm infection in dogs. *Chieron* 9, 198-199.

Lindo, J.F., Atkins, N.S., Lee, M.G., Robinson, R.D. and Bundy, D.A. (1996) Short report: long-term serum antibody isotype responses to *Strongyloides stercoralis* filariform antigens in eight patients treated with ivermectin. *American Journal of Tropical Medicine and Hygiene* 55, 474-476.

Lindsay, D.S. and Blagburn, B.L. (1995) Practical treatment and control of infections caused by canine gastrointestinal parasites. *Veterinary Medicine* May, 441-455.

Little, M.D., Halsey, N.A., Cline, B.L. and Katz, S.P. (1983) *Ancylostoma* larva in muscle fiber of man following cutaneous larva migrans. *American Journal of Tropical Medicine and Hygiene* 32, 1285-1288.

Ljungström, I. and Knapen, F. van. (1989) An epidemiological and serological study of *Toxocara* infection in Sweden. *Scandinavian Journal of Infectious Diseases* 21, 87-93.

Lloyd, S. (1998a) Toxocarosis. In: Palmer, S.R., Lord Soulsby and Simpson, D.I.H. (eds) *Zoonoses*. Oxford University Press, pp. 841-854.

Lloyd, S. (1998b) Occasional and miscellaneous zoonoses and opportunistic infections In: Palmer, S.R., Lord Soulsby and Simpson, D.I.H. (eds) *Zoonoses*. Oxford University Press, pp. 921-933.

Lloyd, S. and Soulsby, E.J.L. (1983) Prenatal and transmammary infections of *Toxocara canis* in dogs: effect of benzimidazole-carbamate anthelmintics on various developmental stages of the parasite. *Journal of Small Animal Practice* 24, 763-768.

Loukas, A., Croese, J., Opdebeeck, J. and Prociv, P. (1992) Detection of antibodies to secretions of *Ancylostoma caninum* in human eosinophilic enteritis. *Transactions of the Royal Society of Tropical Medicine and Hygiene* 86, 650-653.

Magnaval, J.F. (1995) Comparative efficacy of diethylcarbamazine and mebendazole for the treatment of human toxocariasis. *Parasitology* 110, 529-533.

Magnaval, J.F., Fabre, R., Maurières, P., Charlet, J.P. and Larrard, B. de (1991) Application of the Western-blotting procedure for the immunodiagnosis of human toxocariasis. *Parasitology Research* 77, 697-702.

Mak, J.W., Navaratnam, V., Grewel, J.S., Mansor, S.M. and Ambu, S. (1993) Treatment of subperiodic *Brugia malayi* infection with a single dose of ivermectin. *American Journal of Tropical Medicine and Hygiene* 48, 591-596.

Maleewong, W., Wongkham, C., Intapan, P., Mahaisavariya, P., Danseegaew, W., Pipitgool, V. and Morakote, N. (1992) Detection of circulating parasite antigens in murine gnathostomiasis by a two-site enzyme-linked immunosorbent assay. *American Journal of Tropical Medicine and Hygiene* 46, 80-84.

Mansfield, L.S. and Schad, G.A. (1992) Ivermectin treatment of naturally acquired and experimentally induced *Strongyloides stercoralis* infections in dogs. *Journal of the American Veterinary Medicine Asscociation* 201, 726-730.

Marmor, M., Glickman, L., Shofer, F., Faich, L.A., Rosenberg, C., Cornblatt, B. and Friedman, S. (1987) *Toxocara canis* infection of children: epidemiologic and neuropsychologic findings. *Journal of Infectious Diseases* 149, 591-597.

Marty, P. (1997) Human dirofilariasis due to *Dirofilaria repens* in France. A review of reported cases. *Parasitologia* 39, 383-386.

Marty, H., Haji, H.J., Savioli, L., Chwaya, H.M., Mgeni, A.F., Ameir, J.S. and Hatz, C. (1996) A comparative trial of a single-dose ivermectin versus three days of albendazole for treatment of *Strongyloides stercoralis* and other soil-transmitted helminth infections in children. *American Journal of Tropical Medicine and Hygiene* 55, 477-481.

Masdeu, J.C., Tantulavenich, S. and Gorelick, P.P. (1982) Brain abscess caused by *Strongyloides stercoralis*. *Archives of Neurology* 39, 62-63.

Matoff, M. and Komandarev, S. (1963) Comparative studies on the migration of the larvae of *Toxascaris leonina* and *Toxascaris transfuga*. *Zeitschrift für Parasitenkunde* 23, 538-555.

McTier, T.L., McCall, J.W., Dzimanski, M.T., Raynaud, J.P. and Strickland, J.E. (1994) Use of melarsomine dihydrochloride (RM 340) for adulticidal treatment of dogs with naturally acquired infections of *Dirofilaria immitis* and for clinical prophylaxis during re-exposure for 1 year. *Veterinary Parasitology* 55, 221-233.

Measures, L.N. and Anderson, R.C. (1985) Centrarchid fish as paratenic hosts of the giant kidney worm, *Dioctophyma renale* (Goeze, 1782), in Ontario, Canada. *Journal of Wildlife Diseases* 21, 11-19.

Melker, H.E., de Peet, T.E., van der Berbers, G.A.M., Akker, R., van de Knapen, F. van, Schellekens, J.F.P. and Coneyn-van Spaendonck, M.A.E. (1995) Pilot-study for the PIENTER-Project. Report nr. 213675004 National Institute of Public Health and Environmental Protection, Bilthoven, The Netherlands, pp. 37-38.

Migasena, S., Pitisuttithum, P. and Desakorn, V. (1991) *Gnathostoma* larva migrans among guests of a New Year party. *Southeast Asian Journal of Tropical Medicine and Public Health* 22, 225-227.

Miller, A.C., Walker, J., Jaworski, R., Launey, W. de and Paver, R. (1991) Hookworm folliculitis. *Archives of Dermatology* 127, 547-549.

Miller, T.A. (1971) Vaccination against the canine hookworm disease. *Advances in Parasitology* 9, 153-183.

Mims, C.A., Playfair, J.H.L., Roitt, I.M., Wakelin, D., Williams, R. and Anderson, R.M. (1993) *Medical Microbiology*. Mosby, St Louis, Missouri.

Moustafa, M.A. (1997) An evaluation of the modified agar plate method for diagnosis of *Strongyloides stercoralis*. *Journal of the Egyptian Society for Parasitology* 27, 571-579.

Muller, R. (1991) Dracunculus in Africa. In: Macpherson, C.N.L. and Craig, P.S. (eds) *Parasitic Helminths and Zoonoses*. Unwin Hyman, pp. 204-223.

Muller, R. (1999) Slaying the little dragon. *Biologist* 46, 57-60.

Nawa, Y. (1991) Historical review and current status of gnathostomiasis in Asia. *Southeast Asian Journal of Tropical Medicine and Public Health* 22, 217-220.

Nolan, T.J., Genta, R.M. and Schad, G.A. (1998) Strongyloidosis. In: Palmer, S.R., Lord Soulsby and Simpson, D.I.H. (eds) *Zoonoses. Biology, Clinical Practice and Public Health Control*. Oxford University Press, pp. 747-757.

Nopparatana, C., Setasuban, P., Chaicumpa, W. and Tapchaisri, P. (1991) Purification of *Gnathostoma spinigerum* specific antigen and diagnosis of human gnathostomiasis. *International Journal of Parasitology* 21, 677-687.

Nuamtanong, S., Waikagul, J. and Anantaphruti, M.T. (1998) *Gnathostoma* infection in swamp eels, *Fluta alba,* in central Thailand. *Southeast Asian Journal of Tropical Medicine and Public Health* 29, 144-147.

Obwaller, A., Jensen-Jarolim, E., Auer, H., Huber, A., Kraft, D. and Aspöck, H. (1998) *Toxocara* infestations in humans: symptomatic course of toxocarosis correlates significantly with levels of IgE/anti-IgE immune complexes. *Parasite Immunology* 20, 311-317.

Okoshi, S. and Osui, M. (1968a) Experimental studies on *Toxascaris leonina*. V. Experimental infection of dogs and cats with eggs of canine, feline and Felidae strains. *Japanese Journal of Veterinary Science* 30, 81-91.

Okoshi, S. and Osui, M. (1968b) Experimental studies on *Toxascaris leonina*. VI. Experimental infection of mice, chickens and earthworms with *Toxascaris leonina*, *Toxocara canis* and *Toxocara cati*. *Japanese Journal of Veterinary Science* 30, 151-160.

Okoye, S.N., Onwuliri, C.O. and Anosike, J.C. (1995) A survey of prediliction sites and degree of disability associated with guineaworm (*Dracunculus medinensis*). *International Journal for Parasitology* 25, 1127-1129.

Osborne, C.A., Stevens, J.B., Hanlon, G.F., Rosin, E. and Bemrick, W.J. (1969) *Dioctophyma renale* in the dog. *Journal of the American Veterinary Medical Association* 155, pp. 605.

Overgaauw, P.A.M. (1996) Effect of a government educational campaign in the Netherlands on awareness of *Toxocara* and toxocarosis. *Preventive Veterinary Medicine* 28, 165-174.

Overgaauw, P.A.M. (1997a) Aspects of *Toxocara* epidemiology: Toxocarosis in dogs and cats. *Critical Reviews in Microbiology* 23, 233-251.

Overgaauw, P.A.M. (1997b) Aspects of *Toxocara* epidemiology: Human toxocarosis. *Critical Reviews in Microbiology* 23, 215-231.

Panciera, D.L. and Stockham, S.L. (1988) *Dracunculus insignis* infection in a dog. *Journal of the American Veterinary Medical Association* 192, 76-78.

Parsons, J.C. (1987) Ascarid infections of cats and dogs. *Veterinary Clinics of North America* 17, 1307-1339.

Partono, F., Purnomo, Oemijati, S. and Soewata, A. (1981) The long term effects of repeated diethylcarbamazine administration with special reference to microfilaraemia and elephantiasis. *Acta Tropica* 38, 217-225.

Pearson, G.R., Kennedy, S., Taylor, S.M. and Thomson, T.R. (1982) Uncinariasis in kennelled foxhounds. *Veterinary Record* 110, 328-331.

Pegg, E.J. (1977) A new approach to the control of *Toxocara canis* and other parasitic ova on concrete-floored kennel runs. *British Veterinary Journal* 133, 427-431.

Petithory, J.C., Derouin, F., Rousseau, M., Luffau, M. and Quedoc, M. (1987) Serological arguments for multiple etiology of Visceral Larva Migrans. Helminth zoonoses. In: Geerts, S., Kumar, V. and Brandt, J. (eds) *Current Topics Veterinary Medicine Animal Sciences.* Martinus Nijhoff Publishers, pp. 183-191.

Prociv, P. and Croese, J. (1996) Human enteric infection with *Ancylostoma caninum*: hookworms reappraised in the light of a 'new' zoonosis. *Acta Tropica* 62, 23-44.

Prociv, P. (1998) Zoonotic hookworm infections (ancylostomosis). In: Palmer, S.R. Lord Soulsby and Simpson, D.I.H. (eds) *Zoonoses. Biology, Clinical Practice and Public Health Control.* Oxford University Press, pp. 803-822.

Prokopic, J. and Figallova, V. (1982) The migration of larvae of *Toxascaris leonina* (Linstow 1909) in experimentally infected white mice. *Folia Parasitologia (Praha)* 29, 233-238.

Punyagupta, S., Bunnag, T. and Juttijudata, P. (1990) Eosinophilic meningitis in Thailand. Clinical and epidemiological characteristics of 162 patients with myeloencephalitis probably caused by *Gnathostoma spinigerum. Journal of Neurological Science* 96, 241-256.

Quah, B.S., Anuar, A.K., Rowani, M.R. and Pennie, R.A. (1997) Cor pulmonale: an unusual presentation of tropical eosinophilia. *Annuals of Tropical Paediatrics* 17, 77-81.

Quinn, P.J., Donnelly, W.J.C., Carter, M.E., Markey, B.K.J., Torgerson, P.R. and Breathnach, R.M.S. (1997) *Microbial and parasitic diseases of the dog and cat,* Saunders Company Ltd, Baltimore.

Rawlings, C.A. and McCall, J.W. (1996) Melarsomine: a new heartworm adulticide. *Compendium on Continuing Education for the Practicing Veterinarian* 18, 373-379.

Robinson, N.B., Chavez, C.M. and Conn, J.H. (1977) Pulmonary dirofilariasis in man: a case report and review of the literature. *Journal of Thoracic and Cardiovascular Surgery* 74, 403.

Rossi, L. and Bertaglia, P.P. (1989) Presence of *Thelazia callipaeda* Raillietand Henry, 1910, in Piedmont, Italy. *Parassitologia* 31, 167-172.

Rusnak, J.M. and Lucey, D.R. (1993) Clinical gnathostomiasis: case report and review of the English-language literature. *Clinics in Infectious Diseases* 16, 33-50.

Schad, G.A., Hellman, M.E. and Muncey, D.W. (1984) *Strongyloides stercoralis*: hyperinfection in immunosuppressed dogs. *Experimental Parasitology* 57, 287-296.

Schad, G.A., Aikens, L.M. and Smith, G. (1989) *Strongyloides stercoralis*: is there a canonical migratory route through the host? *Journal of Parasitology* 75, 740-749.

Schad, G.A., Smith, G., Megyeri, Z., Bhopale, V.M., Niamatali, S. and Maze, R. (1993) *Strongyloides stercoralis*: an initial autoinfective burst amplifies primary infection. *American Journal of Tropical Medicine* 48, 716-725.

Schantz, P.M. (1981) Zoonotic toxocariasis: dimensions of the problem and the veterinarian's role in prevention. *Proceedings of the United States Animal Health Association* 85, 396-398.

Schantz, P.M. (1989) *Toxocara* larva migrans now. *American Journal of Tropical Medicine and Hygiene* 41, 21-34.

Scheuer, P. (1987) Sensitivity and specifity of IFAT and ELISA for determination of impatent infections with ascarides and anncylostomides in the dog. *PhD Thesis* University of Hannover.

Schmutzhard, E., Boongird, P. and Vejjajiva, A. (1988) Eosinophilic meningitis and radiculomyelitis in Thailand, caused by CNS invasion of *Gnathostoma spinigerum* and *Angiostrongylus cantonensis*. *Journal of Neurosurgery and Psychiatry* 51, 80-87.

Schnieder, T., Heideman, R. and Epe, C. (1994) Investigations into the efficacy of doramectin on reactivated somatic larvae of *Ancylostoma caninum* in pregnant bitches. *Journal of Veterinary Medicine* 41, 603-607.

Schnieder, T., Kordes, S., Epe, C., Kuschfeldt, S. and Stoye, M. (1996) Investigations into the prevention of neonatal *Toxocara canis* infections in puppies by application of doramectin to the bitch. *Journal of Veterinary Medicine B* 43, 35-43.

Schrey, C.F. (1996) Epidemiological prevalence survey and clinical aspects of canine heartworm disease in Germany. PhD Thesis, Free University of Berlin.

Schrey, C.F. and Trautvetter, E. (1998) Canine and feline heartworm disease. Diagnosis and therapy. *Waltham Focus* 8, 23-30.

Shenoy, R.K., Varghese, J., Kuttikkal, V.V. and Kumaraswami, V. (1998a) The efficacy, tolerability and safety of diethylcarbamazine-fortified salt in the treatment of the microfilaraemias of brugian filariasis: an open, hospital-based study. *Annals of Tropical Medicine and Parasitology* 92, 285-293.

Shenoy, R.K., George, L.M., John, A., Suma, T.K. and Kumaraswami, V. (1998b) Treatment of microfilaraemia in asymptomatic brugian filariasis: the efficacy and safety of the combination of single doses of ivermectin and diethylcarbamazine. *Annals of Tropical Medicine and Parasitology* 92, 579-585.

Smith, H.V. (1993) Antibody reactivity in human toxocariasis. In: Lewis, R.M. and Maizels, R.M. (eds) *Toxocara and Toxocariasis, Clinical, Epidemiological and Molecular Perspectives*. British Society for Parasitology and Institute of Biology, London, pp. 91-109.

Sprent, J.F.A. (1959) The life history and development of *Toxascaris leonina* (von Linstow 1902) in the dog and the cat. *Parasitology* 49, 330-371.

Stehr-Green, J. and Schantz, P.M. (1987) The impact of zoonotic diseases transmitted by pets on human health and the economy. *Veterinary Clinics of North America* 17, 1-16.

Stoye, M., Meyer, O. and Schneider, T. (1989) Effect of ivermectin on reactivated somatic larvae *of Ancylostoma caninum* Ercolani 1859 (Ancylostomidae) in the pregnant bitch. *Journal of Veterinary Medicine* 36, 271-278.

Strickland, K.N. (1998) Canine and feline caval syndrome. *Clinical and Technical Small Animal Practice* 13, 88-95.

Stürchler, D., Weiss, N. and Gassner, M. (1990) Transmission of Toxocariasis. *Journal of Infectious Diseases* 162, 571.

Subrahmanyam, B., Reddy, Y.R. and Paul, S. (1976) *Dracunculus medinensis* (guinea worm) infestation in a dog and its treatment with 'Flagyl'. A case report. *Indian Veterinary Journal* 53, 637-639.

Sun, T., Turnbull, A., Liebermann, P.H. and Sternberg, S.S. (1986) Giant kidney worm (*Dioctophyma renale*) infection mimicking retroperitoneal neoplasm. *American Journal of Surgery and Pathology* 10, 508-512.

Tan, J.S. (1997) Human zoonotic infections transmitted by dogs and cats. *Archives of Internal Medicine* 157, 1933-1943.

Taylor, M.R.H. (1993) Toxocariasis in Ireland. In: Lewis, R.M. and Maizels, R.M. (eds) *Toxocara and Toxocariasis, Clinical, Epidemiological and Molecular Perspectives*. British Society for Parasitology and Institute of Biology, London, pp. 71-80.

Taylor, M.R.H., Keane, C.T., O'Connor, P., Girdwood, R.W.A. and Smith, H. (1987) Clinical features of covert toxocariasis. *Scandinavian Journal of Infectious Diseases* 19, 693-696.

Todd, K.S. and Howland, T.P. (1983) Transplacental transmission of *Dirofilaria immitis* microfilariae in the dog. *Journal of Parasitology* 69, pp. 371.

Velikanov, B.P. (1984) A case of *Dracunculus medinensis* infection in a dog in Turkmenia. [In Russian] *Izvestiya Nauk Turkamanskoi SSR, Biologicheskikh Nauk* 1, 64-65.

Vilella, J.M., Desmaret, M.C. and Rouault, E. (1986) Capillariose caused by *Capillaria aerophila* in an adult? *Médecine et Maladies Infectieuses* 1, 35-36.

Wan, W.L., Cano, M.R., Pince, K.J. and Green, R.L. (1991) Echographic characteristics of ocular toxocariasis. *Opthalmology* 98, 28-32.

Weinmann, C.J. (1977) Thelaziasis. In: Steele, J.H. (ed.) *CRC Handbook Series in Zoonoses*, Vol II. CRC Press, Boca Raton, Florida, pp. 289-292.

Weinmann, C.J., Anderson, J.R., Rubtzolf, P., Connolly, G. and Longhurst, W.M. (1974) Eyeworms and face flies in California. *Californean Agiculture* 28, 4.

Chapter Nine

Dogs and Ectoparasitic Zoonoses

Cathy F. Curtis

The domestication of the dog has undoubtedly been of great benefit to humans over the centuries but, inevitably, the invitation into our homes has inadvertently been extended to a number of canine ectoparasite species. Our warm, sheltered environment enhances the survival of these 'unwanted guests' and in some cases (e.g. the cat flea *Ctenocephalides felis felis*), promotes the establishment of their own sustainable 'indoor' ecosystem, at their host's expense. As the ectoparasite population increases, the associated risk of infestation of non-host species becomes greater and human members of the household may be targeted. This chapter will describe the biology and clinical aspects of the four major canine ectoparasitic infections and associated zoonotic disease and will discuss current methods of control.

Insecta

Fleas

Biology

Fleas are brown, wingless insects of approximately 3-4 mm in length. Their polyxenous nature dictates that dogs may become infested with several different flea species such as *Ct. f. felis* (the cat flea), *Ctenocephalides canis* (the dog flea), *Archeopsylla erinacei* (hedgehog flea), *Spilopsyllus cuniculi* (rabbit flea), *Echidnophaga gallinacea* (poultry flea) and even *Pulex irritans* (human flea) (Kalkofen and Greenberg, 1974a; Kalkofen and Greenberg, 1974b; Chesney, 1995; Dryden and Rust, 1997.)

In many parts of the world, *Ct. f. felis* is the commonest species found on domestic dogs (Figure 9.1). This insect's life cycle is an example of complete metamorphosis comprising oval, larval, pupal and adult stages. Adult *Ct. f. felis* acquire a host and rapidly commence feeding on blood taken directly from capillaries (Dryden, 1990). Females begin to produce eggs within 24-36 hours of this first blood meal and following multiple matings, may lay up to 50 eggs per day at peak production (Dryden, 1989). The majority of eggs fall from the host's coat within 8 hours (Rust, 1992) and the developing first-stage larvae emerge a few days later, depending on environmental temperature and relative humidity, with optimal conditions of approximately 27°C and 75%, respectively (Silverman *et al.*, 1981). The first larval instar (L_1) moults twice to L_2 and L_3. All three stages are negatively phototactic and positively geotactic, hence they accumulate deep in the carpet pile or in cracks between floorboards (Byron, 1987).

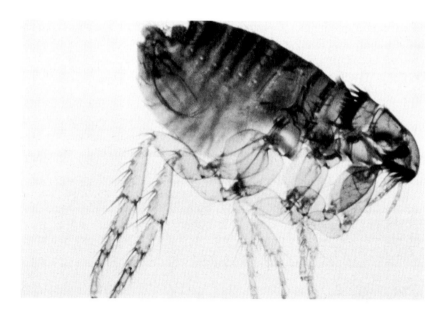

Figure 9.1. Microscopic appearance of adult *Ctenocephalides felis felis* (400x magnification, suspended in liquid paraffin).

Larval development is again dependent on environmental conditions, particularly temperature and can take as little as 8 days in optimal conditions (Silverman and Rust, 1983). The third larval instar then spins a silk cocoon, pupates and becomes a pre-emerged adult. At 26.6°C, adult females and males emerge from the cocoon 5-8 days and 7-10 after pupation, respectively (Hudson and Prince, 1958) and emergence is delayed at lower temperatures. This temperature-dependent mechanism, coupled with a reduced metabolic rate and the protective effect of the cocoon, allow the pre-emerged adults to survive for several weeks to months within the cocoon until a time when environmental conditions are favorable and a suitable host is in the vicinity. The major triggers for emergence are heat and mechanical pressure (Silverman and Rust, 1985). The emerged adults locate their host using visual and thermal detection systems and experimentally have been shown to be attracted to light (particularly intermittent sources) and heat (Osbrink and Rust, 1985). Air currents and carbon dioxide generated by a passing host stimulate jumping behavior and despite a preference for dogs and cats, adult *Ct. f. felis* will readily feed on humans. In dogs, type I, type IV, late-phase immediate and cutaneous basophil hypersensitivities can all be induced by flea bites, resulting in moderate to marked pruritus characterized by papules, alopecia and erythema typically affecting the rump, caudal ventral abdomen and caudal thighs (Scott *et al.*, 1995).

Zoonotic implications

In humans, penetration of the skin by the flea's mouthparts and the subsequent injection of saliva during feeding typically causes irritation and mild to moderate pruritus, characterized by urticarial, papulocrustous lesions. Bites are often in small groups of two or three, described by some as the flea's "breakfast, lunch and dinner". Individuals who sensitize to one or more of the proteins contained within the saliva may become intensely pruritic once bitten, developing large erythematous wheals and in extreme cases, bullous lesions or even erythema multiforme (Wilson and King, 1999). Lesions are most commonly found on the feet, ankles and calves as the newly emerged adult fleas jump up from the floor, but as a true zoonosis may also occur in "contact sites" such as the trunk, upper legs and arms if fleas are transmitted directly from an infested dog. In addition to causing dermatological disease, *Ct. f. felis* poses an additional potential threat to human health as a vector for a number of infectious diseases such as *Bartonella henselae* (cat scratch disease (Jameson *et al.*, 1995)), *Rickettsia typhi* (murine typhus (Farhang-Azad *et al.*, 1984)), *Dipylidium caninum* (intestinal cestode in children (Marx, 1991)) and *Yersinia pestis* (bubonic plague (Pollitzer, 1960)). Fortunately *Xenopsylla cheopis* (the rat flea) and *Pulex irritans* (the human flea), which are more frequently implicated in the transmission of bubonic plague, are much less commonly isolated from dogs.

Control

The success of any flea control program relies upon the simultaneous treatment of both host and environment. Ideally, the products employed should have low mammalian toxicity, possess residual activity, be easy to apply and, in some ways most importantly, be affordable to the purchasing pet-owner. The last decade has witnessed the advent of several such products and their incorporation into "spot-ons", in-feed liquid and tablets, pump-sprays and neck-collars has greatly facilitated their use.

Adulticides (e.g. the nicotinic receptor antagonist imidacloprid, the γ- amino butyric acid receptor inhibitor fipronil, the centrally neurotoxic synthetic pyrethroids and the anticholinesterase organophosphates and carbamates) must be regularly and repeatedly applied to the host and all in-contact animals that are capable of harboring adult *Ct. f. felis* (e.g. cats, rabbits, ferrets and small rodents). A rapid knockdown effect is desirable as this not only offers relief from the irritant effects of fleas, but also may help prevent oviposition if newly emerged females can be killed within 24-36 hours of host acquisition. Provided the owner competently applies the adulticide in accordance with the manufacturer's directions, adult fleas reaching the dog should be swiftly and efficiently killed.

Many of the problems associated with flea control however, arise from the difficulties involved in clearing the environment of the immature forms of the parasite. The manufacturers of some adulticidal preparations claim that hairs and skin debris shed from dogs treated with their product will exert some larvicidal effect in the environment (Hunter *et al.*, 1996; Hopkins *et al.*, 1997). However, most authorities would recommend the concurrent use of products with specific ovicidal and/or larvicidal properties. Currently, the most popular group in this class are the insect growth regulators (IGRs) such as lufenuron, cyromazine, methoprene and pyriproxyfen. These compounds act at various points of the life cycle to inhibit maturation and development of L_1 through L_3. Lufenuron and cyromazine are benzoylphenyl urea compounds available in oral and aerosol spray formulations, respectively, which interfere with the synthesis of exoskeletal chitin and L_1-L_2 stage ecdysis. Methoprene and pyriproxyfen are juvenile hormone analog (JHA) that prolong larval development, preventing their natural progression through the three larval stages and ultimately killing them (Rust and Reierson, 1985). Both are widely available in aerosol preparations for environmental use and are often combined with a synthetic pyrethroid such as permethrin for the control of newly emerged adults. If applied correctly at sufficiently high concentration, the JHAs in these sprays may last for over 12 months (Kawada and Hirano, 1996), offering a convenient and effective method of environmental control. In some countries, they are available in the form of sprays and impregnated collars for on-animal use, exerting an ovicidal effect if newly hatched eggs come into contact with treated hair (Palma *et al.*, 1993).

Outdoor flea control may be necessary in countries with climates capable of sustaining flea development. Microencapsulated chlorpyrifos and diazinon have been shown to kill > 90% of adult fleas for more than a week (Metzger *et al.*, 1996) and pyriproxyfen, fenoxycarb and methoprene applied to turf, inhibited adult emergence for up to 11, 6 and 1 month(s), respectively (Hinkle, 1992). Protracted periods of dry and/or cold conditions can be lethal to all life-cycle stages, with survival times of only 1-10 days at 3°C (Rust and Dryden, 1997). Hence, at northernmost and southernmost latitudes, the harsh winter months will effect a natural "cull" on outdoor fleas. Indoor control measures should continue year-round however, as fleas are believed to be surviving in more traditionally flea-free areas such as Scandinavia, as a result of improved indoor heating methods.

Arachnida

Mites: *Sarcoptes scabiei* var. *canis*

Biology

Sarcoptes scabiei var. *canis* is a common canine ectoparasite, belonging to the Family Sarcoptidae. Adults are globose, measure 200-400 µm in length and have short legs. Mating occurs on the host's skin surface and, following fertilization, female *Sarcoptes* mites burrow into the skin and tunnel through the outer epidermal layers at a rate of 2-3 mm per day, laying eggs at the turning points in their zig-zag course (Sokolova, 1991). The eggs hatch within a few days and after moulting through 6-legged larval and two, 8-legged nymphal stages, they emerge on the skin surface as adults to complete the life cycle, a process taking 14-21 days depending on environmental conditions. The mites are obligate parasites, but can survive for limited periods away from the host. Females and nymphs appear hardier than males and larvae, but all stages have been shown to be capable of surviving for 2-6 days at 20-25°C (Arlian *et al.*, 1989). Scabies is highly contagious, with the majority of mites being transmitted by direct contact with an infested dog or fox, although indirect infestation via fur or fomites has also been reported (Bornstein, 1991). The mites are attracted by the host's body temperature and odour, are positively phototaxic and have a preference for certain cutaneous lipids, properties which may explain their anatomical distribution and host predilections (Arlian *et al.*, 1989; Arlian and Vyszenski-Moher, 1995). Studies in dogs and humans have demonstrated that mites applied to the skin can penetrate within 30 min and that they have a circadian rhythm of activity. From 9 am to 6 pm the mites are inactive, with the majority of tunneling occurring between 6 pm and 9 pm, a pattern of activity which correlates with the degree of pruritus perceived by the subject (Sokolova, 1991). Feeding, oviposition and deposition of feces within the skin exposes the host to mite allergens, which in the majority of dogs induces both humoral and cell-mediated immunological responses (Bornstein and Zakrisson, 1993; Arlian *et al.*, 1996). These host defense mechanisms can lead to spontaneous resolution of the disease after a few months (Bornstein, 1991). Most dogs develop a moderate to intensely pruritic dermatosis initially affecting the pinnal margins, elbows, hocks and ventrum, which in time progresses to involve the entire body surface (Figure 9.2 and 9.3).

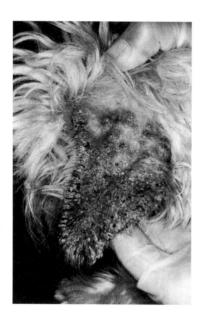

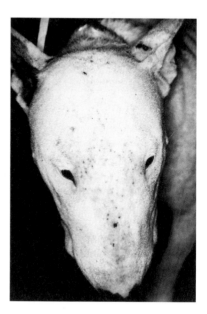

Figure 9.2. Severe crusting of the dorsal pinnal surface of the pinna and pinnal margins in a Lhasa Apso with sarcoptic acariasis.

Figure 9.3. Papulocrustous dermatosis affecting the facial skin of an English Bull Terrier with sarcoptic acariasis.

Zoonotic implications

S. scabiei var. *canis* is quite commonly transmitted from dogs to humans, with estimated human infestation rates of 10-50% (Griffin, 1993). Reverse zoonosis may also occur, but this is very rare (Anderson, 1979). Typically, a combination of pruritic papular, vesicular, crusting lesions develop in areas which are in-contact with the affected dog such as the trunk, arms and upper legs (Charlesworth and Johnson, 1974). These lesions develop within hours to days of contagion, suggesting the pruritus may be a consequence of both the physical effects of mite burrowing (Estes *et al.*, 1983) and a hypersensitivity to mite allergens (Norins, 1969). The majority of human infestations with *S. scabiei* var. *canis* are self-limiting and resolve within days once the affected dog has been treated with a suitable acaricide (see below). However, mites have occasionally been known to propagate in human hosts, producing ova and successive generations of mites (Norins, 1969; Estes *et al.*, 1983), hence persistent cases may require concurrent medical treatment of both dogs and humans (Meijer and van Voorst Vader, 1990).

Control

A number of different acaricidal products are effective against *S. scabiei* var. *canis*. Those used most commonly are the topical "sponge-on" formulations containing monoamine oxidase inhibitors (e.g. amitraz) or organophosphates (e.g. phosmet) which need to be applied weekly or fortnightly, respectively, until clinical cure is achieved. In the US, a 2.5% lime sulfur dip is also available, which has the advantage of a wider safety margin in small mammals; however, its foul odor and potential for staining light-colored coats make it unpopular with some owners (Scott *et al.*, 1995).

Fipronil spray has been used to control an outbreak of scabies in a litter of puppies (Curtis, 1996), but in the author's opinion should be prescribed only for early cases or for those individuals in which the use of more potent products is contra-indicated (e.g. puppies less than 12 weeks of age and pregnant or nursing bitches). To facilitate topical treatment, dogs with long coats may need to be clipped prior to dipping or spraying. Systemic therapy is obviously more pleasant and convenient for the operator. Two macrocyclic lactones, ivermectin and milbemycin oxime, have been used successfully for the treatment of canine scabies. The avermectin compound ivermectin is effective if administered orally or subcutaneously at 200-400 µg per kg, every 7-10 days. However, care must be taken as ivermectin is not licensed for this use in dogs and at these dosages may cause central nervous system (CNS) disease and potentially fatal neuropathies in this species, particularly in collies, sheepdogs and their crosses (Pulliam and Preston, 1989). Milbemycin oxime is also unlicensed for the treatment of scabies, but has been reported to be effective in 71-100% of cases when used at 2 mg per kg once weekly for 2-3 weeks (Miller *et al.*, 1996; Bergvall, 1998). This drug has not been associated with CNS toxicity in collie and sheepdog breeds at this dose, but some collies were found to be sensitive to higher dosages (Tranquilli *et al.*, 1991). Hence drug dosages must always be calculated carefully and owners should be informed of the risks associated with the use of these drugs.

During the treatment period, all dogs known to have been in recent contact with the affected animal should be treated concurrently and grooming equipment, bedding and the domestic environment should be treated with an appropriate acaricidal spray (e.g. permethrin) to prevent possible re-infestation from these sources. Attempts should be made to limit socialization and mixing with other dogs and foxes, and persistently affected humans should consult their doctor to assess whether they themselves require scabicidal therapy.

Cheyletiella spp.

Biology

Cheyletiellidae are relatively large (400-500 μm), white, "fiddle-shaped" mites with long legs terminating in setae and a pair of crescent-shaped hooks on the accessory mouthparts (Figure 9.4). The mites live on the surface of the skin, partly protected by the scale produced in response to infestation, and feed on tissue fluid and lymph obtained by piercing the epidermis. Following mating, adult females lay eggs which they bind to hairs with a silken thread. Larvae emerge and undergo three ecdyses through two nymphal stages before emerging as adults, a process taking approximately 3-4 weeks in total. The mites are obligate parasites but are capable of surviving away from the host for up to 10 days in suitable environmental conditions (Scott et al., 1995).

Cheyletiella yasguri is the species most frequently isolated from dogs, but as a family these mites are not believed to be host specific and may readily transfer between dogs, cats and rabbits although *Cheyletiellidae blakei* and *Cheyletiellidae parasitovorax* are most commonly associated with the latter host species, respectively (Cohen, 1980). Infested dogs typically develop erythema and moderate-to-severe scaling along the dorsum. On closer inspection, particularly against a dark coat or surface, this scale may appear mobile as a result of mite activity, giving rise to the alternative name for the disease "walking dandruff" (Figure 9.5). Although mites can be isolated from dogs of any age, puppies appear to be at increased risk. The degree of pruritus associated with infestation is variable and may be absent to intense.

Zoonotic implications

Humans in contact with dogs carrying *Cheyletiella* are at risk of becoming transiently infested themselves, producing an uncomfortable, pruritic dermatosis. Papular lesions appear on the arms, legs, trunk, buttocks and rarely the face, which in time become vesicular and pustular. The lesions are often damaged as a result of self-trauma and may become crusted or necrotic (Scott and Horn, 1987). Occasionally urticarial and bullous lesions may develop (Hewitt *et al.*, 1971). In one study of 14 patients, more women than men were affected, particularly in the winter months. This may be attributable to closer contact between pet and owner during periods of cold weather (Lee, 1991). As *Cheyletiella* are not capable of reproducing on humans, appropriate treatment of the pet host (see below) should prevent further infestation making human acaricidal therapy unnecessary.

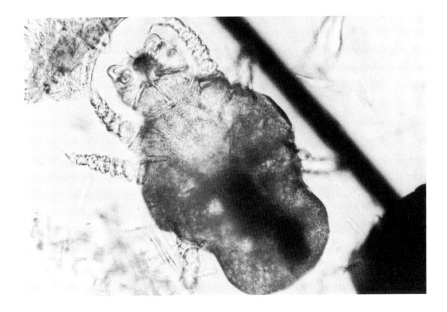

Figure 9.4. Microscopic appearance of *Cheyletiella yasguri* (400x magnification, suspended in liquid paraffin).

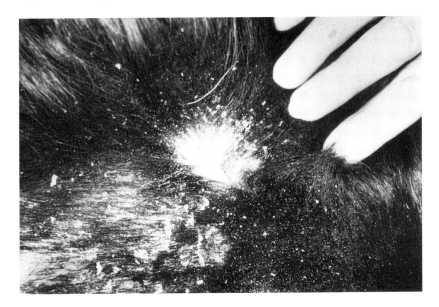

Figure 9.5. Heavy scale ("walking dandruff") in the coat of a Newfoundland dog with cheyletiellosis.

Control

There are currently no veterinary licensed products specifically indicated for the treatment of Cheyletiellosis. However, several of the insecticidal/acaricidal sprays, shampoos and dips available are effective and weekly application of lime sulphur, pyrethrins or amitraz, in conjunction with regular treatment of the environment, is recommended. The author has also had some success with selenium sulfide shampoo applied weekly for 3 weeks, and a recent report described the control of two separate outbreaks using a single application of fipronil spray (Chadwick, 1997). Dogs which resist or do not tolerate topical therapy can be treated systemically with injectable or oral ivermectin at 200-300 μg per kg at 7-10 day intervals, provided the associated risks of adverse reaction are considered (see *S. scabiei*, Control section above) and the owner gives informed consent. All dogs, cats and rabbits which have been in contact with the affected animal should be included in the treatment protocol and care should be taken when selecting an appropriate acaricide for the latter two host species, as they are particularly sensitive to the toxic effects of pyrethrins and amitraz. Bedding and grooming equipment, as potential sources of re-infestation, should be treated or discarded. Washable fabrics should be cleaned in water reaching at least 55°C and then sprayed along with the rest of the environment with a product containing pyrethroids, carbamates or organophosphates. All animals should be re-examined following initial therapy to screen for residual mites and eggs. Treatment should continue until clinical cure, when multiple tape strippings and superficial skin scrapings fail to reveal any evidence of ectoparasites when examined microscopically.

Otodectes cynotis

Biology

Otodectes cynotis belongs to the family Psoroptidae (Figure 9.6). Known colloquially as the "ear mite", it is an obligate parasite which inhabits the vertical and horizontal ear canals of dogs and cats, although other species such as ferrets may become infested. The mites are non-burrowing and live on the surface of the ear canal lining. Adult females lay eggs from which larvae emerge in approximately 4 days. The larvae feed for 3-10 days and then complete three additional ecdyses through protonymphal and deutonymphal stages, to complete the life cycle in approximately 3 weeks (Scott *et al.*, 1995). The mites have an average life span of 2 months and are capable of surviving for several weeks to months away from the host (Larkin and Gaillard, 1981), therefore the environment must always be included in the control program. Dogs infested with *O. cynotis* most commonly develop otitis externa characterized by erythema and a dark brown, ceruminous otic exudate. These signs result from the mites' feeding activity, during which the host becomes exposed to mite antigens. In cats, this has been shown to induce a reaginic hypersensitivity response in some individuals who may subsequently develop immunity to the mite proteins (Powell *et al.*, 1980). This acquired immunity may explain why puppies and kittens appear to be most susceptible to otocariasis. In addition to otitis, mites escaping the ear canals may also cause lesions on the head, neck and tail head (Scott and Horn, 1987).

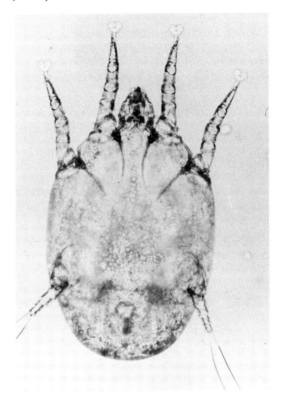

Figure 9.6. Microscopic appearance of larval *Otodectes cynotis* mite (400x, suspended in liquid paraffin).

Zoonotic implications

O. cynotis is not particularly host specific and has been known to infest humans on occasion (Herdwick, 1978; Suetake *et al.*, 1991; Lopez, 1993). The mites usually produce pruritic vesicular, papular lesions and/or wheals on areas of the body that are in contact with an infested pet, such as the arms and torso (Scott and Horn, 1987). However, natural and experimental infestations of human ear canals have also been reported (Suetake *et al.*, 1991; Lopez, 1993). A veterinarian who infested himself with *O. cynotis* described how the mites had regular feeding patterns (being most active between 6 pm and 9 pm and midnight and 3 am) and a tendency to temporarily vacate the ear canal and walk across his face during the night (Lopez, 1993). The degree of pain, pruritus and tinnitus

Lopez experienced was surprisingly intense, but diminished with time. Two subsequent re-infestations induced less severe disease, suggesting some form of acquired immunity.

Another interesting slant on the public health significance of *O. cynotis* stems from the observations of Larkin and Gaillard (1981) who prick tested a group of human atopic patients with a known sensitivity to *Dermatophagoides* mites. They found that all seven patients tested developed positive prick test reactions to both *Dermatopagoides* and *Otodectes* and proposed that there may be a degree of immunological cross-reactivity between the two mite species. Therefore, atopic patients who own or come into contact with infested dogs or cats could potentially become sensitized to *Otodectes* allergens and suffer further as a consequence.

Control

Different preparations are available for the aural treatment of *O. cynotis*. The majority are drops containing acaricides such as thiabendazole, monosulfiram or pyrethroids, which are frequently combined with a variety of local anaesthetic, antimicrobial and/or glucocorticoid drugs. The limited residual action of the acaricides dictates that drops be applied regularly and repeatedly for at least 10 days, to ensure that all ova have hatched and that the newly emerged larvae are exposed to the drug. For dogs that resent aural topical therapy, an alternative protocol of two, 5-day treatment periods separated by a 3-4 day break may improve compliance. Ceruminolytics can be applied to remove otic exudate (e.g. cerumen, blood and epithelial debris) prior to treatment and an acaricide should be applied to the entire body to control any mites that have left the ear canals. All in-contact dogs, cats and ferrets should be included in the ectoparasiticidal program, as should the environment, bedding and grooming equipment, given the potential for survival away from the host (see above). Infested humans should recover once the canine infestation has been controlled.

References

Anderson, R.K. (1979) Canine scabies. *Compendium of Continuing Education for the Practicing Veterinarian* 1, 687-692.

Arlian, L.G. and Vyszenski-Moher, D.L (1995) Response of *Sarcoptes scabiei* var. *canis* (Acari Sarcoptidae) to lipids of mammalian skin. *Journal of Medical Entomology* 32, 34-41.

Arlian, L.G., Vyszenski-Moher, D.L. and Pole, M.J. (1989) Survival of adults and developmental stages of *Sarcoptes scabiei* var. *canis* when off the host. *Experimental and Applied Acarology* 6, 181-187.

Arlian, L.G., Morgan, M.S., Rapp, C.M. and Vyszenski-Moher, D.L. (1996) The development of protective immunity in canine scabies. *Veterinary Parasitology* 62, 133-142.

Bergvall, K. (1998) Clinical efficacy of milbemycin oxime in the treatment of canine scabies: a study of 56 cases. *Veterinary Dermatology* 9, 231-233.

Bornstein, S. (1991) Experimental infection of dogs with *Sarcoptes scabiei* derived from naturally infected wild red foxes (*Vulpes vulpes*): Clinical observations derived from. *Veterinary Dermatology* 2, 151-159.

Bornstein, S. and Zakrisson, G. (1993) Humoral antibody response to experimental *Sarcoptes scabiei* var. *vulpes* infection in the dog. *Veterinary Dermatology* 4, 107-110.

Byron, D.W. (1987) Aspects of the biology, behaviour, bionomics and control. Siphonaptera of immature stages of the cat flea, *Ctenocephalides felis felis* (Bouche) (Siphonaptera: Pulicidae) in the domiciliary environment. PhD thesis. Virginia Polytech Institute State University, Blacksburg, pp. 135.

Chadwick, A.J. (1997) Use of a 0.25% fipronil pump spray formulation to treat canine Cheyletiellosis. *Journal of Small Animal Practice* 38, 261-262.

Charlesworth, E.N. and Johnson, J.L. (1974) An epidemic of canine scabies in man. *Archives of Dermatology* 110, 572-574.

Chesney, C.J. (1995) Species of flea found on cats and dogs in southwest England: further evidence of their polyxenous state and implications for control. *Veterinary Record* 136, 356-358.

Cohen, S.R. (1980) *Cheyletiella* dermatitis (in rabbit, cat, dog, man). *Archives of Dermatology* 116, 435-437.

Curtis, C.F. (1996) Use of a 0.25% fipronil spray to treat Sarcoptic mange in a litter of five-week-old puppies. *Veterinary Record* 139, 43-44.

Dryden, M.W. (1989) Host association, on-host longevity and egg production of *Ctenocephalides felis felis*. *Veterinary Parasitology* 34, 117-122.

Dryden, M.W. (1990) Blood consumption and feeding behaviour of the cat flea, *Ctenocephalides felis felis* (Bouche, 1835). PhD thesis. Purdue University, West Lafayette, Indiana, 128.

Dryden, M.W. and Rust, M.K. (1997) The biology, ecology and management of the cat flea. *Annual Review of Entomology* 42, 451-473.

Estes, S.A., Kummel, A.B. and Arlian, L. (1983) Experimental canine scabies in humans. *Journal of the American Academy of Dermatology* 9, 397-401.

Farhang-Azad, A., Traub, R., Safi, M. and Wisseman, C.L. (1984) Experimental murine typhus infection in the cat flea, *Ctenocephalides felis* (Siphonaptera: Pulicidae). *Journal of Medical Entomology* 21, 675-680.

Griffin, C.E. (1993) Scabies. In: Griffin, C.E., Kwochka, K.W. and Macdonald, J.M. (eds) *Current Veterinary Dermatology*. Mosby, St Louis, pp. 85-89.

Herwick, R.P. (1978) Lesions caused by canine ear mites. *Archives of Dermatology* 114, 130.

Hewitt, M., Walton, G.S. and Waterhouse, M. (1971) Pet animal infestations and human skin lesions. *British Journal of Dermatology* 85, 215-225.

Hinkle, N.C. (1992) Biological factors and larval management strategies affecting cat flea (*Ctenocephalides felis felis Bouche*) populations. PhD thesis, University of Florida, Gainesville, 181.

Hopkins, T.J., Woodley, I. and Gyr, P. (1997) Imidacloprid topical formulation: Larvicidal effect against *Ctenocephalides felis* in the surroundings of treated dogs. *Compendium on Continuing Education for the Practicing Veterinarian* (Supplement) 19, 4-10.

Hudson, B.W. and Prince, F.M. (1958) A method for large scale rearing of the cat flea, *Ctenocephalides felis felis* (Bouche). *Bulletin of the World Health Organisation* 19, 1126-1129.

Hunter, J.S., Keister, D.M. and Jeannin, P. (1996) The effect of fipronil treated dog hair on the survival of the immature stages of the cat flea *Ctenocephalides felis*. *Proceedings of the 14th Annual Veterinary Medical Forum, ACVIM*, May 1996, San Antonio, Texas, pp. 730.

Jameson, P., Greene, C., Regnery, R., Dryden, M., Marks, A., Brown, J., Cooper, J., Glaus, B. and Greene, R. (1995) Prevalence of *Bartonella henselae* antibodies in pet cats throughout regions of North America. *Journal of Infectious Disease* 172, 1145-1149.

Kalkofen, U.P. and Greenberg, J. (1974a) *Echidnophaga gallinacea* infestations in dogs. *Journal of the American Veterinary Medical Association* 165, 447-448.

Kalkofen, U.P. and Greenberg, J. (1974b) Public health aspects of *Pulex irritans* infestations in dogs. *Journal of the American Veterinary Medical Association* 165, 903-905.

Kawada, H. and Hirano, M. (1996) Insecticidal effects of the insect growth regulators methoprene and pyriproxyfen on the cat flea. *Journal of Medical Entomology* 33, 819-822.

Larkin, A.D. and Gaillard, G.E. (1981) Mites in cats ears, a source of cross antigenicity with house dust mites. Preliminary report. *Annals of Allergy* 46, 301-303.

Lee, B.W. (1991) Cheyletiella dermatitis: a report of 14 cases. *Cutis* 47, 111-114.

Lopez, R.A. (1993) Of mites and man (letter to editor). *Journal of the American Veterinary Medical Association* 203, 606-607.

Marx, M.B. (1991) Parasites, pets and people. *Primary Care* 18, 153-165.

Meijer, P. and van Voorst Vader, P.C. (1990) Canine scabies in man. *Nederlands Tijdschrift voor Geneeskunde* 134, 2491-2493.

Metzger, M.E., Rust, M.K. and Reierson, D.A. (1996) Activity of insecticides applied to turf grass to control adult cat fleas. *Journal of Economic Entomology* 89, 935-939.

Miller, W.H., de Jaham, C., Scott, D.W., Cayatte, S.M., Bagladi, M.S. and Buerger, R.G. (1996) Treatment of canine scabies with milbemycin oxime. *Canadian Veterinary Journal* 37, 219-221.

Norins, A.L. (1969) Canine scabies in children. *American Journal of Diseases of Children* 117, 239-242.

Osbrink, W.L.A. and Rust, M.K. (1985) Cat flea (Siphonaptera: Pulicidae): factors influencing host-finding in the laboratory. *Annals of the Entomology Society of America* 78, 29-34.

Palma, K.G., Meola, S.M. and Meola, R.W. (1993) Mode of action of pyriproxyfen and methoprene on eggs of *Ctenocephalides felis* (Siphonaptera: Pulicidae). *Journal of Medical Entomology* 30, 421-426.

Pollitzer, R. (1960) A review of recent literature on plague. *Bulletin of the World Health Organisation* 23, 313-400.

Powell, M.B., Weisbroth, S.H., Roth, L. and Wilhelmson, C. (1980) Reaginic hypersensitivity in *Otodectes cynotis* infestation of cats and mode of mite feeding. *American Journal of Veterinary Research* 41, 877-882.

Pulliam, J.D. and Preston, J.M. (1989) Safety of ivermectin in target animals. In: Ed Campbell, W.C. (ed.) *Ivermectin and Abamectin.* Springer-Verlag, New York, pp. 157-161.

Rust, M.K. (1992) Influence of photoperiod on egg production of cat fleas. (Siphonaptera: Pulicidae) infesting cats. *Journal of Medical Entomology* 29, 301-305.

Rust, M.K. and Dryden, M.W. (1997) The biology, ecology and management of the cat flea. *Annual Review of Entomology* 42, 451-473.

Rust, M.K. and Reierson, D.A. (1985) Factors influencing pest management strategies with IGRs against cat fleas. *Proceedings of the First IGR Symposium*, Dallas, Texas, pp. 7-24.

Scott, D.W. and Horn, R.T. (1987) Zoonotic dermatoses of dogs and cats. *Veterinary Clinics of North America* 17, 117-144.

Scott, D.W., Miller, W.H. and Griffin, C.E. (1995) Parasitic skin diseases. In: *Muller and Kirk's Small Animal Dermatology*, 5th edn. W.B. Saunders Company, Philadelphia, pp. 392-468.

Silverman, J. and Rust, M.K. (1983) Some abiotic factors affecting the survival of the cat flea *Ctenocephalides felis* (Siphonaptera: Pulicidae). *Journal of Medical Entomology* 18, 78-83.

Silverman, J. and Rust, M.K. (1985) Extended longevity of the pre-emerged adult cat flea (Siphonaptera: Pulicidae) and factors stimulating emergence from the pupal cocoon. *Annals of the Entomology Society of America* 78, 763-768.

Silverman, J., Rust, M.K. and Reierson, D.A. (1981) Influence of temperature and humidity on survival and development of the cat flea, *Ctenocephalides felis* (Siphonaptera: Pulicidae). *Journal of Medical Entomology* 18, 78-83.

Sokolova, T.V. (1991) Experimental study of the formation of burrows in human scabies. *Vestnik Dermatologii I Venerologii* 12, 14-23.

Suetake, M., Yuasa, R. and Saijo, S. (1991) Canine ear mites *Otodectes cynotis* found on both tympanic membranes of an adult woman causing tinnitus. *Tohoku Rosat Hospital; Practicing Otology of Kyoto* 84, 38-42.

Tranquilli, W.J., Paul, A.J. and Todd, K.S. (1991) Assessment of toxicosis induced by high-dose administration of milbemycin oxime in collies. *American Journal of Veterinary Research* 52, 1170-1172.

Wilson, D.C. and King, L.E. (1999) Arthropod bites and stings. In: Freedberg, I.M., Eisen, A.Z., Wolff, K., Frank Austen, K., Golsmith, L.A., Katz, S.I. and Fitzpatrick, T.B. (eds) *Fitzpatrick's Dermatology in General Medicine*, 5th edn. McGraw Hill, London, pp. 2685-2695.

Chapter Ten

Zoonoses and Immunosuppressed Populations

Robert A. Robinson

Canine zoonotic infections encompass a wide range of viral, bacterial, fungal and parasitic infections as described in the previous chapters. Given the WHO definition (WHO, 1959) of zoonoses as "those diseases and infections which are naturally transmitted between vertebrate animals and man", it is useful to review the concept of a "chain of infection" as shown in Box 10.1.

Box 10.1. Chain of infection.

> A zoonotic agent
> An immediate source or reservoir of the agent
> A method of escape from the source or reservoir
> A method of transmission
> A method of entry into the human host
> A susceptible human or population

For a zoonotic infection to occur in humans, all links in the above chain must be completed. Successful control and prevention efforts are usually focused on the weakest link. The role of the immune system is especially important in both the reservoir hosts and humans. Immunological defects in either may increase the likelihood of infection becoming established in the reservoir species or increase the likelihood that humans will become infected if exposed.

Zoonoses are both emerging and re-emerging. Infections that were once thought to be controlled are now manifesting themselves again especially as some established surveillance systems gradually decline (Berkelman *et al.*, 1994). Some of the factors leading to the emergence of zoonotic disease include natural selection and evolutionary progression of the agents, changes in individual host determinants (i.e. immunity), and societal population and environmental determinants, i.e. climate (Murphy, 1998). In this chapter, the focus will be immunosuppression as a risk factor for the development and transmission of zoonoses or in some cases the recrudescence of chronic subclinical zoonoses as a result of the host becoming immunosuppressed. In this latter situation it may be difficult to distinguish this phenomena from a reinfection. Zoonotic infections that result in immunosuppression, i.e. certain viral infections, will not be discussed in this chapter.

Role of the immune system in relation to zoonotic agents

The various components of the immune system function according to strict regulatory mechanisms. The immune system's response to an antigenic challenge is diverse and results in a chain of events that lead to the production of either specifically activated effector T-cells (cell-mediated response) or B-cells (humoral or antibody response) or both. In contrast to normal hosts where many infectious diseases are usually self-limiting, immunocompromised patients developing such infections have the potential of becoming life-threateningly ill. Certain so-called "opportunistic pathogens", which are widely distributed in the environment, rarely cause serious illness in immunocompetent hosts (St Georgiev, 1997).

Viruses

Immune resistance to viral infections is primarily by cell-mediated immunity. Antibodies also play a minor role by preventing virus from attaching to cell receptors. Thus patients with defects in cell-mediated immunity are more likely to develop serious viral infections, and those with antibody deficiencies are more likely to develop life-threatening bacterial infections.

Bacteria

Bacterial pathogens are an extremely diverse group but can be categorized into two general types: those causing intracellular or extracellular infections. The former, i.e. *Brucella* spp., avoid being killed after phagocytosis and resistance to these agents is primarily cell-mediated. The extracellular infectious agents survive by avoiding phagocytosis. Extracellular pathogens present a surface that minimizes the opsonic and lytic effects of antibody and complement. If phagocytosed, they are readily inactivated. Typical extracellular bacterial pathogens include both gram-negative bacteria such as some strains of *Escherichia coli* and gram-positive bacteria such as *Clostridium tetani.*

Fungi

Cell-mediated immunity (CMI) appears to be the most important immunological factor in resistance to these organisms. Intense granulomatous reactions occur in tissues infected with fungi, and these infections are also associated with depressed immune reactions of the delayed hypersensitivity leading to opportunistic infections.

Protozoa

The mechanism of protection against protozoal infections depends upon the location of the agent in the host. They may be located intracellularly or extracellularly in organs, blood or in the gastrointestinal tract. Intracellular zoonotic pathogens such as *Leishmania* spp. are eliminated by delayed (Type IV) hypersensitivity reactions, for example, limited focal inflammatory skin lesions. If delayed hypersensitivity is lost, dissemination of the organisms may occur. The role of antibodies in the immune response to zoonotic protozoa remains unclear.

Helminths

The response to endoparasites depends on the location of the infestation. Those located in the gastrointestinal tract generally provoke no protective immunologic response, while parasites with larval forms that invade tissues do stimulate an intense response. Eosinophils attack parasites by antibody-dependent cellular cytotoxicity. IgE anaphylactic antibodies are also frequently associated with helminth infestations.

Immunosuppression in dogs

The potential risks of zoonotic infection must be considered when immunodeficient animals and immunosuppressed humans interact. While there is little published evidence to show how much greater risk such an association may pose, it is likely that this risk is increased specifically if the dog fails to mount a satisfactory immune response to a vaccine such as rabies. Alternatively if the dog manifests a severe infection with a zoonotic agent it probably will excrete organisms at a much higher level than an immunocompetent dog, e.g. a 2-month old puppy with acute Salmonella diarrhea following a decrease in maternal immunity

Immunodeficiencies in dogs can be divided into those that are (a) primary, i.e. inherited or genetic and (b) secondary, i.e. acquired as a result of interference in host defense mechanisms. Secondary immunodeficiencies may occur in relation to malnutrition, certain infectious diseases, metabolic disturbances, intoxications, and drug therapies.

A number of important clinical signs may suggest an immunodeficiency in dogs; these include:

- A recurrent or protracted course of an infection.

- An infection with microorganisms usually considered non-pathogenic (i.e. opportunistic). Examples include bacteria such as *Citrobacter* spp., *E. coli* and *Staphyococcus intermedius*.
- Unusually severe signs of the disease.
- A poor response to antimicrobial therapy.
- An adverse or poor response to vaccines, especially live products.

Some medical problems commonly implicated in immunocompromised dogs include: recurrent skin and mucosal infections, neonatal sepsis and mortality, vasculitis, arteritis, polyarthritis, recurrent bacteremia, granulomatous infections, chronic hypersensitivity reactions, and autoimmune diseases. A recent study of 238 dogs with various infectious and parasitic diseases found 62 (26%) with marked immunodepression (Toman *et al.*, 1998).

Primary (hereditary) immunodeficiencies in dogs

At least 20 primary immunodeficiencies of dogs have been collated by Greene (1990). The mode of inheritance (if known), breed predisposition, defect, and clinico-pathological presentation are described. Some immunodeficiencies lead to massive infections and death within the first few weeks of life, whereas others may not be consistently associated with any marked predisposition to infection. The majority of serious deficiencies manifest before 1 year of age, though not all puppies in a litter may be affected. Some deficiencies predispose certain breeds to infection by specific microorganisms. Defects involving the skin and mucous membrane surfaces occur and are often associated with infections of certain organs. Disorders of the immune system especially the phagocytic and complement systems can lead to pyogenic and granulomatous infections.

Secondary (acquired) immunodeficiencies

Initially the immune system of animals that develop secondary immunodeficiences are intact and functional, but following a disease, exposure to certain chemicals or treatments, secondary immunodeficiencies may occur. A partial list of diseases or exposures resulting in immunodeficiencies is as follows:

- Organ disorders such as diabetes mellitus, skin, pulmonary and gastrointestinal diseases, and cancer.
- Barrier damage resulting from burns, catheterization, endoscopy, splenectomy.
- Whole body radiation.
- Immunosuppressive viral agents such as canine distemper, parvovirus and retrovirus.
- Other infections such as demodicosis, ehrlichiosis, and protracted bacterial infections.
- Chemical and drug-induced suppression such as cytotoxic agents,

chloramphenicol, and griseofulvin.
- Antibiotic and antacid usage for gastrointestinal diseases.
- Nutritional disorders such as protein-calorie restriction (malnutrition), vitamin A and E deficiency.

Puppies are especially susceptible to infection in the first few weeks of life as their immune systems are not completely developed. Colostrum deprivation in puppies does not appear to have the same serious sequelae as in many other species if they are kept in clean and well-managed kennels. A temporary hypoglobulinemia occurs at 2-4 months of age as maternal immunity wanes and these animals may be more susceptible to infections. A decline in both T- and B-cells occurs as dogs age, which may be an explanation for their increased susceptibility to infections and neoplasia. While protein and/or calorie malnutrition can lead to thymic atrophy and decreased immune responses, obese dogs have also been reported to increase susceptibility to infections. Lastly there is some degree of immunosuppression associated with the later stages of pregnancy, which may influence susceptibility to zoonotic pathogens in dogs.

Assessment of the canine immunologic status

Dogs showing clinical signs and a history of an underlying immunological problem such as recurrent infections, fevers of unknown origin, a failure to thrive, signs of autoimmune or allergic diseases, and cancer, should be subject to a preliminary laboratory work-up. This should include a complete blood count (CBC) with both total and differential white cell counts, urinalysis, blood chemistry panel, and any organ system specific tests as indicated. As mentioned earlier, animals with T-cell defects are more likely to have severe viral, mycotic or protozoal infections while those with B-cell defects will be most affected by bacterial infections.

Evaluation of the immune system is generally carried out by examination of the four component parts as follows:

- Humoral immune system: This can be done by quantifying the major immunoglobulin classes of IgG, IgM, and IgA levels, quantifying B-cell numbers in the peripheral blood, measuring the Ig response to specific antigens, and identifying the types of bacteria causing recurrent infections.
- Cellular immune system: T-cell functions can be evaluated by quantitation of a stimulation index in response to T-cell mitogens, a peripheral blood lymphocyte count, and quantitation of total T-cells by immunofluorescence.
- Complement system: Tests are available to detect the absence of components of complement such as C3.
- Phagocytic system: Tests to determine the adequacy of cell numbers, chemotaxis, phagocytosis, and killing are available.

Specific samples are needed for the above tests and readers should consult with laboratories prior to collection. For detailed information on these and other tests to evaluate the immune system the reader is referred to Gershwin (1992).

Immunosuppression in humans

As in dogs, humans suffer from both primary and secondary immunodeficiencies. Characteristics of infections associated with immunodeficiency diseases in humans include: increased frequency, increased severity, prolonged duration, unexpected complications, unusual manifestations, infection with agents with low infectivity.

There have been at least 70 different kinds of primary immunodeficiencies in humans identified involving B- and T-cells, phagocytic cells and complement proteins. Essentially three major primary immune deficiencies occur: combined antibody and CMI, antibody alone, or CMI alone. Some of these diseases are inherited by autosomal recessives, some are linked to the X chromosome, while others remain unknown (Sell, 1996).

Secondary immunodeficiencies in humans may result from naturally occurring disease processes or subsequent to the administration of an immunosuppressive agent. "Opportunistic" infections occur with microorganisms not usually pathogenic for healthy individuals. Some typical diseases include sarcoidosis, tuberculosis, measles, diabetes, neoplasia and HIV/AIDS infections (see later). Immunosuppressive agents include radiation, steroids, alkylating agents, folic acid antagonists, some antibiotics and anti-rejection drugs following transplantation, e.g. cyclosporine A.

Some infants may exhibit a temporary and transient hypogammaglobulinemia. This is associated with an abnormal delay in the onset of immunoglobulin synthetic capacity by the baby. This deficiency usually terminates between 9 and 18 months of age.

Pregnancy has been known for some time to be associated with "physiological" depression of selective aspects of CMI that permit fetal retention, but also may interfere with resistance to specific infectious and neoplastic agents. (Weinberg, 1984). Total white cell counts are also significantly increased in pregnancy. Both total T-cells and activated T-cells fell and mitogen activity was significantly increased during pregnancy (MacLean *et al.*, 1991). Some infections, including zoonotic infections such as Toxoplasmosis may be reactivated during pregnancy, especially if the mother's CD4 lymphocyte count is very low (Biedermann *et al.*, 1995).

Throughout the world, the most common form of immunodeficiency is probably that which is secondary to malnutrition. In protein-energy malnutrition, most of the host defense mechanisms are breached, primarily cell-mediated immunity. The actual mechanisms involved are difficult to identify since deficiencies usually involve multiple dietary factors, e.g. macro and micronutrients such as zinc, iron, vitamins and specific amino acids.

The human immunodeficiency virus (HIV), first identified in 1983, as the cause of acquired immunodeficiency syndrome (AIDS) is now recognized as the most significant infectious depressor of the immune system, and thus clearly a risk factor for many other infections including zoonoses. HIV infection is characterized by the depletion of the CD4+ helper/inducer subset of T-lymphocytes. It has been estimated that today between 40 and 100 million people have been infected worldwide. HIV is transmitted by sexual contact, by parenteral exposure to blood or blood products, during pregnancy or the perinatal period and by breast-feeding. The median time between primary HIV infection and the development of AIDS is approximately 10 years. The case fatality rate of AIDS is very high, especially in developing countries, with 90% of persons dying within 3-5 years. In recent years more effective anti-retroviral therapy and prophylactic drugs to prevent opportunistic infections have significantly prolonged survival. In developing countries however, where the incidence of HIV infection continues to increase, therapy is usually unavailable.

In summary, those individuals at greatest risk from zoonotic infections acquired directly from dogs would include the very young, the elderly, pregnant women, and the immunocompromised. In the USA this segment of the population represents almost 20% and is expected to increase as people both live longer, immunocompromised patient populations increase following transplantation and cancer therapy, and the relentless spread of HIV infection. The population of immunosuppressed individuals worldwide, and especially in developing countries, will also increase in the coming decades, mainly due to the HIV pandemic.

Human contact with dogs

Obviously this is going to vary greatly with the region, country, rural versus urban domicile, as well as religious and social attitudes toward keeping dogs as companion animals. Based on 1996 US data (AVMA, 1997). A total of 53 million dogs were in 31.6% of households with the lowest rates being in the large cities. Cities now usually have regulations designed to reduce biting incidents through stricter controls, and also requirements for fecal collection by owners. Middle to older aged persons, those with higher incomes and larger household sizes, and those owning their own homes were more likely to have dogs. Although the rate of dog ownership and the number of households owning dogs has decreased in recent years, the total dog population remains stable as the percentage of households owning more than one dog keeps increasing. There has been a trend also in recent years for the elderly to have more contact with dogs through either visiting or live-in animals in geriatric institutions. The use of service dogs to assist physically and mentally handicapped persons is also increasing. In developing countries dogs are often seen as a protective measure for a household rather than as a companion, but close contact albeit under less hygienic conditions is still common.

A 1993 survey of 408 adults with AIDS at three local health departments in Florida, USA revealed that 46% were or had been living with a companion animal during the last 5 years (Conti *et al.*, 1995), Approximately 30% of these people had one or more dogs. There were no significant differences with regard to sex, race/ethnicity, age group, HIV transmission mode, employment status, education, or living situation between pet owners and non-pet owners.

Canine zoonotic diseases of special concern for immunosuppressed populations

Risk factors for zoonotic infections in dogs include:

- Use such as companions, service, hunting, herding, guarding, research, etc.
- Degree of confinement, ranging from a single dog totally confined to free-ranging feral dogs in packs.
- Diet, including complete commercial foods, raw meat, scavenging, hunting.
- Water source and water contact.
- Region of the world and recent travel.
- Degree of immunosuppression.
- Immunity, either natural or vaccination-induced.
- Breed. This may be a surrogate for "use", or a breed at high risk of developing a primary immunodeficiency disease.

Some human risk factors for exposure to canine zoonoses include: occupation, recreational activities, age and sex, pregnancy, personal hygiene, residence or recent travel, immune status including vaccination, degree of immunosuppression, degree of contact with dogs either direct or indirect.

Direct contact with a dog may involve a bite, lick, scratch, and spray from urine, inhalation of respiratory droplets from sneezing or coughing, contact with reproductive discharges, or feces or just handling the animal. Indirect contact includes contact with an arthropod vector (flea, tick or mite) or an inanimate object on which the zoonotic agent survives (bedding or toilet areas), or ingestion of contaminated food or water.

It should be emphasized that in some instances dogs and humans may be infected with the same agent but actual transmission has not occurred. Rather both have been exposed to the same source of infection. For example, although blastomycosis has been transmitted by a bite from an infected dog (Gnann et al., 1983), this is a very rare event in most. In a few instances dogs may acquire an infection from humans such as Mycobacterium tuberculosis, thus the dog may serve as a monitor for undetected human infections.

From time to time articles appear both in the popular press and the scientific literature suggesting that certain human diseases are associated with an animal reservoir. These reports often generate a great deal of public concern. Although patients with these diseases, such as multiple sclerosis, rheumatoid arthritis and the leukemias, may have underlying immunological problems, the methods used to define animal exposure have often been imprecise. An accurate method of detecting and measuring exposure, particularly to animals shedding a specific agent, should be used to avoid misclassification in epidemiologic case-control and cohort studies. Problems in selective recall of exposure need to be addressed also as persons with chronic diseases may exaggerate exposure potential. Some of these methods for measuring exposure include: residence in a household keeping animals, exposure to diseased animals, exposure to a specific animal pathogen, bite exposures, and exposure as a member of a high risk group.

In assessing the risks of various canine zoonotic infections for persons with primary or secondary immunodeficiencies, we have to rely on a variety of information sources. There are numerous case reports, for example, of HIV/AIDS patients with zoonotic infections such as enteric bacterial infections (*Salmonella* spp. and *Campylobacter* spp.) and also enteric protozoal infections (*Cryptosporidium* spp.). In virtually all of these instances the course of the disease is more severe and the case-fatality rate higher than in otherwise healthy individual persons infected with the same pathogen. For many zoonotic diseases there are multiple sources and routes of transmission and there may be no direct animal contact involved. In other instances, a case series of AIDS patients with a zoonotic agent may state that they had animal exposure, but there was either no attempt made to test the hypothesized animal source, nor was there any attempt at molecular "fingerprinting" of animal and human isolates to suggest zoonotic transmission. The Florida study described above (Conti *et al.*, 1995) showed that specific AIDS-defining diseases that might be common to animals and humans were just as likely to occur in pet owners as in non-pet owners.

Nevertheless canine-origin zoonotic infections can occur in immunosuppressed populations and the following section summarizes the current state of knowledge of the more important diseases.

Salmonellosis

Case reports indicate that *Salmonella* spp. are important agents in AIDS patients (Celum *et al.*, 1987). These authors showed that the average annual incidence of salmonellosis in men with AIDS was 384/100,000 compared to 20/100,000 in men without AIDS. The median age was similar in both groups. *Salmonella* bacteremia was more common in AIDS patients. Also the distribution of serotypes differed in that AIDS patients had twice as many *Salmonella typhimurium* and *Salmonella dublin* isolates as those without AIDS. There was no difference in the survival time of AIDS patients with or without salmonellosis. The authors concluded that salmonellosis was a severe but treatable pathogen in patients with AIDS. Given the increase in multiple antibiotic resistance in many *Salmonella* isolates over the last decade this conclusion might be premature. Recurrent *Salmonella* bacteremia is more likely in HIV infected persons who do not receive maintenance antimicrobial therapy presumably is the result of incomplete clearance of the primary infection because of impaired cellular immunity. Persons receiving prior antimicrobial treatments are also at risk of infection from both antimicrobial sensitive and resistant strains of *Salmonella* spp. (Pavia *et al.*, 1990).

Salmonellosis is primarily transmitted via the fecal-oral route, and food and water are the major sources. The source of most *Salmonella* infections for HIV infected persons is likely to be very similar to that for the rest of the population. This includes contaminated food both of animal and non-animal origin, raw or inadequately cooked food, or those foods cross-contaminated during preparation (Angulo and Swerdlow, 1995).

The role that companion animals play as a direct source of *Salmonella* spp. particularly for sporadic cases is unclear. An older source cites data suggesting that pets are a risk factor for about 3% of outbreaks (CDC, 1996; 1997). The frequency of *Salmonella* isolates from fecal samples of both healthy and hospitalized dogs ranges from 1-36% (Greene, 1990) but the actual prevalence may well be higher especially in certain subpopulations. Dogs not properly supervised or confined are exposed through coprophagia and scavenging. Even commercially prepared dog food is occasionally contaminated with *Salmonella* spp.

The usual presenting clinical signs of salmonellosis in dogs are gastroenteritis, with young and old animals showing the most severe signs. Diarrheic animals excrete much higher numbers of bacteria than asymptomatic animals. The majority of dogs do recover from the clinical disease, though fecal excretion continues for at least 6 weeks (Greene, 1990). Salmonella organisms may also be present in oral secretions. While antimicrobial therapy to treat severe clinical disease is indicated, its use to eliminate fecal excretion is problematical. In some instances excretion may actually be prolonged, and there is the increased risk of antibiotic resistance.

In order to protect the immunocompromised human population with companion dogs from *Salmonella* infection, strict measures should be taken with the canine diet, contact with other animals should be limited, and dogs should be supervised appropriately to prevent access to environmental sources of the bacteria.

Campylobacteriosis

Campylobacteriosis is now regarded as one of the most common causes of enteric illness in the USA and many other countries. A study in Los Angeles County, California showed that the average annual incidence rate of campylobacteriosis among AIDS cases was 519/100,000, which is approximately 40 times the crude population rate of 13.3/100,000 (Sorvillo *et al.*, 1991). *Campylobacter jejuni* is the most common type isolated. Female AIDS patients were at significantly higher risks than male patients of having campylobacteriosis. Patients with AIDS and *Campylobacter* infections had higher rates of bacteremia and hospitalization than patients infected with *Campylobacter* without AIDS. As with salmonellosis, there are many potential sources of infection for *Campylobacter* spp. but inadequate hygiene when preparing or eating undercooked chicken, and drinking raw milk are clearly risk factors. Case reports and case control studies indicate that human infections in the general population show that recently acquired puppies from pet stores or kennels suffering from diarrhea or even asymptomatic have been a source of infection (Blaser *et al.*, 1980). A recent study suggests that about 6% of human cases can be attributed to diarrheic animals (Saeed *et al.*, 1993), but the role of companion animals as a source for HIV-infected persons is unclear at this stage.

Campylobacter infections have been detected in from < 0.5% to > 45% of dog fecal specimens (Glaser *et al.*, 1994), indicating a wide range of asymptomatic carriage. Clinical disease, when it occurs, is most often seen in dogs less than 6 months of age. Animals stressed by hospitalization, concurrent disease, pregnancy, travel, and surgery appear to be at risk for clinical disease (Greene, 1990). As with people, a wide range of signs are seen ranging from mild to bloody mucoid diarrhea of up to 15 days or even longer duration. Therapy with erythromycin has been the usual drug of choice for dogs. Prevention of canine *Campylobacter* infections would seem to be similar to salmonella infections with particular emphasis on avoidance of any chicken sources.

Yersiniosis

Yersiniosis (*Yersinia enterocolitica*) is an infection primarily manifested by enteritis causing significant morbidity and occasional mortalities. Although most human infections are acquired through contaminated food or water there is some evidence that direct transmission can occur. For example in one instance a 4-month-old baby developed severe yersiniosis. Prior to this a number of puppies in the home developed a wasting illness and some died. The same serotype of *Y. enterocolitica* was isolated from both the baby and the remaining dogs (Wilson *et al.*, 1976).

Bartonellosis

HIV-infected persons, particularly those who are severely immunosuppressed, are at high risk for developing disease due to infection with *Bartonella henselae*. This agent is one of the causes of bacillary angiomatosis as well as cat scratch disease or fever. Until very recently, this zoonotic infection was believed to be only associated with cats. However, a recent report suggests that *B. henselae* may occur in dogs also (Tsukahara *et al.*, 1998). A study of 52 dogs of unknown origin found four seropositive for *B. henselae*, three PCR positive on blood, and 5/9 positive on both oral swabs and nail clippings. Further research is needed to clarify the actual canine dimension of this infection.

Bordetellosis

Bordetella bronchiseptica has been isolated from a number of persons with AIDS (Woodward *et al.*, 1995; Dworkin *et al.*, 1999). Some of these individuals had contact with dogs either as companions or an occupational exposure. Healthy dogs may carry small numbers of this bacterium in their oropharynx for variable lengths of time. Exposure to high doses of bacteria together with stress may result in tissue invasion in dogs and development of so-called "kennel cough". While vaccination of dogs is recommended where they may be heavily exposed as in a large kennel for example, vaccination has not been shown to prevent colonization. However, its use could be justified in high-risk situations as long as other hygienic measures were undertaken to prevent cross-infection from dogs to humans.

Mycobacterial infections

Human tuberculosis primarily due to *M. tuberculosis* is emerging as one of the more important diseases affecting those with HIV/AIDS as well those undergoing immunosuppressive therapy, following organ transplants and primary immunodeficiencies (St Georgiev, 1997). Also with the spread of AIDS, *Mycobacterium bovis* infections have been recorded in this population. Many of the isolates have been the BCG human vaccine strain but multidrug-resistant strains of *M. bovis* have been recorded in a nosocomial outbreak (Bouvet *et al.*, 1993). The *Mycobacterium avium* complex (MAC) is also a very significant cause of death in AIDS patients with between 30 and 50% of patients showing evidence of disseminated MAC at death. Infections with MAC tend to occur later in the course of AIDS when immunosuppression is more advanced. In general the primary environmental source of MAC is natural waters. Even hot-water systems in hospitals have been shown to be persistently contaminated with MAC bacteria (von Reyn *et al.*, 1994). Animals, including dogs, do not appear to be an immediate source of MAC infections for humans.

M. tuberculosis infections in dogs have been recorded (Cordes *et al.*, 1963), especially those in close contact with an infected person. The epidemiological evidence suggests that this is "reverse zoonosis" and the dog should therefore be seen as an indicator rather than a source for people. Dogs are also susceptible to *M. bovis* infections acquired primarily from drinking raw milk or eating offal from infected cattle. *M. avium* infections occur rarely in dogs and the granulomatous lesions are indistinguishable from those caused by the mammalian tubercle bacteria (Greene, 1990). The source of these infections may be poultry or swine, but an environmental source is equally likely given the long persistence of these organisms. Tuberculosis in dogs is usually sub-clinical. Presenting signs are referable to pulmonary disease with coughing, fever, anorexia and weight loss. Diagnosis of tuberculosis in dogs can be attempted using both tuberculin skin tests and serology. None of these tests have been sufficiently evaluated to give the user a high degree of confidence, and attempted bacteriological isolation from biopsy, exudate, oropharyngeal fluids or urine is a better approach.

Treatment of dogs may be undertaken in exceptional circumstances, but euthanasia is the safest course of action, especially as many strains of pathogenic mycobacteria are now resistant to a wide range of drugs.

Rabies

In rabies endemic countries, the primary source of infection for humans is a domestic or feral dog bite where the animal is excreting virus in its saliva. The dog may or may not be exhibiting clinical signs at the time of the bite. Fatal human rabies cases have been documented in HIV seropositive individuals but this probably represents a random association (Adle-Biassette *et al.*, 1996). Rabies is endemic in many of the countries where AIDS is spreading. There is no legitimate reason why immunocompromised persons should not receive complete post-exposure rabies treatments including vaccines and antisera as soon as possible after proven or suspected exposure. However, Wilde *et al.* (1989) notes those persons with chronic diseases, alcoholics and drug addicts may have an impaired immune response to postexposure rabies vaccines. Postexposure vaccination of pregnant women appears to be safe and efficacious (Chutivongse and Wilde, 1989). Pre-exposure rabies immunization with human diploid cell vaccine has resulted in variable immune responses in some persons in developing countries. Current recommendations include not taking chloroquine antimalarial chemoprophylaxis at the same time as rabies immunizations in case immunosuppression occurs (Benenson, 1995). Alternatively rabies antibody titers should be measured in immunosuppressed persons.

Cryptosporidiosis

Cryptosporidiosis is an enteric coccidian protozoan pathogen that is an important cause of diarrhea in persons with AIDS. It has been estimated in the USA that 10-15% of persons with AIDS develop crytosporidiosis, and in some the severe diarrhea persists until death (Peterson, 1992). The organism is widely found in the gastrointestinal tracts of many mammals, birds, reptiles and fish. Based on morphology and site of infection, at least six species exist, with *Cryptosporidium parvum* being the most common in mammals. Epidemiological evidence shows that this infection is clearly a zoonosis with emphasis on cattle as likely sources for humans. Molecular techniques are now being used to detect intraspecific variations in *C. parvum* and a recent study shows that several genotypes can be distinguished. Most human epidemics appear to be caused by human genotypes (Sulaiman *et al.*, 1998).

A recent study of *Crytosporidium* genotypes from HIV-infected individuals revealed four distinct types: a human genotype, a bovine genotype, a type identical to *Cryptosporidium felis* (a bovine type), and one identical to a *Cryptosporidium* isolate from a dog (Pieniazek *et al.*, 1999). An epidemiological case-control study by Glaser *et al.* (1998) evaluated HIV-infected persons with and without crytosporidiosis. Dog ownership as a risk factor reached borderline statistical significance, whereas surface water ingestion, rural exposure, travel or contact with diarrheic individuals did not.

Cryptosporidium spp. were detected in 2% of 200 stray dogs in San Bernardino County, California, USA in 1991 (El-Ahraf *et al.*, 1991). Experimental infection of healthy puppies results in shedding of the oocysts without obvious clinical signs (Greene, 1990). Cryptosporidiosis has also been described in both immunosuppressed dogs with distemper and apparently immunocompetent dogs also (Greene, 1990). Given the persistence of these organisms in the environment, as well as the paucity of effective chemotherapy, it is difficult to prevent this infection in dogs apart from rigorous attention to hygiene and disinfection with ammonia solutions or boiling water. The concerns over human water-borne outbreaks of cryptosporidiosis have led to evaluation of alternate methods of ensuring freedom from oocysts such as membrane filtration. Immunocompromised persons should ensure that their dog has access to the same quality of water they are recommended to drink. Extrapolating from other species such as cattle where calves are most at risk of infection, it would appear wise to acquire puppies of at least 6 months of age.

Giardiasis

Giardiasis is one of the more common causes of diarrhea in HIV-infected persons (Glaser *et al.*, 1994). This protozoan parasite is ubiquitous and is probably the most common pathogenic intestinal parasite of humans worldwide. Children are at especial risk. Transmission is primarily via the fecal-oral route and both water-borne and food-borne outbreaks have been described. The zoonotic significance of *Giardia* spp. has been somewhat controversial, but most authorities now regard *Giardia* infection as a zoonosis (Thompson, 1998). A molecular study of *Giardia* from humans and dogs in northern Australia where the prevalence is high suggested that zoonotic transmission was infrequent (Hopkins *et al.*, 1997). However, from the point of view of immunosuppressed populations, all precautions to prevent transmission from dogs and other hosts should be undertaken. Surveys have shown up to 50% of dog feces contain *Giardia* cysts or trophozoites. Younger dogs appear to shed more organisms than do older dogs. Overt disease in dogs appears to be rare, although signs such as diarrhea and malabsorption may occur especially in young animals in kennel situations. Metronidazole is the drug of choice for treatment.

Vector-borne zoonoses

Leishmaniasis

Human leishmaniasis, a vector-borne disease, occurs as either cutaneous, mucocutaneous or visceral forms (see Chapter 5). It is widespread in many areas of the world. The disease is more likely to be seen in rural areas and children are especially at high risk in certain areas such as the Mediterranean littoral including Spain, France and Italy. Both cutaneous and visceral leishmaniasis is being increasingly seen in HIV-positive individuals and also following renal transplantation (Fenech, 1997). Using isoenzyme typing at least nine different zymodemes have been identified. All dog isolates appear to be of the same type. The exclusive presence of certain zymodemes in some immunocompromised patients and their absence in dogs suggests that there may be an anthroponotic pattern of disease spread by intravenous drug use (Jimenez *et al.*, 1995).

 Canine leishmaniasis is widespread in both wild canidae and domestic dogs, which are considered the major reservoir with sandflies being the vector. The disease has a long and variable incubation period and presents in dogs as skin lesions, weight loss, local or generalized lymphadenopathy, ocular lesions, renal or liver failure, chronic diarrhea, or lameness. Smears from bone marrow or lymph nodes and serology can be used to confirm a diagnosis together with clinical signs. Treatments are usually not rewarding, and euthanasia of infected dogs is recommended or even required in some countries.

Prevention of canine infections by vaccination is currently not practicable. Elimination of infected dogs alone is unlikely to be useful unless their programs also control unowned or feral dog populations together with strategic vector control (see also Chapter 5).

Human ehrlichoses are recently recognized tick-borne zoonotic infections. Several species have been identified including *Ehrlichia ewingii*, also a cause of arthritis and chronic infection in dogs (Greig *et al.*, 1996). This species was shown to be a cause of illness in four persons, all who had been exposed to ticks and had contact with dogs shortly before developing symptoms. In addition, three were receiving immunosuppressive therapy (Buller *et al.*, 1999). Whether prior immunosuppression is a risk factor for other tick-transmitted infections such as Lyme disease (Borreliosis), and Rocky Mountain Spotted fever is unclear at this stage. Nevertheless, dogs can serve as important carriers of infected ticks that can transmit the organisms to humans as well as other dogs, and continual efforts need to be made to ensure that ticks as well as other potential vectors are not introduced into the environment of an immunosuppressed individual.

Canine zoonotic helminth infestations

Strongyloides stercoralis infestation is commonly seen in tropical and subtropical countries with occasional fatal outcomes in malnourished children. Persons on corticosteroid therapy, transplant recipients, chronic infections, or suffering from protein-calorie malnutrition are at higher risk of developing systemic strongyloidiasis. Although there is a high prevalence of HIV seropositivity in *S. stercoralis*-infected persons, the actual occurrence of disseminated strongyloidiasis is not widespread in these patients (St Georgiev, 1997). The main source of infection for humans is soil contaminated by feces, either human or animal. The role of the dog in the perpetuation of human infections is a subject of some debate, but dogs in contact with vulnerable persons should be examined and treated if found to be infected.

Currently there is no evidence that other canine zoonotic helminths such as *Echinococcus granulosus*, *Taenia multiceps*, *Dipylidium caninum*, *Toxocara canis*, *Ancylostoma* spp., occur at higher rates or result in more severe disease in AIDS patients than those without AIDS (Schantz, 1999, personal communication).

Canine zoonotic dermatoses

Dermatophyte infections acquired from dogs occur sporadically and are usually caused by *Microsporum canis*, *Microsporum gypseum*, and *Trichophyton mentagrophytes*. Both localized ringworm and *Tinea capitis* are seen, as well as exudative secondary bacterial infections. Relapsing *Tinea capitis* caused by *M. canis* has recently been described in an immunosuppressed renal transplant patient. More prolonged therapy was required in this type of situation (Virgilli and Zampino, 1998).

Human scabies has been recorded in association with AIDS and other immunosuppressive diseases. As their immune responses deteriorate, they become more vulnerable to generalized hyperkeratosis (St Georgiev, 1997). Human scabies contracted from dogs has been reported frequently, especially over pet-contact areas (see Chapter 9).

Injuries

Dog bites are a major cause of human injuries worldwide. Many, especially in adults, are not reported to the public health authorities and reliance on those seen by physicians especially in hospital emergency rooms and/or requiring rabies post-exposure prophylaxis is used to generate national data. For example, based on dog bite injuries treated in emergency departments in the USA, a rate of 12.9/10,000 persons was calculated, with the rate in boys 5-9 years being 60.7/10,000 (Weiss *et al.*, 1998).

Bacteriological studies of dog bites would usually show that *Pasturella* spp. (primarily *Pasturella multocida*) are the most common isolates, but usually there are a mixture of aerobic and anaerobic bacteria found as well. *Capnocytophaga canimorus* (DF-2) has been isolated from victims of bite wounds and although it is an opportunistic pathogen of low virulence, the case fatality rate has been as high as 25% (McCarthy and Zumla, 1988). This bacterium seems to favor those immune systems that are suppressed, especially those who have had splenectomies, are alcoholics, or who have chronic respiratory disease. Fortunately both this organism and *Pasturella* spp. are sensitive to most antibiotics, including penicillin.

Blastomycosis is increasingly being recognized as a serious infection in immunocompromised persons, including those with AIDS, undergoing long-term corticosteroid use, malignancy and pregnancy. The case fatality rate in these high-risk individuals can exceed 30% (Pappas, 1997). Although blastomycosis is usually acquired from an environmental source, there are a number of reported cases following dog bites (Gnann *et al.*, 1983).

Perceived and actual risks of dog ownership for immunosuppressed persons

It is doubtful if many people go through a formal risk assessment procedure before acquiring or relinquishing a companion animal. In most cases it is likely that the strength of the human-animal bond outweigh any disease risks or even the potential for causing injury. Immunosuppressed individuals and especially the parents of immunosuppressed children do, however, have many questions regarding not only the risks of pet ownership, but also the preventive care needed if they assume or continue ownership.

From an epidemiological perspective, risks generated from case-control or cohort studies are preferred over descriptive case reports or a series of cases. In preparing this review it became obvious that there are few robust studies comparing the zoonotic infection in terms of rates and severity between immunocompromised and immunocompetent persons. The causes of immunosuppression are so diverse that case definitions become unwieldy unless a specific syndrome such as pregnant versus non-pregnant women or specific infections such as HIV/AIDS versus non-HIV/AIDS patients are compared. However, on general principles it has to be assumed that prior immunosuppression is a risk factor for many zoonoses, albeit small and manageable. Possession or close contact with a dog assumes that the concern relates to direct transmission, whereas some zoonoses have multiple routes of transmission, many of which are indirect.

Unfortunately physicians and veterinarians appear to hold divergent views on the risks involved. A recent comparison of physicians and veterinarians in Wisconsin, USA (Grant and Olsen, 1999) showed that when asked to "list the two zoonotic pathogens they believed should be of greatest concern for immunocompromised individuals" physicians named *Toxoplasma gondii* and *Salmonella* spp., whereas veterinarians identified *Salmonella* spp. and *C. parvum* as the highest risks. For both *Salmonella* spp. and *T. gondii*, contact with companion animals is not the only, nor even the most important source of human infection. *Salmonella*-contaminated foods are clearly the most common vehicle and undercooked meats especially lamb and pork are a high risk for *Toxoplasma* infection. Both groups identified diseases such as Lyme disease, histoplasmosis, blastomycosis and *Pneumocystis carinii* infections as zoonotic risks, but these are shared infections transmitted from a common environmental source. Some physicians even listed Cytomegalvirus as a zoonose, when there is clearly no evidence to support this. Adult dogs were rated by physicians as posing the highest risk for immunocompromised patients, while in reality kittens, puppies, and reptiles actually pose a higher risk. One of the more disturbing features of the study was that clearly neither profession was communicating with each other on zoonoses.

Veterinarians have a critical role to play in providing factual advice both to individual dog owners as well as through public health and community agencies with regard to actual risks of zoonotic diseases and how they can be managed. Unfortunately, many veterinarians have not been very proactive in assuming these human health responsibilities, despite the fact that many people who are immunocompromised have questions about pet ownership and diseases. For example, one study (Spencer, 1992) showed that less than 1% of HIV-infected persons had obtained health information about their pets from veterinarians but rather from the news media, friends, associates and health care workers. The same study also revealed that 45% of HIV-infected persons owned pets, of whom 60% had been told they should not. Very few actually take heed of this advice. Presumably there is a very strong animal-human bonding, especially for these persons who may have feelings of isolation and rejection. A recent study has clearly shown that persons with AIDS who owned pets reported less depression than persons with AIDS who did not own pets (Siegel *et al.*, 1999).

Veterinarians are encouraged to provide expanded services to persons who may have immunological problems. One way to encourage this is to have available a sign, brochure, or newsletter announcing that if clients have cancer, kidney or liver diseases, transplants, HIV/AIDS, or are undergoing immunosuppressive therapy, they should seek assistance especially if they are considering relinquishing their dog (Angulo *et al.*, 1994).

In the USA a number of active voluntary groups have developed in the last few years, primarily to provide information and "at home" support for immunocompromised people who wish to keep their dogs and other companion animals. These individuals often may have extended unanticipated hospitalization, or physical or financial limitations, but one of the most pressing needs is to ensure they receive accurate and prompt health information and care for their dog. Veterinarians, veterinary technicians and veterinary students can assist the organizations providing these services as well as liaising with other health caregivers and professionals. Several organizations in the USA provide educational material and other resources for immunocompromised people as well as for the elderly in nursing homes and children in hospitals (Appendix).

Preventive health care of dogs for immunocompromised persons

Assuming that many immunosuppressed persons with dogs will keep their animals, and also others may wish to acquire dogs or use them in a visitation schedule, and the actual risks of a zoonotic infection are small, some general recommendations are summarized. These are based on published recommendations (Angulo *et al.*, 1994; Scheck *et al.*, 1996; Greene, 1998). The US Public Health Service and the Infectious Diseases Society of America publish annual guidelines for the prevention of opportunistic infections in persons infected with HIV. These consensus recommendations include specific information on pet-related exposures and preventive measures. They can be obtained electronically via the Internet at: www.hivatis.org. Probably the two most important issues for all immunocompromised persons are that they must maintain a clean personal environment and also intact mucocutaneous barriers.

General recommendations

Dog selection

It is recommended that only dogs at least 6 months of age be acquired, as puppies are more susceptible to infection especially enteric bacteria and nematode infections. Avoid obtaining dogs from a source where there is poor hygiene, or the facilities are crowded. Dogs should be temperament tested and any with a tendency to aggressive behavior should be avoided. It is useful to obtain a dog on the condition that it does pass a veterinary examination prior to actual purchase. Veterinarians can often assist in suggesting suitable and safe sources.

Diet

Dogs should be fed a high-quality commercial diet that is appropriate for their age and body condition. The assumption is that this food will be free of pathogenic microorganisms. If owners want to supplement their dog's diet with other food such as eggs or meats these should always be well cooked. Only pasteurized dairy products should be used. Dogs should have access to water that is provided for human use and should not be allowed to drink from surface water, or out of toilet bowls. Dogs should also be confined wherever possible, and when walked be leashed so they cannot eat garbage, hunt or indulge in coprophagia.

Hygiene

The owner must be meticulous in handwashing especially before eating and after handling their dog or if they inadvertently have contact with feces or urine. Children's handwashing should be supervised. Wear gloves, preferably disposable, when picking up dog feces in a plastic bag, as many communities require this to be done. Preferably persons other than the immunosuppressed should remove feces. This also applies to any blood, saliva or urine. Hands should be thoroughly washed after gloves are removed. If an animal is diarreahic another person should be asked to remove the feces. Contact with the dog's mouth should be avoided as saliva contains potentially infectious bacteria. The dog's skin and coat should be kept in good condition by weekly bathing, brushing, trimming of matted hair as well as trimming of the nails if indicated.

Dog-related injuries

If an immunosuppressed person is bitten or scratched, it is especially important to take immediate first aid procedures such as washing with soap and clean water, followed by disinfection using dilute organic iodine or quaternary ammonium disinfectants. Medical consultation for antibiotic prophylaxis and any other treatment is strongly recommended. Some authorities recommend that all persons with a history of asplenia, alcoholism, or hematologic malignancy receive antibiotic prophylaxis following animal bites (Goldstein, 1992).

Veterinary preventive care and vaccination

All dogs should receive routine annual veterinary examinations which includes both a careful clinical examination and history taking for the previous 12 months, standard immunizations at intervals and routes recommended by the manufacturer including the following:

- Viral vaccines including canine distemper, adenovirus, parainfluenza, and parvovirus.
- *Leptospira* vaccines may be given if there is likelihood of exposure. These are inactivated products and may not necessarily prevent development of the carrier state. Thus their role in preventing human infections is equivocal.
- Rabies virus vaccines in countries or regions where the disease is endemic.
- Lyme disease. *Borrelia burgdorferi* vaccine may be administered if the owner lives in, or is travelling to an endemic area. There is no data to demonstrate that vaccination of dogs with this product provides protection for their owners. It has been shown that infected dogs can transmit the bacteria to immature ticks, and this may serve to increase the risk of exposure to *B. burgdorferi*-infected adult ticks (Mansfield, 1996).
- *B. bronchiseptica* vaccine. This vaccine is specifically recommended where dogs may be boarded, exhibited, or housed with other dogs.

While post-vaccination serological testing of poultry and swine is used to monitor their immune status, it has not been widely used or recommended for individual companion animals. In the case of viral vaccines where immunity is primarily cell-mediated, it probably has limited value, but could be undertaken following bacterial vaccination to determine the immune status (Tizzard and Ni, 1998).

Diagnostic testing

Provided the animal is not showing signs of diarrhea, there is probably limited value in the routine testing of fecal samples to isolate bacteria such as *Salmonella* spp. or *Campylobacter* spp. or identify protozoan pathogens such as *Cryptosporidium* spp. or *Giardia* spp. It may be warranted if the person is severely immunocompromised. For example if the client has a CD4 count below 200 cells per µl. If the animal is showing signs of diarrhea, fecal samples should be tested for the above pathogens and the animal held in isolation until the results are known. If infected, the animal should be treated appropriately and monitored for efficacy. *Campylobacter* infections usually respond to erythromycin treatment and *Giardia* infections to metronidazole or albendazole.

There are no recognized treatments for cryptosporidiosis, although fecal excretion is believed to be of fairly short duration. Dogs with a *Salmonella*-associated diarrhea and no obvious systemic signs are probably best treated symptomatically only, as antibiotics are likely to prolong excretion. Testing for the presence of *Leishmania* spp. may be indicated in endemic areas. Both lymph node smears and serology can be used.

Ectoparasitic zoonoses

Ectoparasites of dogs can either infect humans directly or act as vectors for zoonotic diseases (see above and Chapter 9). Among the former, fleas, *Cheyletiella*, sarcoptic and demodectic mites and various tick species can all affect humans. In many instances the clinical signs in humans may be minimal, but for the immunosuppressed person this is an unnecessary risk. Excellent ectoparasiticides are now available for routine treatments of dogs. Flea control should involve regular bathing and/or dipping with insecticide and also intensive environmental treatment of the area where the dogs sleeps. Flea collars, powders, sprays or topical application of insecticides are also indicated. Dogs in endemic areas should be checked daily for ticks and especially when leaving tick-infested areas. Tick removal should be carried out carefully using gloves and forceps. The major emphasis should be ensuring that exposures from infested dogs or other species is kept to an absolute minimum.

Endoparasite control and prevention

Routine treatments should be based on the endemicity and exposure potential for the various canine zoonotic parasites as discussed earlier. Testing and treating for *S. stercoralis* is certainly indicated. Given the widespread prevalence of zoonotic endoparasites in dogs as well as the availability of broad spectrum anthelmintics, government agencies and scientific associations in the USA are now recommending repeated monthly treatments to prevent environmental accumulation of infective eggs and larvae (CDC, 1996; also see Chapter 8). Where an intermediate host is involved such as in echinococcosis, dietary control is the obvious measure to ensure freedom in addition to anthelmintic treatment.

Conclusions

While a number of zoonoses can be transmitted directly from dogs to immunosuppressed persons, adherence to simple guidelines involving preventive health care, diet and management of the dog will reduce these risks to a minimum. Overall the benefits of maintaining the human-animal bond clearly outweigh in most instances the risks of contracting these infections. Veterinarians have a responsibility to diagnose, treat, and advise the owner or caregiver on zoonotic diseases. In addition they have a major role to play as a member of the health team in ensuring that physicians and other health professionals are given accurate and current information on the risks for their patients and practical advice on how to minimize infections occurring.

References

Adle-Biassette, H., Bourhy, H., Baudrimont, M., Gisselbrecht, M., Chretien, F., Wingertsmann, L., Rotivel, Y., Godeauu, B. and Gray, F. (1996) Rabies encephalitis in a patient with AIDS: a clinicopathological study. *Acta Neuropathologica* (Berlin) 92, 415-420.

American Veterinary Medical Association Center for Information Management (1997) *U.S. Pet Ownership and Demographics Sourcebook*. Schaumburg, USA.

Angulo, F.J. and Swerdlow, D.L. (1995) Bacterial enteric infections in persons infected with Human Immunodeficiency Virus. *Clinical Infectious Diseases* 21 (Supplement), S84-S93.

Angulo, F.J., Glaser, C.A., Juranek, D.D., Lappin, M.R. and Regnery, R.L. (1994) Caring for pets of immunocompromised persons. *Journal of the American Veterinary Medical Association* 205, 1711-1718.

Benenson, A.S. (1995) *Control of Communicable Diseases Manual*, 16th edn. American Public Health Association. Washington D.C., USA.

Berkelman, R.L., Bryan, M.T., Osterholm, M.T., LeDuc, J.W. and Hughes, J.M. (1994) Infectious disease surveillance: A crumbling foundation. *Science* 264, 368-370.

Biedermann, K., Flepp, M., Fierz, W., Joller-Jemelka, H. and Kleihues, P. (1995) Pregnancy, immunosuppression and reactivation of latent Toxoplasmosis. *Journal of Perinatal Medicine* 23, 191-203.

Blaser, M.J., LaForce, F.M., Wilson, N.A. and Wang, W.L.L. (1980) Reservoirs for human campylobacteriosis. *Infectious Diseases* 141, 665-670.

Bouvet, E., Casalino, E., Mendoza-Sassi, G., Lativen, S., Valee, E., Pernet, M., Gottot, S. and Vachon, F. (1993) A nosocomial outbreak of multidrug-resistant *Mycobacterium bovis* among HIV-infected patients: a case-control study. *AIDS* 7, 1453-1459.

Buller, R.S., Arens, M., Hmiel, S.P., Paddock, C.D. and Sumner, J.W. (1999) *Ehrlichia ewingii*, a newly recognized agent of human Ehrlichiosis. *New England Journal of Medicine* 341, 148-155.

CDC (1996) How to prevent transmission of intestinal roundworms from pets to people. Publication No. MS F22 Division of Parasitic Diseases, Centers for Disease Control and Prevention, Atlanta, Georgia.

CDC (1997) *Salmonella* Surveillance. Annual Summary. US Department of Health, Education and Welfare. Public Health Service.

Celum, C.L., Chaisson, R.E., Rutherford, G.W., Barnhart, J.L. and Echenberg, D.F. (1987) Incidence of Salmonellosis in patients with AIDS. *Journal of Infectious Diseases* 156, 998-1002.

Chutivongse, S. and Wilde, H. (1989) Postexposure rabies vaccination during pregnancy: experience with 21 patients. *Vaccine* 7, 546-548.

Conti, L., Lieb, S., Liberti, T., Wiley-Bayless, M., Hepburn, K. and Diaz, T. (1995) Pet ownership among persons with AIDS in three Florida counties. *American Journal of Public Health* 85, 1559-1561.

Cordes, D.O., Robinson, R.A. and Bailey, B.H. (1963) A case of Tuberculosis (human strain) in a dog. *New Zealand Veterinary Journal* 12, 111-113.

Dworkin, M.S., Sullivan, P.S., Buskin, S.E., Harrington, R.D., Olliffe, J., MacArthur, R.D. and Lopez, C.E. (1999) *Bordetella bronchiseptica* infection in human immunodeficency virus-infected patients. *Clinical Infectious Diseases* 28, 1095-1099.

El-Ahraf, A., Tacal, J.V. Jr., Sobih, M., Amin, M., Lawrence, W. and Wilcke, B.W. (1991) Prevalence of Cryptosporidiosis in dogs and human beings in San Bernardino County, California. *Journal of the American Veterinary Medical Association* 198, 631-634.

Fenech, F.F. (1997) Leishmaniasis in Malta and the mediterranean basin. *Annals of Tropical Medicine and Parasitology* 91, 747-753.

Gershwin, L.J. (1992) Immunologic assessment of the small animal patient. In: Kirk, R.B. (ed.) *Current Veterinary Therapy, XI Small Animal Practice.* W.B. Saunders Company, Philadelphia, pp. 1346.

Glaser, C.A., Angulo, F.J. and Rooney, J.A. (1994) Animal associated opportunistic infections among persons infected with the Human Immunodeficiency Virus. *Clinical Infectious Diseases* 18, 14-24.

Glaser, C.A., Safrin, S., Reingold, A. and Newman, T.B. (1998) Association between *Cryptosporidium* infection and animal exposure in HIV-infected individuals. *Journal Acquired Immune Deficency Syndrome and Human Retrovirology* 1, 79-82.

Gnann, J.W., Bressler, G.S., Bodet, C.A. and Avent, C.K. (1983) Human Blastomycosis after a dog bite. *Annals Internal* 98, 48-49.

Goldstein, E.J.C. (1992) Bite wounds and infection. *Clinical Infectious Diseases* 14, 633-640.

Grant, S. and Olsen, C.W. (1999) Preventing zoonotic diseases in immunocompromised persons: The role of physicians and veterinarians. *Emerging Infectious Diseases* 5, 159-163

Greene, C.E. (1990) *Infectious Diseases of the Dog and Cat.* W.B. Saunders Company, Philadelphia.

Greene, C.E. (1998) *Infectious Diseases of the Dog and Cat*, 2nd edn. W.B. Saunders Company, Philadelphia.

Greig, B., Asanovich, K.M., Armstrong, P.J. and Dumler, J.S. (1996) Geographic, clinical, serologic, and molecular evidence of Granulocytic Ehrlichosis, a likely zoonotic disease, in Minnesota and Wisconsin dogs. *Journal of Clinical Microbiology* 43, 44-48.

Hopkins, R.M., Meloni, B.P., Groth, D.M., Wetherall, J.D., Reynoldson, J.A. and Thompson, R.C.A. (1997) Ribosomal RNA sequencing reveals differences between the genotypes of *Giardia* isolates recovered from humans and dogs living in the same locality. *Journal of Parasitology* 83, 44-51.

Jimenez, M., Ferrer-Dufol, M., Canavate, C., Gutierrez-Solar, B., Molina, R., Laguna, F., Lopez-Velez, R., Cercenado, E., Dauden, E. and Blazquez, D. (1995) Variability of *Leishmania infantum* among stocks from immunocompromised, immunocompetent patients and dogs in Spain. *FEMS Microbiology Letter* 131, 197-204.

MacLean, M.A., Wilson, R., Thomson, J.A., Krishnamurthy, S. and Walker, J.J. (1991) Changes in immunologic parameters in normal pregnancy and spontaneous abortion. *American Journal of Obstetrics and Gynecology* 165, 890-895.

Mansfield, P.D. (1996) Vaccination of dogs and cats in veterinary teaching hospitals in North America. *Journal of the American Veterinary Medical Association* 208, 1242-1247.

McCarthy, M. and Zumla, A. (1988) DF-2 Infection may follow dog bites and be hazardous to the immunosuppressed. *British Medical Jorurnal* 297, 1355-1356.

Murphy, F.A. (1998) Emerging Zoonoses. *Emerging Infectious Diseases* 4, 429-435.

Pappas, P.G. (1997) Blastomycosis in the immunocompromised patient. *Seminars Respiratory Infection* 12, 243-251.

Pavia, A.T., Shipman, L.D., Wells, J.G., Puhr, N.D., Smith, J.D., McKinley, T.W. and Tauxe, R.V. (1990) Epidemiological evidence that prior antimicrobial exposure decreases resistance to infection by antimicrobial sensitive salmonella. *Journal of Infectious Diseases* 161, 255-260.

Peterson, C. (1992) Cryptosporidiosis in patients infected with the human immunodeficency virus. *Clinical Infectious Diseases* 15, 903-909.

Pieniazek, N.J., Bornay-Llinares, F.J., Slemenda, S.B., da Silva, A.J., Moura, I.N.S., Arrowood, M.J., Ditrich, O. and Addiss, D.G. (1999) New cryptosporidium genotypes in HIV-infected persons *Emerging Infectious Diseases* 5, 444-449.

Saeed, A.M., Harris, N.V. and Di Giacomo, R.F. (1993) The role of exposure to animals in the etiology of *Campylobacter jejuni/coli* enteritis. *American Journal of Epidemiology* 137, 108-114.

Scheck, J., Lewis, L.A. and Lane, T.J. (1996) A model program for assisting pet owners infected with human immunodeficiency virus. *Journal of American Veterinary Medical Association* 208, 483-484.

Sell, S. (1996) *Immunology, Immunopathology and Immunity*, 5th edn. Appleton and Lange, Stamford.

Siegel, J.M., Angulo, F.J., Detels, R., Wesch, J. and Mullen, A. (1999) AIDS diagnosis and depression in the Multicenter AIDS Cohort Study: the ameliorating impact of pet ownership. *AIDS Care* 11, 157-170.

Sorvillo, F.J., Lieb, L.E. and Waterman, S.H. (1991) Incidence of Campylobacteriosis among patients with AIDS in Los Angeles County. *Journal of Acquired Immune Deficency Syndromes* 4, 598-602.

Spencer, L. (1992) Study explores health risks and the human/animal bond. *Journal of American Veterinary Medical Association* 201, pp. 1669.

St Georgiev, V. (1997) *Infectious diseases in immunocompromised hosts*. CRC Press, Boca Raton.

Sulaiman, I.M., Xiao, L., Yang, C., Escalante, L., Moore, A., Beard, C.B., Arrowood, M.J. and Lal, A.A. (1998) Differentiating human from animal isolates of *Cryptosporidium parvum*. *Emerging Infectious Diseases* 4, 681-686.

Thompson, R.C.A. (1998) *Giardia* infections. In: Palmer, S.R., Lord Soulsby and Simpson, D.I.H. (eds) *Zoonoses*. Oxford University Press, Oxford, UK, pp. 545-561.

Tizzard, I. and Ni, Y. (1998) Use of serologic testing to assess immune status of companion animals. *Journal of American Veterinary Medical Association* 213, 54-60.

Toman, M., Svoda, M., Rybnicek, J., Krejci, J. and Svobodova, V. (1998) Secondary immunodeficency in dogs with enteric, dermatologic, infectious, or parasitic diseases. *Zentralbl Veterinarmed (B)* 45, 321-334.

Tsukahara, M., Tsuneoka, H., Lino, H., Ohno, K. and Murano, I. (1998) *Bartonella henselae* infection from a dog. *Lancet* 352, 1682.

Virgili, A. and Zampino, M.R. (1998) Relapsing tinea capitis by *Microsporum canis* in an adult female renal transplant recipient. *Nephron* 80, 61-62.

von Reyn, C.F., Maslow, J.N., Barber, T.W., Falkinham III, J.O. and Arbeit, R.D. (1994) Persistent colonisation of potable water as a source of *Mycobacterium avium* infection in AIDS. *Lancet* 343, 1137-1141.

Weinberg, E.D. (1984) Pregnancy-associated depression of cell-mediated immunity. *Review Infectious Diseases* 6, 814-831.

Weiss, H.B., Friedman, D.I. and Coben, J.H. (1998) Incidence of dog bite injuries treated in Emergency departments. *Journal of American Medical Association* 279, 51-53.

WHO (1959) Second report of a joint WHO/FAO expert committee on zoonoses. Technical report Series, No. 169.

Wilde, H., Choomkasien, P., Hemachudha, T., Supich, C. and Chutivongse, S. (1989) Failure of rabies postexposure treatment in Thailand. *Vaccine* 7, 49-52.

Wilson, H.D., McCormick, J.B. and Feeley, J.C. (1976) *Yersinia enterocolitica* infection in a 4-month old infant associated with infection in household dogs. *Journal of Pediatrics* 89, 767-769.

Woodward, D.R., Cone, L.A. and Fostvedt, K. (1995) *Bordetella bronchiseptica* infection in patients with AIDS. *Clinical Infectious Diseases* 20, 193-194.

Appendix

Examples of organizations offering support and information for immunocompromised persons

These organizations provide information, brochures, and home support for immunocompromised persons wishing to keep their pets in a number of US states.

Pets are Wonderful (PAWS), Los Angeles, California USA
7327 Santa Monica Blvd, West Hollywood, 90046-6615 USA
Website: www.pawsla.org Email: pawsla@earthlink.net
Tel: 323-876-7297 Fax: 323-876-0511

Delta Society, 289 Perimeter Road East, Renton, WA 98055-2569 USA
Website: www.deltasociety.org Email: info@deltasociety.org
Tel: 206-226-7357 Fax: 206-235-1076

Chapter Eleven

Dog Population Management

Joy Leney and Jenny Remfry

Why dog population management is necessary

Some people love dogs. Some people hate them. Some dogs are man's best friend. Others, or sometimes the same ones, are sources of injury, accident, disease and pollution. Dogs can breed and multiply their numbers very quickly. They are also subject to fatal diseases which can cause them much suffering and reduce populations drastically. In most parts of the world, dogs are valued for their role in the guarding of property, the herding of livestock and in hunting, and yet in some of these countries they may also be seen as unclean. These contradictions cause tensions, and they need to be understood before policies can be developed which will encourage the happy co-existence of most dogs with most people.

How problems arise

Traditionally, the number of dogs in rural areas is mainly controlled by the owners of the dogs, who do not permit all their bitches to breed and who kill any pups which are born surplus to their requirements. It was, and is, important that no unowned dogs live in rural areas, because of their natural inclination to chase and injure livestock. Traditional methods used for killing puppies: exposure - leaving the puppies in an exposed place so that they die of starvation or cold, or are taken by predators; by drowning; or by breaking the neck. In places where there is access to substances such as chloroform, these methods are still sometimes used.

In urban areas, these traditions tend to break down, and unwanted puppies may be left in the street in the hope that somebody will take care of them. If the puppies are given some protection by humans, they may survive. If not, most will die of disease or starvation, or be killed in road accidents. Those that live will join a street population which is made up of dogs which are lost, stray, abandoned or which were born there, and survive by scavenging. These may be given protection as neighborhood or community dogs, or they may be treated as outcasts.

Any dog that is not under the control of its owner may cause a nuisance by scavenging for food, causing road accidents, biting people, fouling public places and transmitting disease. A pack of uncontrolled dogs, particularly a group of males in excited pursuit of an estrous female, can be dangerous. In tourist areas such dogs will frighten visitors and lead to great concern about the risk of injury and disease, particularly rabies, if a dog should bite a visitor.

Animal protection societies differ in their views on how dog and cat populations should be managed, but most accept sterilization (castration or neutering of males and ovariectomy or spaying of females) as a vital part of population control. Most reluctantly accept that the humane destruction (euthanasia) of healthy animals may sometimes be unavoidable.

Unsuccessful methods of control

When people complain to their Local Authorities about problems caused by straying dogs, the authorities have to take action. For many years and in most parts of the world, this action has been to employ dog-catchers to capture the dogs and take them to a municipal dog-pound, or to kill them on the street by shooting or poisoning. Impounded dogs that are not reclaimed by their owners are killed, often by methods selected to be quick and cheap rather than painless. In some countries where there is no legislation to prevent it, dog-catchers may be encouraged to capture pedigree dogs and sell them to new owners, and to sell long-haired dogs to fur dealers, whilst in other countries the law requires dog-pounds to send dogs to laboratories for experimentation (WSPA, 1992a).

If the purpose of these measures is to reduce the number of stray dogs on the streets, they are remarkably unsuccessful. Statistics show that the number of dogs caught or killed each year often rise instead of falling (see the case history of Taiwan, below) and the effects of even a major campaign to remove dogs from the streets are only temporary. Dog populations return to their previous levels within a few years unless the campaigns are maintained.

Animal lovers whose dogs are captured by the dog-catchers, or who see animals in the agony of strychnine poisoning, become distressed and angry. Many animal protection societies respond to the activities of the local authorities and their dog-catchers in a confrontational way, and accuse the authorities of being deliberately cruel to animals.

The effects on tourism can be devastating. In 1993, attempts were made to eliminate stray dogs on a beach in Lanzarote by laying poison. The hotel guests heard about this and refused to take their children onto the beach for fear of them picking up the poison. Word spread, and soon tourists had ceased to book into hotels in that town. It set back the tourist industry of the island for 3 years. This was reported at a press conference in Crete in 1995 by the representative of the German tour company concerned (Leney, WSPA, 1998, personal communication).

The development of dog control policies

The role of WHO

An important long-term aim of WHO is to reduce the risk of transmission of communicable diseases, particularly rabies, from dogs to humans. Plans developed by WHO to prevent and control transmission have always included activities aimed at reducing stray dog populations. At first they encouraged the methods involving impounding and killing, but data soon accumulated which showed that these methods did not actually reduce the dog population in the long run. They were moreover very expensive because they require vehicles for transportation of the dogs and buildings for housing them, as well as the personnel for catching the dogs and feeding them.

It has been suggested that studies of dog populations using the methods of ecology might lead to better long-term solutions (WHO, 1984). Such studies were later initiated in South America, Asia and Africa. They all showed that most dogs regarded as "stray" by the authorities were in fact dependent on an owner or family for food and shelter and that this "referral household" could be identified. A smaller proportion of dogs had been abandoned by their owners but were given food and shelter by a number of families in the neighborhood. The smallest proportion were those dogs that were given no direct human support but scavenged at markets, abattoirs and rubbish dumps. These dogs were genuinely ownerless. Their reproductive rate was poor, and their population was maintained by immigration of other abandoned and rejected dogs (see Chapter 2). These studies clarified the relationship between dogs and their environment. Dogs have a high reproductive potential and could in theory treble their population every year. Populations in fact stabilize either through the intervention of humans, who control the reproduction of their own dogs, or through the natural processes of disease, starvation and accident. The actual number of dogs at the equilibrium point will depend on the availability of food, water and shelter. The habitat of street dogs will offer a certain amount of these essentials, sufficient to support a certain number of dogs, and the density of the dog population will always tend towards that carrying capacity. If some dogs are removed through death or capture, there will be a rapid compensation through better survival of the dogs, which remain, and by immigration of new ones.

The WHO/WSPA guidelines for dog population management

The World Society for the Protection of Animals (WSPA) had protested to WHO about some of the methods of killing dogs recommended in the 1984 Guidelines, particularly the use of strychnine. In 1986 a working group of scientists, animal control professionals and animal protectionists met to provide recommendations for controlling surplus populations of dogs (WHO/WSPA, 1990). The recommendations urged governments to study the pattern of dog populations and the traditions of dog management in their areas in order to work out effective management strategies. In particular, they were urged to give greater encouragement to the identification and to the neutering of household dogs; to do more to reduce the carrying capacity of the habitat. Controlling street food vendors and clearing up rubbish dumps; and to educate animal owners in order to make them more responsible in their attitudes to animal ownership could do this. If this worked, they would then be able to spend less money on catching and housing stray dogs.

The message was reinforced by the 8th Report of the Expert Committee on Rabies (WHO, 1992) which concluded that the removal and destruction of dogs should no longer be carried out on a large scale, as no impact on the spread of rabies had been demonstrated. Local authorities may still find it necessary to impound dogs to remove nuisance, but rabies control could no longer be given as a prime reason. The new strategies require better legislation, surer systems for identification of dogs, better animal control equipment, education about sterilization, and drugs for euthanasia which are often not available in the countries which most need them. They also require educational materials which the animal protection societies are in a better position to provide. Good working co-operation with the local animal protection societies is often difficult because of past histories of confrontation. All these problems have to be surmounted. It was in response to this challenge that WSPA set up its Pet Respect Campaign in 1994, with the aim of assisting governments, veterinarians and animal protection societies to manage and control animals humanely and efficiently. Pet Respect has now been introduced into 20 countries.

Case histories

Not all the dog population management programs of WSPA and other organizations have been successful and those that are proving successful are taking several years to achieve their objectives. However, by learning from the failures it is now possible to see the essential features required for success. These are highlighted in the case histories below.

Taiwan

A country which had no legislation to protect animals in spite of a Buddhist culture which teaches respect for all life and where a booming economy produced unforeseen problems of surplus dogs. Here, adverse publicity forced the municipal authorities to bring in animal protection legislation and humane methods of control. Population numbers are still not under control but good progress is being made.

In 1994, a representative of WSPA went to Taiwan to look at the stray dog problem in the capital, Taipei, at the request of the Life Conservationist Association (LCA) of Taipei.

The problem

Government statistics showed the scale of the problem: the number of dogs being caught by the Environmental Protection Agency in Taipei alone had risen from 6944 in 1992 to 7941 in 1993 and 13,862 in 1994. The rate at which dogs were being removed from the streets of the city was obviously not keeping pace with the rate at which they were being abandoned. This reflected the growing fashion for buying pedigree dogs bred from imported stock amongst the newly rich of Taiwan and the activities of professional and amateur dog breeders working to meet the new demand. There appeared to be a dissatisfaction with the local breeds and a tendency to reject them and also rejection of pedigree dogs which did not live up to the expectations of their owners.

The Life Conservationist Association (LCA) found that dogs roaming the streets, whatever their breed and condition, were caught by city employees using wire loops which cut into the animals' necks and were then taken to dirty, over-crowded dog pounds where they were given little or no care. Many died of starvation. There was no animal protection legislation, and dogs were officially regarded as "moving objects". The dog pounds were usually sited in or adjacent to rubbish dumps and straying dogs were indeed regarded by the local authorities as a form of rubbish. The result was that great suffering was caused to these unfortunate animals. WSPA reported the situation to the international press, and the world was shocked that a country like Taiwan, which had become so economically successful, should treat its animals in such an inhumane way.

Looking for a solution

WSPA and the LCA approached the problem by holding a Stray Animal Welfare Management Policy Conference in Taipei to which government employees of all levels were invited. In 1995, experts from Europe visited Taiwan and explained how dog populations should be managed, and WSPA put together a list of ten suggestions for the Government to follow:

- Draw up legislation to protect animals from cruelty and abandonment.
- Use humane methods to catch the dogs.
- Work out other methods of control as alternatives to "catch and kill".
- Construct better facilities and introduce better management at official dog pounds.
- Register all owned dogs.
- Identify all owned dogs.
- Promote population control through neutering programs.
- Introduce humane education into the schools.
- Mount a public awareness campaign to educate the general public about dog ownership.
- Commit the Government to finding humane solutions to problems caused by stray animals.

Making dog pounds into dog shelters

In 1996, WSPA sent an expert on kennel design to advise the Taipei city authorities on improvements to their dog pounds. Some changes had already been made: plastic-covered nooses had replaced the wire loops for catching the dogs. The bars forming the floor of the cages had been partially covered with plastic-coated sheeting, and this provided the animals with greater comfort, as well as preventing newborn puppies from falling through, or legs being trapped. WSPA made these further recommendations:

- Reduce overcrowding of cages.
- Give treatments for worms and skin disease.
- Do not give dogs access to rubbish.
- Separate the males from the females, and bitches with puppies from the rest.
- Separate the healthy from the diseased.
- Identify the seriously ill or injured, and those suffering severe pain, so that they can be humanely killed.
- Instruct staff to inspect the cages twice a day to remove any dead animals.
- Put solid floors in the cages.
- Give food and water in such a way that all the animals can eat and drink.
- Forbid all methods of killing except those recommended in the WHO/WSPA Guidelines, that is, carbon monoxide gas or injection of barbiturates.

In 1997, 15 officials from the Environmental Protection Bureau in Taipei came to Europe and included a visit to the Battersea Dogs' Home, London, where they were able to see how a large number of dogs can be housed comfortably in a small space in a built-up area without causing stress to the animals or the spread of disease.

Education

In 1997, an international team co-ordinated by LCA went to Taiwan to give workshops on humane education for teachers, to help local experts prepare a training manual on dog shelter management procedures, and to give practical demonstrations on dog handling and the injection techniques used in barbiturate euthanasia. There were also discussions on how to use carbon monoxide without causing explosions or poisoning the operators.

Euthanasia

It was found that there was resistance amongst some of the LCA volunteers and shelter staff to the idea of killing dogs, even when it was done to stop the animals' suffering. The Director of the LCA was a Buddhist and he had been criticized for stressing the need for euthanasia as part of a dog population management program. Even veterinarians were reluctant to kill dogs; however, this was probably largely because pentobarbitone sodium was not available, so they were not familiar with the "putting to sleep" method of euthanasia used in the West. When it was made available to them in a practical demonstration, most of them willingly participated.

Legislation

In 1994, an Animal Protection law had been drafted at the instigation of the LCA. The preamble stated that the purpose of the law was to show respect to living things and to protect them. It applied to all captive vertebrates and made it an offense to cause unnecessary suffering or to abandon an animal. Killing an animal would be permitted to alleviate suffering, but it would have to be carried out by a veterinarian except in an emergency. "Surplus" animals could be killed by a competent authority. Pets would have to be registered and wear an identity tag issued by the local authority. Animal shelters would be authorized. This law came into effect in November 1998, and already there has been a successful prosecution for causing suffering by organized dog-fighting.

Follow-up

In 1998, there was a follow-up survey of the 65 previously-visited facilities, and 10 further ones. It was found that the worst dog pounds had been closed down, including one where the dogs had been kept in a hole in the ground. At most of the others, food and water was available to all dogs; hygiene was improved; the sexes were separate; there was less over-crowding; the staff showed greater sensitivity. There was increased veterinary involvement, although it was not well organized. The importance of good house-keeping was beginning to be understood and the need for management training was beginning to be recognized. Unfortunately the methods used to catch the dogs were still poor.

The latest statistics from the Environmental Protection Agency in Taiwan show that the number of dogs caught in Taipei is not yet falling, because the sterilization programs are not yet in place and no attempt has been made to control the breeding of dogs for sale. In 1998, WSPA was assured by the Council of Agriculture in Taipei that all the ten points suggested by WSPA in 1995 would be implemented within 5 years.

Conclusions

Thanks to the local efforts of the LCA of Taipei, the international pressure brought to bear through WSPA, and the practical advice given by animal protection experts, conditions for dogs removed from the streets of Taiwan are improving. There is not a strong tradition of keeping dogs as companion animals in Taiwan, but this is now changing and people are ready to learn what responsible ownership means. WSPA hopes that soon an unwanted dog will be seen as a sentient being and not as an item of rubbish. Full details of this WSPA Pet Respect Campaign are in WSPA Reports (1996, 1997a, 1998).

Castel Volturno

A small town in southern Italy, where new animal protection legislation, although not enforced nationally, was harnessed to the efforts of a local animal protection society. A novelty here was that street dogs were returned to their streets after sterilization and marking. This prevented the "vacuum effect", where removal of animals leads to the filling of the site by immigration from other areas (the "neuter-and-return" method is used in many parts of the world for feral cats). The program in Castel Volturno described below has been published (Friz, 1998) and a summary is provided here.

Background

Rome is famous for its stray cats, but Naples and the south of Italy have a real problem with stray dogs. Up to 1989, the municipal authorities of Naples caught 3000 dogs every year, and killed most of them after 3 days. In 1989 the Italian Government passed an animal protection law which forbade the killing of healthy animals, but which made no provision of state funds for neutering. The Naples authorities stopped catching dogs and closed down the dog pound. The number of dogs on the streets did not increase, because the amount of food, water and shelter available to them did not change, but the problems of nuisance, hunger, disease and death of puppies got worse.

The Lega Pro Animale

Dorothea Friz, a German veterinarian, lived and worked in Italy since 1983. She formed an animal protection society - the Lega Pro Animale - and spent several years rescuing and neutering dogs, with very little local encouragement and no official assistance. Her program met with little success in reducing the overall problem and a different strategy was required. In 1991 she started up an integrated dog population management program, selecting the town of Castel Volturno, in southern Italy, in which to do it. This has been successful, because it has involved the local authorities, veterinarians and dog owners.

The problem

The human population of the Castel Volturno district is 11,000 in an area of 77 sq km. The total dog population is not known but may be assumed to be at least 1000. Of these, 430 have been observed and counted while running free. This suggests that a large proportion of the dog population of Castel Volturno live on the street. A local animal protection society tried to help the street dogs by taking them into a refuge. Soon they had over 650 dogs there. Funds were very limited, so the dogs were fed mostly on bread soaked in water and sick animals were rarely given veterinary treatment. The policy of the society was not to kill the old or sick dogs, and not to sterilize. Puppies born rarely thrived and some were eaten by hungry adults. In spite of the efforts of the members of the society, and the undoubted love they had for the animals in their care, the problems of over-crowding and hygiene were overwhelming, and made the kennels an unpleasant place to visit. Very few animals were found new homes.

Starting the program

In 1995, Friz started her program by systematically catching street dogs, looking for their tattoo marks and, if they had one, returning the dog to its owner. If the dog had no tattoo, Friz gave it a clinical examination and euthanized the sick, old, injured and vicious. The healthy ones were wormed, sterilized, vaccinated and tattooed or ear-ringed and then either returned to their street or kept in her kennels for re-homing. This program was accompanied by a large-scale information campaign, so that local people would understand that healthy dogs were not being taken away to be killed. Soon, the people who cared enough for the dogs to give them food started co-operating with the program. Within a few months, the population of street dogs began to fall; dog owners began to lose their prejudice against sterilization and veterinarians all over the area began offering a neutering service.

Co-operation with the veterinary and municipal authorities

Also in 1995, Friz offered the use of her clinic to the state veterinarians for the tattooing and registration of dogs. Between August 1995 and April 1998, 250 dogs were registered. Later that year, the Municipality agreed to pay Friz for kennelling the stray dogs which they caught because of complaints of nuisance. Between 1995 and 1998, 212 dogs were brought in. Of these, most were sick and were euthanized, but 56 were re-homed and 20 are still there waiting for new homes. The catching, neutering and tattooing of street dogs continued. Most of the dogs were returned to their street if the people living there agreed. Seventy-seven dogs were offered homes before they were caught, and so went to their new homes immediately they recovered from their operations. In these cases, the municipality paid for worming and vaccination.

Education

From November 1995, Friz and her colleagues visited schools in Castel Volturno to talk about animals, to show a video on the stray dog problem and to lead discussions on how they should be controlled. This has been a great success in the spreading of information about caring for dogs and cats.

By 1998 it was rare to see a sick dog in the streets of Castel Volturno, and the male dogs no longer formed packs, because there were no oestrous females.

There is so much demand for similar programs in other towns that the *Lega Pro Animale* started up training courses for veterinarians and is planning courses for dog catchers, kennel staff and volunteers. In 1997 they ran the first course for educationalists. Overseas animal welfare organizations have sponsored these courses and WHO has co-operated in aspects of public health education.

Conclusions

This program has shown the importance of combining identification with neutering, the necessity of working with the local authorities and the local veterinarians, the importance of education not only to gain acceptance for the program but also for the long-term solution to the problem of over-production of dogs and cats. The program also illustrated the fact that a well-organized program can attract sponsorship and support from other organizations.

"Neuter and return"

Returning sterilized dogs (or cats) to the street can be controversial, particularly in those countries which have laws against the abandonment of animals. It is important that animals are returned only to sites where systems, people and rotas are in place for supervising the health and welfare of the animals and for feeding them regularly. Local animal lovers must be made aware of these systems, and asked to co-operate if this is appropriate. Local authorities must be asked to recognize marked animals as part of a management program and take care to exclude them from poisoning campaigns. It is important that these authorities should be involved in the planning of the program so that their employees can co-operate in it. New legislation needs to be drafted in such a way that sterilized animals which are healthy and not aggressive can be returned to supervised sites, such as the streets from which they came. These animals should be given the same protection as owned animals. WSPA regards this method as appropriate in the early, transitional, stages of a dog population management program, particularly in hot countries where there is a strong tradition of dogs living in the street. It is not ideal, and can lead to suffering to dogs and humans through road traffic accidents. The long-term aim, particularly in European countries, should be to reduce the street population to zero.

Dundee

Dundee was one of the first British cities to introduce animal wardens (animal control officers) with an educational as well as dog-catching role. Animal wardens are now employed by local authorities throughout Britain, with excellent results. They often depend on the co-operation of an animal welfare society to train its officers and to re-home some of the impounded animals.

Background

In the UK dogs are required by law to wear a collar whenever they are in a public place. The collar must carry a means of identification, such as a tag with the owner's name and address. Until 1990, the police were responsible for stray dog control. Members of the public had the duty of reporting lost or stray dogs to the police, who then tried to return the dogs to their owners. The success of this arrangement depended on owners complying with the law requiring dogs to wear a collar and tag. Unidentified and unclaimed dogs were made available for adoption (re-homing). This service was, in theory, financed by dog owners paying an annual license fee, but no efforts were made to enforce payment.

The problem

In Dundee, as in many other large cities with new housing estates, the system of dog control broke down and the police became more and more reluctant to fulfil their role. The problem arose because families moved into the new apartment blocks with their animals and then let the dogs out to run during the day while they were at work. Many of the families found that they could not cope with their dogs in their new living conditions and abandoned them. Many complaints were received from the public about the problems caused by stray dogs.

In 1981, the City of Dundee Environmental Health Department employed two dog wardens (animal control officers) to take over the duties of the police, and to collect the stray dogs to take them to the dog pound. Each year, about 2400 dogs were taken in and a third of them had to be killed because they were not reclaimed by their owners. The complaints from the public continued.

The solution

In 1988, the Department began to include sterilization in its program: impounded bitches were ovario-hysterectomized (spayed) before re-homing, and owned bitches in the community who were recognized as persistent re-breeders were brought in for spaying. This was followed by a subsidized spaying service to encourage all owners of bitches to bring them in for surgery. The number of straying dogs collected fell to one half within 5 years, and the number of puppies collected fell dramatically. The packs of dogs which once roamed the estates are a thing of the past. The statistics show the story (Table 11.1).

In 1990, there was a change in the law with the introduction of the Environmental Protection Act. This gave all local authorities the responsibility for dealing with stray dogs and they were advised to employ animal wardens who were good at dealing with the public as well as with animals and who could be used to educate animal owners. In particular they were to explain the necessity for dogs to carry identification and even to offer them free collars with metal tags, and to encourage owners to have their animals sterilized. The wardens could then make their own registers of dogs living in the area. License fees for dogs were abolished and the service was paid for out of local taxes, supplemented by charging owners fines for allowing their dogs to stray, and fees if the dogs had spent any time in the dog pound.

Table 11.1. Changes in the numbers of dogs and puppies collected or euthanized in Dundee between 1988 and 1998 (WSPA, 1994; Dundee City Council, 1998, personal communication).

	1998	1993	1998
Number of dogs collected	2314	1390	948
Euthanized	866	181	82
Adopted	542	649	464
Number of puppies collected	447	73	21
Euthanized	232	5	1

Dundee now employs five animal control officers who deal not only with stray dogs but with the problems of barking, biting and fouling of public places. The service is partly financed by the sale of healthy, unclaimed dogs.

The spread of the animal warden service

Within a year of the new Environmental Protection Act, 200 local authorities had some kind of animal warden service and several of them were offering a free or subsidized sterilization service. Today many offer a service to insert subcutaneous microchips for permanent identification, including registration on one of the voluntary registration schemes now available in the UK. Some supply scoops and plastic bags to deal with the problem of dogs fouling footpaths and public paths. Others run dog training classes. In some local authorities the animal wardens have become the victims of their own success, with their employers no longer seeing a problem with straying dogs, and so no longer wishing to employ them. Many of the animal wardens were trained by animal welfare societies, notably the College of Animal Welfare at the Wood Green Animal Shelter, Godmanchester. Most boroughs and districts depend on the co-operation of societies such as The Battersea Dogs' Home, Wood Green Animal Shelters and the RSPCA for the re-homing of unclaimed animals.

Methods for dog population management

Warning

It may be seen from the case-histories presented that there is no quick-fix solution to the problem of surplus dogs, and that no single agency, whether it be a local authority or an animal welfare society, can do it alone. Before deciding on the strategy for control the problem and its sources need to be understood. The traditions of the country need to be taken into account and a consideration of what could become acceptable if dog owners were given education in responsible ownership. The process may be speeded up by accepting the advice of experts. A successful solution will contain the following elements: assessment of the problem, legislation, humane methods of dealing with dogs, availability of euthanasia and sterilization and education in responsible dog ownership.

Assessment of the problem

Estimating dog populations

The first question asked by an authority or organization is usually "how many dogs are there?" The estimates given by worried local people are often greatly exaggerated and should not be accepted without checking. For example, a group of stray dogs may gather to feed at several points and so be counted several times over by people who are not familiar with them.

To understand the nature of the problem, the numbers of straying dogs, ownerless and feral dogs need to be known as percentages of the total dog population, which will also include the owned and supervised population.

Estimating the dog population of an area is not easy. The methods are described in Chapter 2. To get a clear picture, it is usually necessary to use questionnaires as well as counting methods, in order to include dogs kept on private property as well as those in the streets, and to calculate what percentage of the dogs in the streets have identifiable owners. The results of the studies carried out in certain South American, Asian and African countries show that total dog populations in many different parts of the world are similar if calculated in relation to human populations, being somewhere in the range of one dog to ten humans and one dog to six humans. However, there are some countries where, because of the religious and socio-cultural background, there are fewer dogs than this. Examples are Syria, Jordan and Yemen. Within one country there may be wide differences between rural, peri-urban and urban areas. In Tunisia, for example, the ratio varies between one dog per three inhabitants to one dog for 25 or 40 people. In the UK in 1988 there was a human population of about 58 million and about 7 million owned dogs; half a million dogs were loose in the streets or the countryside at any one time, and half of those had known owners (London School of Economics, 1989). The statistics produce a dog:human ratio of about 1:8. Since 1988, the number of dogs kept in the UK has fallen slightly. This has been associated with changing life-styles, such as smaller households and more women going out to work (Pet Food Manufacturers' Association, 1998).

The composition of the dog population also needs to be considered, particularly the proportion of males to females and of juveniles to adults. A high proportion of juveniles suggests a high mortality rate amongst adult dogs coupled with a high reproductive rate amongst the adults which survive. To differentiate between dogs which live more-or-less permanantly in a particular area and those which are passing through, it is necessary to draw up a register with the help of local people through questionnaires. Once the size of the problem has been defined and sub-divided in this way, it becomes less daunting and priorities can be set for dealing with it. Estimates can also be made of the number of dogs which may need to be impounded and for which kennels will have to be provided.

Supply and demand

It is useful to know where people get their dogs from. Well-bred dogs with good pedigrees are expensive, and many people will look for cheaper sources. This gives encouragement to owners of non-pedigree bitches to allow them to breed, and opportunities for commercial breeders and pet shops. A successful program to reduce the number of dogs straying in an area can lead to the unfortunate consequence that irresponsible owners will lose their dogs, fail to reclaim them and then go out to buy new ones.

In several countries, including the UK, there is now a recognized problem of "puppy farming", where people will keep several bitches for the sole purpose of breeding. They may be housed in poor, unhygienic conditions with no control over the spread of disease. Moreover, the puppies may not be given the handling when young which is required to socialize them - that is, to make them confident and trusting of people and thus safe as future companion animals. Such puppies will require a lot of time and patience from their new owners, which the owners may not be prepared to give. The animal may develop unsuitable behavior such as timidity, aggression, fear of being left alone or destructiveness, which may lead to the owner abandoning the animal and the animal being difficult to re-home successfully.

Sources of dogs which can cause problems

Possible sources of dogs causing a nuisance are:

- owned but unsupervised dogs, or those let out to scavenge for food
- dogs lost or abandoned, e.g. after the departure of their owners
- dogs accompanying people migrating from rural to urban areas
- lost or straying dogs attracted into particular areas by availability of food
- dogs rejected because of behavioral or other problems
- community or neighborhood dogs given inadequate supervision
- unsupervised dogs breeding in the feral state.

Problems caused by the dogs

Complaints received, whether by the local authority, tourist authority or animal protection society, can usually be put into one of these categories:

- sick puppies or dogs needing attention

- animals scrounging or scavenging for food
- dogs biting
- dogs forming packs and roaming
- dogs fouling public places
- dogs causing road accidents
- dogs barking.

The causes of dogs behaving in unacceptable ways will depend largely on the tradition of dog ownership in the area. For example, it may be usual for owners to let their dogs roam unsupervised and to scavenge for food instead of providing them with adequate food at home. Stalls in the street selling food, or the rubbish tips in the area may be very attractive to dogs, and encourage them to stray. Owners may make no attempt to keep their estrous bitches indoors and thus encourage pack formation amongst the males.

Legislation

Before a dog population management scheme can succeed, legislation must be in place to support it and to make provision for the enforcement of some elements of it. The pressure for new legislation to protect animals will often come from the animal protection societies. They can be a useful source of information about current abuses of animals and the sort of laws that are necessary to prevent those abuses. Other laws are necessary for the enforcement of control measures and for the control of dangerous dogs. The necessary legislation is in four parts, as below.

1. Laws to protect animals against cruelty

The first part of the necessary legislation is to protect animals against cruelty, in order to instill a sense of respect for animals amongst the human population in general and to state clearly the responsibilities of an owner towards their own animals. Cruelty is usually defined as the infliction of unnecessary suffering and includes terrorizing an animal as well as inflicting physical pain. Neglect is also a form of cruelty. For example, failing to provide food, water and shelter to the animal and failing to provide care and treatment if the animal is sick or injured. It is also the responsibility of the owner to permit the euthanasia of their animal if it is suffering from pain that cannot be relieved. Abandonment of an animal is a form of neglect. Owners should be encouraged to take their unwanted animals to a specified place such as a state veterinary clinic or animal refuge.

The use of cruel poisons such as strychnine, or methods of capture which cause injury to the animals, would be forbidden in this law and it would apply to private persons and to people employed to deal with stray dogs. Humane methods of control would therefore have to be adopted by local authorities. This law could also specify the standards to be maintained in dog pounds and lay down the minimum statutory periods that the dogs must be kept to allow owners to come and reclaim them. An animal protection law may also forbid certain mutilations, such as the cropping of ears or the docking of tails. Exceptions would have to be made for the surgical act of sterilization and any agreed method of marking the animal to signify that it has been sterilized.

The question of killing animals may also be dealt with here. In most countries, an owner has the right to kill his own animals, but the methods to be used may be stipulated. Normally, a veterinarian should carry out the killing by a method of euthanasia but there are occasional emergencies, such as road accidents, where a more direct method such as a sharp blow to the head, may be permitted. The methods used to kill unwanted dogs that have been impounded would also be subject to this law. In recent years, several countries have introduced legislation that forbids the killing of healthy stray dogs. Such legislation is not helpful to the animals or the authorities unless other measures are in place to ensure that humane methods are being developed to deal with surplus dogs, such as subsidized sterilization and encouragement of re-homing.

2. Control through identification and registration

The second part of the necessary legislation is to make it compulsory for owners to give their animals a form of identification and to register them if a register is thought necessary such as for disease control purposes. In countries where rabies is endemic, a register could assist in the identification of a dog that has bitten a human, and in knowing whether or not it has been vaccinated against rabies. A registration system could also be combined with other veterinary procedures such as de-worming and sterilization. In developed countries it could be combined with an insurance scheme to indemnify the owner for damage caused by his dog. Once identification has been made compulsory, it is possible to employ animal control officers to re-unite straying dogs with their owners and to impound those that cannot be identified. No method of identification of dogs is perfect, but these are the ones that have withstood the test of time:

- Wearing a collar to which is attached a metal plate or disc bearing the name and address of the owner, or a registration number. This is the most convenient method, but the collars are sometimes lost through theft or accident.
- Tattooing of a registration number or code on the inside of the ear or the inside of the thigh. Trained personnel can carry this out without anaesthetizing the animal, and the mark persists for several years.
- Implanting a microchip subcutaneously bearing a registration number. This has the advantage of being permanent and tamper-proof, but the disadvantage of not being obvious and requiring a special scanner to read and decode the information. This method is now routinely used by the Battersea Dogs' Home and the RSPCA so that they can keep track of the animals re-homed from their shelters.

If registration numbers are used instead of names and addresses in any of these methods, it must be easy to consult the register or to contact the registrar at most times of the day and most days in the year, in order to obtain the information necessary to re-unite the dog with its owner. If the dog has to be re-registered every year, a color-coded disc or tag could be worn in addition to the microchip. If the prime purpose of identification is to show that the animal has been vaccinated against rabies, it may be sufficient to fit a color-coded collar or tag (disc) at the time of vaccination or re-vaccination. The collar could be made of cheap but tough material such as woven nylon, with a fastening which is not easily undone. Care must be taken not to fit the collar too tightly if the dog is still growing. Color-coded ear tags could be used for the same purpose.

International registers

When the aim is to develop an internationally-recognized register, the implantable microchip offers the most practical solution. In the past, a disadvantage of the microchip system has been the incompatibility between the microchips and readers produced by different manufacturers. To overcome this problem, an international standard which uses the FDX-B microchip was agreed by some international bodies, such the Federation of European Companion Animal Veterinary Associations and the World Small Animal Veterinary Association in 1997. It incorporates ISO 11784 and 11785, which require a 15-digit coding sequence incorporating a country code and a unique identification code, and describes the electronic and radio frequency technology which controls how information is exchanged between reader and microchip. In the UK, the register is kept on the Petlog database, which is run jointly by the Kennel Club, the RSPCA and the Scottish Society for the Prevention of Cruelty to Animals. It can link up with registers in other countries, and so is particularly useful for animals that travel outside their own countries. Information is available from the RSPCA (see Appendix). In other countries, the local Veterinary Association should be able to supply information.

3. Legal control of supply of animals

The third part of the necessary legislation should deal with commercial breeders and pet shops, which can be important sources of surplus animals. There should be a licensing system in which inspectors ensure that good standards of animal health and welfare in breeding premises and in pet shops are set and maintained. In the UK, this is done through the Breeding of Dogs Acts 1973 and 1991. Recent concern about the use of agricultural premises for the breeding of puppies on a large scale ("puppy farming") has led to a tightening of the existing licensing system through The Breeding and Sale of Dogs (Welfare) Act 1999. This law will make it illegal for commercial breeders to mate bitches before they are 12 months old, or to allow a bitch to have more than six litters in her lifetime, or to have more than one litter in a 12-month period. Pet shops must be licensed and sell puppies only from licensed breeders. This measure should reduce the number of dogs subsequently abandoned by their owners on grounds of poor conformation, poor health or poor behavior. Legislation of this type could be used for the licensing and inspection of establishments for boarding dogs and cats, and perhaps also for animal protection society shelters. In most countries operating a licensing system, it is the Department of the Environment that is responsible for its administration. In the Gdansk area of Poland, micro-chipping is proving a useful way of eliminating bad puppy-farmers. All dogs have to be micro-chipped and registered at 2 months and no dog can be sold at a street market or pet shop unless it is registered. The sources of diseased or deformed puppies can thus be traced and prosecuted. Any unregistered dog offered for sale is sent to an animal welfare shelter, where it is given a permanent identification before treatment and re-homing (Animal Protection Society of Gdansk, 1998, personal communication).

4. Dangerous dogs

The fourth part of the necessary legislation should deal with the protection of humans and their livestock against dangerous dogs. A law should allow that any dog which has been shown to be dangerous by attacking people and causing serious injury, or by killing livestock, may be shot dead by a police marksman. The owner should also be punished for allowing a dangerous dog outside his premises without close supervision. Certain breeds could be outlawed, for example those specially bred for dog-fighting such as pit-bull terriers. In the UK it has been found to be difficult to identify these breeds with certainty, which makes enforcement of the law difficult. More detailed suggestions may be found in WSPA (1994) and in WHO-WSPA (1990).

Humane methods of dealing with dogs

Methods used to capture dogs

Animal control officers should be trained to use a gentle approach. It is often possible to catch tame stray dogs using only a little meat or biscuit as bait and a loop of rope to pass through the collar or round the neck. The dogs can then be lifted into a vehicle for transport to the dog pound and attached to a hook by a lead from the collar. Sometimes it is advisable to put a muzzle on the dog. More timid dogs may need to be caught with specialized equipment such as a semi-rigid slip-lead (e.g. the Nimrod produced by MDC products Ltd) or a dog grasper (a loop at the end of a rigid pole) or a net. For this, it may be necessary to coax them into an enclosed area. In the vehicle, they should be placed in a cage or carrier for transport to the dog pound. This cage should then be lifted out and carried, and the dog not released into its pen until it has been examined and registered.

Dogs in open spaces that cannot be cornered should be caught using a cage trap. This may require patience and the use of baits for a few days to accustom the dog to the cage before the trap is set. The dog should be transported in the trap and not released into a pen until it has been examined and registered. Dangerous dogs should not be approached unless the handler is wearing protective clothing. Dogs in inaccessible places or suspected of being rabid may be immobilized using dart guns or blowpipes. The necessary equipment and expertise may be available at wildlife parks or zoos. For details of the equipment available and the methods of use, see WSPA (1999), and the publications of the Humane Society of the US. Suppliers include Animal Care Equipment and Services (ACES) and MDC (see Appendix).

Dog pounds

In many countries, impounded dogs must be put into quarantine for 2 weeks to ensure that they are free from rabies. All countries should have a statutory length of time during which the animal must be kept to allow its owner to come and reclaim it; this is usually 1 week. It is therefore necessary to have kennel accommodation available.

In the UK and many other countries, the local authorities often depend on the animal protection societies to provide some of this accommodation and to organize the re-homing of healthy and suitable unclaimed animals, in return for a set scale of fees. Each of the London Boroughs has short-term kennels close by, where they take impounded dogs as soon as they have caught them, but after a few days they are sent on to animal shelters which are run by animal protection societies where the dogs can be housed in greater comfort. The Boroughs pay a fee to the charities for providing this service.

Impounded dogs should be housed separately and not mixed until they have undergone veterinary examination, endo- and ecto-parasite treatment and vaccination. Then, females must be kept separate from males and young dogs from adults. Each animal should be able to move freely and have a bed area where it can lie comfortably. Pens must be designed so that kennel staff can get in easily to clean them without endangering themselves. Impervious surfaces are necessary for good hygiene. Every kennel and shelter should be clear about its maximum capacity, beyond which it is not possible to accept more animals if good standards of animal care and hygiene are to be maintained. Kennels need to be carefully planned and managed (see WSPA, 1992b; RSPCA, 1996; Association of British Dogs' Homes, 1998). Advice is also available from other animal protection organizations, notably the Humane Society of the US, the American Society for the Prevention of Cruelty to Animals, the Massachusetts Society for the Prevention of Cruelty to Animals and the Universities Federation for Animal Welfare (see Appendix).

Euthanasia

Definition of euthanasia

A method of euthanasia, or humane killing, is one that causes rapid loss of consciousness, which is then followed by cardiac arrest and death.

Indications for euthanasia

In a dog population management program there are always some dogs which are suffering and should be humanely killed. A service to provide a gentle, painless death to such animals can be a valuable part of the program. Ideally, a service should be available to all owners who have animals they can no longer care for at home, or unwanted litters of puppies.

Euthanasia can be an emotive topic, particularly in animal protection societies. Conflict may be avoided if each organization works out its policies on euthanasia before the program begins, by compiling a list of the indications or situations in which they would wish animals to be euthanized, with the criteria to be applied. These criteria should be known to the other organizations co-operating in a program, so that they may work together amicably, with each respecting the views of the others.

A local authority should employ a veterinarian to examine dogs before a decision to euthanize is made and the decision should be taken according to agreed criteria. The indications and criteria for euthanasia may include any of the following. Severe injury which is causing long-term or severe pain which cannot be relieved. Incurable illness which is causing distress to the animal or a risk to other animals. Serious illness which cannot be treated for reasons of cost or difficulty in handling the animal. Disease communicable to man which cannot be effectively treated. Behavior making the animal unsuitable for re-homing, such as aggression. Dangerous behavior which is putting personnel in the dog pound at risk. Old age or other factors which will make the animal unlikely to attract a new owner. An animal protection society will often be prepared to put more effort into treating and rehabilitating animals than a municipal dog pound and so have different criteria for euthanasia.

Animal shelters run by societies that refuse euthanasia for any animal have only limited value in a dog population management program. If the society prefers to let dogs live even though they are suffering, their shelters will almost inevitably be over-crowded, with the problems of finance and hygiene that follow. The leaders of such a society may change their minds when they see a method of euthanasia sympathetically carried out. The training of veterinarians in euthanasia techniques is of great importance. In a program with many dogs, the local authority may need to run its own kennel with a pro-euthanasia policy and only pass on homeable dogs to an animal protection society when it is known that the society's shelter has space available. If there is no animal protection society shelter willing to co-operate, then the local authority will have to euthanize all unclaimed animals after an agreed period of time. This period may be as short as 3 days, but should be at least 14 days to give owners a chance to reclaim their animals and to prepare the dogs for possible re-homing.

Availability of materials for euthanasia

The substances recommended for euthanasia are normally available only to veterinarians, because of national or local regulations restricting the use of dangerous drugs. Administration of these substances should be carried out only by veterinarians or by people working under their supervision who have been trained and are known to be competent. Fire-arms are normally available only to licensed or authorized persons and must be kept under conditions of security.

Physical restraint

Any pain or anxiety felt by the animals is likely to be caused by the method of holding or restraining the animal. It is thus important that all personnel involved in euthanasia should be trained in methods of restraint. This includes ways of holding the animal during intravenous injection procedures and how to use muzzles, dog graspers and nets to enable the veterinarian to give injections accurately by other routes, or for fire-arms to be used safely.

Chemical restraint

Nervous animals can be calmed by giving them tranquilizers such as acepromazine by mouth or injection before euthanasia. The handling of difficult animals has been greatly simplified by the availability of anesthetic drugs which cause deep sedation. The most widely used is ketamine, which is a non-barbituric, non-narcotic dissociative anesthetic which can be administered by intra-muscular or sub-cutaneous injection. For dogs, it is best used in combination with xylazine, by the intramuscular route. The animal is held with a grasper or cornered in its pen and injected with a long-reach hypodermic syringe. Metomidine is also effective but more expensive. Smaller dogs can be transferred into special squeeze or crush cages from their traps and injected through the wire mesh (see WSPA, 1997b). Once anesthetized and thus unconscious, the animal can be killed by the injection of a lethal dose of one of the substances listed below.

Recommended substances for euthanasia

Barbiturates

The drugs of choice are the barbiturate anesthetics given as an over-dose. The most commonly used are:

- Pentobarbitone or pentobarbital sodium, which is available as a soluble powder or as a ready-made solution. It can be injected by the intravenous or intraperitoneal routes in adult animals. In puppies it is administered intra-peritoneally. It is bitter to the taste but can be administered orally in the form of capsules.

- Thiopentone sodium, a faster-acting anaesthetic, which can be given only intravenously. This drug is more expensive than pentobarbitone, but sometimes more easily available because it is used in human surgery. Care must be taken in its use, because animals can recover consciousness after an apparently lethal dose.
- Phenobarbitone, a tasteless powder which can be administered by mixing with food. It causes death in 1-2 hours if taken in sufficient quantity (see Instituto Dex, Seville, in Appendix).
- T 61, a mixture of a general anesthetic, a local anesthetic and a paralyzing agent. When administered intravenously, it causes loss of consciousness and death. It is sometimes available in countries where barbiturates are not permitted and so can be used as a substitute. If it is administered at the wrong speed, it can cause muscle paralysis in the conscious animal and, because of this risk, the drug has been banned in several countries.

Substances which can be used in the anesthetized animal

Once the dog has been anesthetized, e.g. with ketamine or by inhalation of a gaseous anesthetic, it can be killed by the intravenous or intracardiac injection of barbiturate. If barbiturates are not available the following could be administered intravenously in the unconscious animal. Magnesium sulfate $MgSO_4$ (Epsom salts), as a concentrated solution. This should be carried out in a place which is easy to clean, because the injection often causes evacuation of the bowels. Potassium salts, e.g. KCl, KNO_3 (saltpetre), KSO_4 as concentrated solutions.

Air

Inhalation of gaseous anesthetic

A dog can be anaesthetized using an agent such as ether, halothane or nitrous oxide mixed with oxygen. Once the animal is unconscious, the oxygen supply can be cut off so that the animal dies of anoxia, or an injection can be given as above.

Carbon monoxide gas

CO is a highly toxic gas, which is present in petrol engine exhaust fumes. It can be used for the euthanasia of individual or large numbers of animals if no other method is available, preferably by using the pure compressed gas from a cylinder. It is dangerous: safety precautions must be taken to protect personnel from inhaling it and to prevent explosions (see AVMA, 1993).

Firearms

A dog may be shot with a pistol firing either a free bullet or a captive bolt. The animal should be firmly restrained, then the open end of the pistol placed firmly against the animal's head, between the eyes and the ears. A free bullet should penetrate the brain and kill the animal; care must be taken in case it passes right through the head and penetrates the operator's foot or ricochets against the floor or wall. A captive bolt only stuns the animal and makes it unconscious. The unconscious animal must be killed by pithing or exsanguination. A rifle or revolver may also be used, with the open end held at 3-5 cm from the animal's head.

Methods no longer recommended

RSPCA Chloroform Chamber

Special chambers for the anesthesia and euthanasia of puppies using chloroform have been widely used in the past. Their manufacture was discontinued when it was discovered that chloroform is toxic and that operatives using the boxes frequently were at risk of liver damage.

Electrocution

Cabinets designed to pass an electric shock through the brain and then the body of the dog, to render it first unconscious and then to arrest the heart, are in use in some parts of the world. They are humane if correctly used. They are no longer manufactured.

Cyanide

Cyanide is an effective but highly dangerous drug and cannot be recommended.

Drowning

This is a traditional method of killing puppies. It causes distress to the animals and is not recommended.

Curariform drugs

These drugs cause death by paralyzing the respiratory muscles of the conscious animal. It is known from human experience that this is a terrifying experience, and they should not be used.

Strychnine

Taken by mouth as a poison strychnine causes a painful death, and because it is toxic in small quantities it is also dangerous to other animals which may eat it by mistake. Its action is more rapid if administered by injection, but it still causes convulsive seizures. WSPA recommends that strychnine should never be used to kill dogs.

Methods for use in emergencies

In emergencies where it is not possible to obtain the services of a veterinarian or other authorized person, an animal can be killed by physical methods, such as a hard blow to the back of the head or by breaking the neck.

Disposal of carcasses

The signs of death are the cessation of respiration and heart beat. Animals do sometimes revive from a state of apparent death. It is important that animals should not be assumed to be dead until rigor mortis has set in. Only then should the carcasse be disposed of. The usual methods of disposal are burial and incineration. If neither of these is practicable, the local authorities should be consulted about the use of rubbish tips. Animals which have been euthanized by administration of anesthetics will contain residues of those substances and should not be eaten by other animals, and nor should animals which have died of disease. This could make the use of public rubbish tips dangerous.

For a complete overview, see the 1993 Report of the AVMA Panel on Euthanasia. Guidelines on euthanasia have been produced by the RSPCA (Phillips, 1997). For recommendation on the use of firearms, see Humane Slaughter Association, 1998 and 1999.

Neutering (sterilization)

Control of reproduction

Reducing the number of puppies born is a vital part of a dog population management program. Owners of dogs often need to be educated in the importance of controlling the reproduction of their animals. Animal pounds and shelters must have clear policies on when the dogs in their care will be sterilized, and whether unsterilized animals will be made available for adoption or re-homing. Education is important, because there are sometimes psychological barriers that need to be broken down. Owners may want their dogs to produce puppies to replace absent children; or they may see "taking their sex away" as incompatible with animal rights. Some owners may think that religious objection to contraception in humans also applies to animals. Such owners need to consider their responsibilities towards the animals they allow to be born; the burden that unwanted animals place on society and the misery caused to abandoned animals.

Physical control

Bitches usually come into season (estrus) twice a year and are fertile for several days each time. Owners may try to prevent their bitches from being mated by keeping them indoors but this usually fails because estrous animals show great determination in escaping. One also needs to consider the distress caused to an estrous bitch and to the dogs attracted to her, by being prevented from mating.

Chemical control

Many chemical substances have been tested for their effect on reproduction in animals and research is still continuing to find the perfect product. None has yet replaced the well-established synthetic progestational steroids, such as megestrol acetate, which are used for the temporary sterilization of bitches. They are available from veterinarians and are useful for owners who wish to rest their breeding bitches or to postpone surgery. WSPA does not recommend their use for non-breeding animals and considers that they should not be used for stray dogs except under exceptional circumstances.

Surgical methods

Surgical methods have the advantage of being permanent. They also have useful secondary effects. Male dogs which have been castrated show modifications in behavior, such as reduced aggression and reduced tendency to roam. Females which have been ovariectomized show a reduced tendency to roam. Behavior is not modified after vasectomy or destruction of the epididymis in males, or in ligation of the fallopian tubes in females. This may be seen as an advantage in guard dogs but not in other cases. To sterilize females, most veterinarians prefer to remove the uterus as well as the ovaries (ovario-hysterectomy) to prevent the development of pyometra later in life. Removal of the ovaries alone (ovariectomy) is quicker and may cause less trauma to the animal. It should not be risked if there is a possibility that the animal is pregnant. WSPA recommends that in a dog population management program, as many dogs and bitches as possible be neutered by castration and ovario-hysterectomy. The surgical operations for neutering must be carried out under anesthesia in order to eliminate pain and under sterile conditions in order to prevent the risk of infection. The cost may be a disadvantage unless there is a system of reduced or subsidized costs. A campaign or scheme organized by a local authority or animal protection society may enable local veterinarians to reduce their costs by increasing their throughput. In many countries, animal protection societies offer vouchers to poorer owners that subsidize the cost at the surgery. Ideally, a system like this should be put in place and then extended in order to neuter poorly supervised dogs and community dogs.

Early-age neutering

Surgical castration and ovario-hysterectomy can be carried out on the young animal before the sexual organs reach maturity. The physical and mental development of the animal is not greatly affected and there do not appear to be any harmful side effects. Extra care is needed during anesthesia and precautions taken against hypothermia. The surgical techniques involve smaller-scale instruments than normal, but the procedure is otherwise straightforward (Howe, 1997).

In the USA it is now becoming a common practice to operate on dogs as young as 8 weeks in animal shelters, so that the animals can be offered for adoption already neutered. This has the advantage that the new owner does not have to bring the animal back for neutering later on. Early neutering cannot yet be recommended for animals which are returned to places where they will be poorly supervised and offered little protection, because the effect of the operation on the animals' behavior has not yet been adequately studied.

Marking

Dogs that have been sterilized could be given a distinctive mark, e.g. an ear tag or stud, or a notch in the ear, or a colored collar. This would be particularly useful if they were to be returned to poorly supervised sites, so that their status could be clearly seen.

Veterinary expertise

WSPA's Pet Respect campaigns in developing countries have highlighted the problem of veterinarians who are employed mainly by the state veterinary services to deal with farm animals and who may have been given little training in companion animal medicine and surgery. WSPA can offer opportunities for such veterinarians to develop their practical skills and knowledge through 2-week intensive veterinary development programs.

Education

Children

Children have a natural affinity for animals and are receptive to ideas about caring for them. Talks in school, after-school clubs and illustrated booklets can be used to give them information on basic care, such as feeding, providing shelter, giving training and the dog's need for exercise. The information may be produced and disseminated by animal protection societies, teachers and animal control officers.

Animal-owners

People need information at the time they acquire an animal, on a number of topics, including: vaccinations and anti-parasite treatments, their legal obligations to identify, register and limit the freedom of their dog, advice on feeding and training the dog, the advantages of neutering. This information could be provided by the animal shelter, a veterinarian or an animal control officer. Leaflets are often available from animal feed and medicines companies. Several books are available on the behavior of dogs and how to train them (see Bailey, 1998). Training classes may be needed where owners can take their dogs to learn obedience.

The public

There may be religious or other reasons for people to be fearful of unsupervised dogs, for example because they are considered dangerous or unclean. If so, steps may need to be taken to make people less fearful. For example, owners could be persuaded not to allow their dogs to roam in public places. Methods could be used to identify dogs that have been vaccinated against rabies and so are less dangerous to the public. Owners could be persuaded to de-parasitize their dogs regularly so that there is less risk of them transmitting zoonoses. Particular situations, such as a rabies vaccination campaign or a sterilization campaign, can be publicized through TV, radio and magazine articles, as well as by the societies and the local authorities.

Training animal control officers and animal protection society personnel

Animal control officers and the personnel at animal shelters are likely to be the main source of information to animal owners, so it is important that they are well-trained and knowledgeable in aspects of law and animal care as well as animal control. Animal control officers need to have a good basic education and training courses should be provided for them. In the UK, the number of dogs straying has been significantly reduced by the activities of the animal wardens and this has given them more time to educate dog owners, to run obedience classes and to undertake inspection and licensing of animal breeding and holding premises. Information is available from the National Dog Warden Association (see Appendix).

The human-companion animal bond

The value of companion animals, particularly dogs, to humans is now being studied more systematically (see Chapter 1). The use of dogs in therapy for disturbed and disabled children, their use as guides to the blind and ears to the deaf and their value in giving comfort to the sick and elderly are now more greatly understood and appreciated. This information can be put to practical use in the devising of policies for harmonious co-existence of animals and people in towns. For example, l'Association Francaise d'Information et de Recherche sur l'Animal de Compagnie (AFIRAC) provides an information service and a team of experts to advise on these matters. The Society for Companion Animal Studies (SCAS) provides information on assistance animals, therapy using animals, and bereavement counselling for animal owners (see Appendix).

The cost of dog population management programs

Calculating the cost

The direct costs of dealing with stray dogs can be calculated from the records kept by the police or local authority. They are the costs involved in collecting and kenneling dogs and destroying those that are not reclaimed or rehomed. Included are fees paid to animal shelters who accept healthy unclaimed dogs with a view to finding them new homes. There are also indirect costs which are imposed on society by road accidents caused by dogs, hospital treatments for people injured by dogs, post-exposure rabies vaccination of people bitten by dogs of unknown vaccination status and injury to livestock caused by straying dogs. These are more difficult to calculate but can be very high. In a study commissioned from the London School of Economics by the RSPCA (LSE, 1989), an attempt was made to put figures to some of these categories. The figures were collected when the police were responsible for the control of stray dogs. A later report (Economists Advisory Group, 1998) has collected figures for the years after 1990, when responsibility for stray dog control passed from the police to the Department of the Environment. These figures show the impact made by the employment of animal wardens (Tables 11.2 and 11.3). The fall in the number of dogs straying and being dealt with by the authorities is dramatic and is observable in most areas. The number of road accidents caused by dogs has fallen even more dramatically, so that the cost of employing animal wardens is more than offset by the reduction in costs to the health services. The number of other injuries caused by dogs has not fallen, because most injuries are caused by the owner's own dog at home. There are still costs to the police under the new schemes, because animal wardens work only in the daytime and police still have to take in lost dogs which members of the public bring to them at other times. In the 1998 Report the RSPCA and the Kennel Club conclude that the best way of dealing with the problem of straying dogs is to introduce a national registration scheme, so that lost dogs can be re-united with their owners as quickly as possible. They propose that the registration fee should be set at a level that would cover the cost of the animal warden service.

Table 11.2. Numbers of dogs handled by police and animal wardens in the UK in 1988 and 1996 (Adapted from LSE, 1989; EAG, 1998).

	1988	1996
Number of dogs in the UK	7.4 million	6.9 million
Dogs not identifiable and recorded as stray	240,000	139,000
Dogs claimed by owners	60,000	46,500
Dogs adopted or sent to animal shelter	90,000	51,600
Dogs euthanized	90,000	16,200

Table 11.3. The costs of stray dogs in 1988 and 1996. Figures quoted are in millions of UK pounds. (Adapted from LSE, 1989; EAG, 1998.)

	1988	1996
Costs to police of dealing with stray dogs	6	15
Costs to local authorities of animal wardens	6	11-16
Direct costs of road accidents	> 50	18
Hospital treatments for other injuries by dogs	> 7	9
Injuries to livestock caused by stray dogs	1	2
Total	70	60

In countries such as India, where dogs live in the street as part of the community, successful programs involving collaboration between municipalities and animal protection societies have been developed. For example, the Animal Welfare Board of India (a government organization) is now giving financial support to 12 Animal Welfare Organizations (AWOs) who are carrying out 23 programs in six cities. The programs involve capture, neutering, vaccination against rabies and release. The number of dogs treated in this way in the years 1993-1998 was 97,000. The board gives a grant for each female and each male treated which more than covers the cost of surgery and allows the AWO to give post-operative care. A recent assessment shows that dog populations should be stabilized within 5-7 years so long as the programs are carried out efficiently, with clear identification of the dogs (preferably by making a notch in the ear while anesthetized). Programs also require good record-keeping; vigilance to bring incoming dogs into the program before they start breeding; special training in the necessary techniques for veterinarians and dog-catchers; good co-operation between the agencies involved in the program, and continuous efforts to raise public awareness (Dhanapalan and Thirunavukkarasu, 1999).

Measures of success

For WSPA, a Pet Respect campaign is successful if the host government recognizes the nature of the stray dog problem and is prepared to co-operate with animal welfare societies to implement policies to manage dog populations, in particular by the enforcement of animal protection legislation and by the empowerment of local authorities to deal with stray dogs humanely. For governments, success of a scheme will be visible when the costs of dealing with dogs, and particularly the indirect costs of dealing with problems caused by dogs, are reduced. This may take a few years.

For veterinary authorities administering dog registration schemes, success will be measured by the increasing numbers of owners complying with the regulations and thus becoming accessible for health measures, such as vaccination and worm control. Benefits to human health will follow. For veterinarians in private practice, a successful scheme will result in more owned dogs being presented for neutering and other treatments. For local authorities and tourist authorities, success will be seen in lower numbers of dogs in the streets and on the beaches and a fall in the number of complaints received about dogs. For animal protection societies, success is measured in the improved health of dogs, a reduction in the number of puppies produced and a reduction in the number of dogs needing refuge and care in their shelters. Another success would be better co-operation with the local and veterinary authorities. In general, success will lead to improved public attitudes towards dogs and a greater appreciation of their value to society as companions, helpers and therapists.

Conclusions

Dog population management is still a fairly new concept. The WHO-sponsored studies on dog ecology led the way to the new schemes based on legislation, education, neutering and humane techniques. These have been introduced successfully in countries where animal control officers are employed to implement them. Animal protection societies such as WSPA are learning from these experiences and are now introducing successful schemes into developing countries.

References

American Veterinary Medical Association (1993) Report of the AVMA panel on euthanasia. *Journal of the American Veterinary Medical Association* 202, 229-249. Also available on the Internet from the Animal Welfare Information Center at http://www. nal.usda. gov/ awic/ pubs.

Association of British Dogs' Homes (1998) Code of practice for animal rescue organization caring for cats and dogs. ABDH, c/o The Dogs' Home Battersea, London, pp. 16.

Bailey, G. (1998) *Good Dog Behavior - an Owner's Guide*. Harper Collins, London, pp. 128.

Dhanapalan, P. and Thirunavukkarasu, M. (1999) *Performance Evaluation of Animal Birth Control (ABC) Project of Animal Welfare Board of India*. Report commissioned by The Animal Welfare Board of India. Directorate of Clinics, Tamil Nadu Veterinary and Animal Sciences University, Chennai.

Economists Advisory Group (1998) The cost of stray dogs in the UK and the need for a national registration scheme: a report jointly funded by the RSPCA and the Kennel Club. Available from the RSPCA, Horsham, UK, pp. 38.

Friz, D. (1998) The Italian experience. *Proceedings of an International Companion Animal Conference* held in Bratislava, Slovakia. National Canine Defence League, London, pp.150.

Howe, L.M. (1997) Short-term results and complications of prepubertal gonadectomy in cats and dogs. *Journal of the American Veterinary Medical Assocation* 211, 57-61.

Humane Slaughter Association (1998) *Captive-bolt Stunning of Livestock,* 2nd edn. HSA, Wheathampstead, pp. 23.

Humane Slaughter Association (1999*) Humane Killing of Livestock using Firearms.* HSA, Wheathampstead, pp. 23.

London School of Economics (1989) *The Costs of Stray Dogs and Proposals for a National Dog Registration Scheme.* A report commissioned by the RSPCA. RSPCA, Horsham, pp. 49.

Pet Food Manufacturers Association (1998) *PFMA Profile 1998.* Available from PFMA, 12-13 Henrietta Street, London, WC2E 8LH.

Phillips, J.M. (1997) *Animal Euthanasia.* Guidelines published by the RSPCA, Horsham, pp. 14.

Royal Society for the Prevention of Cruelty to Animals (1996) *Guidelines for the Design and Management of Animal Shelters.* RSPCA, Horsham, pp. 56.

WHO (1984) *Guidelines for Dog Rabies Control.* VPH/83.43. WHO, Geneva.

WHO (1992) *WHO Expert Committee on Rabies,*eighth report. Technical Report Series, No. 824. WHO, Geneva, pp. 84.

WHO and WSPA (1990) *Guidelines for Dog Population Management.* WHO, Geneva. 116 pp in English; also in French: *Guide pour la Gestion des Population Canines,* Fondation Marcel Meriux, Lyon, France, pp. 118. Available from WSPA.

WSPA (1992a) *Proceedings of the 1992 Study Visit for Representatives of Animal Welfare Societies in Central and Eastern Europe.* WSPA, London, pp. 93.

WSPA (1992b) *Planning and Running an Animal Shelter.* WSPA, London, pp. 21.

WSPA (1994) *Stray Dog Control.* WSPA, London, pp. 49.

WSPA (1996) *Disposable Dogs: Made in Taiwan.* Report of an investigation by Joy Leney and David Marks for the WSPA Pet Respect Campaign. WSPA, London, pp. 44.

WSPA (1997a) *Pet Respect Campaign Visit to Taiwan, August 1997.* Report by Joy Leney. WSPA, London, pp. 23.

WSPA (1997b) *Cat Care and Control - a Practical Guide to the Management of Companion, Stray and Feral Cats.* WSPA, London, pp. 37.

WSPA (1998) *Disposable Dogs: Made in Taiwan - a Follow-up Report.* An investigation and survey of government holding facilities for stray dogs in Taiwan by Joy Leney (WSPA) and J.Lloyd Tait (ASPCA) January 1998. WSPA, London, pp. 32.

WSPA (1999) *Animal Control Officer: Dog Control Techniques.* Available as a book, 15pp, or as a video in VHS-Pal 625 or NTSC format, 15 mins. WSPA, London.

Appendix

Animal Care Equipment and Services (ACES),
PO Box 3275, 580 Forest Shade Drive,   Tel: (714) 338-1791
Crestline, CA 92325 USA   Fax: (714) 338-2799

Association of British Dogs' Homes,
c/o The Dogs' Home Battersea,
4 Battersea Park Road, London, SW8 4AA UK

Association Francaise d' Information et de Recherche sur l'Animal de Compagnie, 7 rue du Pasteur Wagner,
75011 Paris France

American Society for the Prevention of Cruelty to Animals,
424 East 92nd Street,
NY 10128 USA

Humane Slaughter Association (HSA)
The Old School, Brewhouse Hill,
Wheathampstead, Hertfordshire, AL4 8AN UK

Humane Society of the United States (HSUS),
2100 L Street NW,
Washington DC 20037 USA

Instituto Dex,
Jaime Balmes 8, 41007 Seville Spain

Massachusetts Society for the Prevention of Cruelty to Animals (MSPCA),
350 S Huntington Avenue,   Tel: 01582 655600
Boston, MA 02130 USA   Fax: 01582 613013

MDC Products Ltd,
35 Hastings Street,
Luton, Bedfordshire, LY1 5BE UK

National Dog Wardens Association,
PO Box 16188, London, NW1 2WN UK

Ritchey Taggs Ltd,
Fearby Road, Masham, Ripon,   Tel: 01765 689541
North Yorkshire, HG4 4ES UK   Fax: 01765 689851

Royal Society for the Prevention of Cruelty to Animals (RSPCA),
Causeway, Horsham,
West Sussex, RH12 1HG UK

Society for Companion Animal Studies (SCAS),
10b Leny Road, Callandar,
FK17 8BA UK

Universities Federation for Animal Welfare,
The Old School, Brewhouse Hill,
Wheathamstead, Hertfordshire, AL4 8AN UK

World Health Organization (WHO),   Tel: 791 21 11
1211 Geneva 27 Switzerland   Fax: 791 07 46

World Society for the Protection of Animals (WSPA),
2 Langley Lane, London, SW8 1TJ UK   Tel: 020 7793 0540
                                          Fax: 020 7793 0208
                                          Email: wspa@wspa.org.uk

Chapter Twelve

Zoonoses Control in Dogs

Francois X. Meslin, Michael A. Miles, J. Alejandro Vexenat and Michael A. Gemmell

As can be seen in the above chapters many diseases whether parasitic, bacterial or viral can be transmitted from dogs to humans. A very small number of them have been recognized as posing a significant public health problem requiring the initiation of large scale prevention and control activities. Two parasitic diseases, namely echinococcosis and leishmaniasis and one viral disease, rabies, fall into this category. Their epidemiological cycles and especially pathways for human infection are quite different. Zoonotic canine leishmaniasis requires the presence of an invertebrate vector, the sandfly, whereas the other two can be transmitted directly to humans. This may be through close contact with an infected dog or via the environment contaminated by eggs in dog feces in the case of cystic echinococcosis and through the bite of a diseased dog in the case of rabies. In all three diseases, dogs are involved as the main source or reservoir of the causal agents and consequently the first measures at hand to combat these diseases aimed at eliminating the most obvious source of the infectious agent. These measures were designed soon after the co-existence of a similar agent or pathological manifestations in humans and dogs could be observed and both a pattern and direction of transmission between the human and canine diseases were suspected.

The link between dog and human rabies was established a long time ago. The systematic implementation of measures aimed at eliminating dogs in rabies outbreaks was first documented during the 18th century and when applied at the national level, it led in a number of countries to the implementation of dog rabies elimination programs at the beginning of the 20th century. Hydatid cysts have been recognized in humans and animals since ancient times. Recognition that the cyst was of animal origin was attributed to Redi in the 17th century. Experimental infection of dogs with the adult worms was followed by the introduction of the first attempt to control the parasite in Iceland during the last part of the 19th century. For rabies and echinococcosis, dog population reduction policies were implemented soon after the link between the dog and human diseases was suspected. Evidence that dogs are the primary host of human visceral leishmaniasis due to *Leishmania infantum* became available only very recently as a result of epidemiological studies and molecular characterization of the agent involved in humans and dogs.

Empirical dog population control activities have since been complemented with new diagnostic tools, biological products, by more scientific methods for disease control based on diagnosis and treatment (echinococcosis and leishmaniasis) and disease prevention by dog immunization (rabies). In addition, data newly acquired on dog populations and their characteristics, particularly in developing countries as well as ethical and animal welfare considerations, have influenced, at least in some countries, control strategies applied to combat these three diseases. Finally, approaches including mathematical models for comparing the effectiveness of the various components of prevention and control strategies for these diseases have been developed and applied. This chapter reviews the past and current situation regarding prevention and control policies/strategies and tries to identify, on the basis of existing research, future trends for control and the feasibility of their elimination.

Dog rabies control

Approximately 40,000 to 60,000 people are believed to die from rabies each year in the world. A large number of mammalian animal species are involved in rabies maintenance and transmission. Many rabies host species are wild animals (e.g. red, arctic and grey foxes, racoons, skunks, coyotes, mongooses, wolves and jackals). Additionally, in the USA, certain South American countries, some European countries, and more recently in Australia many bat species are also involved either as hosts, transmitters or victims of rabies. In terms of public health, owned and ownerless dogs remain the main transmitters of rabies to humans in most developed and developing countries. In the former group of countries, the dog is merely a victim of wildlife-mediated rabies (e.g. fox rabies in Europe); whereas in the latter group, the disease is maintained within the dog population with or without the existence of a wildlife cycle. In both situations, rabid dogs are the most common transmitters of the disease to humans as they belong to the normal human environment and usually maintain a close relationship with people. As almost all human cases are reported in developing countries, dogs in this part of the world require most attention if a program leading to human rabies prevention were to be launched and eventually be successful (WHO, 1997, 1998a).

As is the case with other zoonoses, a number of different strategies can be used to control and possibly eliminate human rabies. These strategies can be divided into those primarily directed at humans (pre-exposure or post-exposure prophylaxis) and those primarily directed at the animals that transmit the disease to humans (population control, parenteral or oral vaccination). The strategies can be used alone or in combination. In this section, we will restrict ourselves to a review of the veterinary measures that were and are applied to dogs to control or eliminate rabies in many different settings, and discuss the prospects and strategies for the elimination of dog rabies in developing countries.

Dog rabies control: historical perspectives

Measures for the prevention of the disease in dogs were carried out as soon as the possible transmission of rabies to humans and animals through the bite of an infected dog was suspected. This happened very early for rabies as the similarity between the animal and human diseases and bites as the major transmission pathway were more easily identified than in most other zoonotic diseases. As a consequence, the Avesta in India already recommended the compulsory muzzling of aggressive dogs, in the 6th century BC. The control of dog movements was recommended by the Talmud in the 4th century AD and the destruction of stray dogs recommended in China 2 centuries BC and in ancient Greece and the Roman Empire (Blancou and Meslin, 2000). It seems that dog movement restriction and depopulation were not applied on a large scale in European countries before the beginning of the 18th century. Dog muzzling became compulsory only at the end of the 19th century (in 1871 in the UK and 1884 in France). It should be borne in mind that no efficacious human treatment after exposure to a rabid dog existed before Pasteur's vaccine was applied for the first time in 1885.

Elimination of rabies in dogs was attempted during the 19th and the beginning of the 20th century and some areas in Europe became free from rabies. Scandinavian countries successfully brought the disease under control in the 19th century through stray dog elimination and quarantining of owned and well-supervised dogs (WHO, 1987). Rabies in dogs was first eliminated from the UK in 1902 when a series of orders requiring dog muzzling, elimination of strays and tracing movements of rabid dogs and their contacts together with the implementation of a strict import regulation policy, eliminated the disease. The disease was reintroduced in the country in 1918 by one dog and eventually eradicated in 1922 (Meldrum, 1988). Mass vaccination of dogs played no role in these first successes.

In 1921, vaccine for mass immunization of dogs was used in Japan but it was not until 1957 that the disease was eliminated (Umeno and Doi, 1921). This rabies-free status has been maintained since then through compulsory dog vaccination campaigns involving more than four million dogs annually and the application of very strict rules for imported susceptible animals as well as restriction on the movement of native dogs.

The veterinary services of Hungary demonstrated by field trials in 1937 that canine rabies could be eliminated by a combination of dog vaccination and classical measures of dog movement control and population reduction (Manniger, 1968). In Malaysia, a rabies control program with compulsory vaccination of all dogs and rigorous destruction of strays was initiated in 1952. The disease was brought under control in 1953 (Tan, 1988). Since 1955, limited outbreaks have been reported only in the buffer zone at the border between peninsular Malaysia and Thailand (WHO, 1998a). In 1996, one isolated, probably imported, dog rabies case was reported outside the buffer zone (Hussin, 1997).

During the second half of the 20th century only a limited number of countries eliminated the disease. These, in addition to those mentioned above, include Taiwan in 1961, Portugal in 1961 and Uruguay in 1983 (WHO, 1987).

Dog rabies control: current trends

Progress has been continuously reported in Latin American countries since the initiation in the early 1980s, of the hemispheric dog rabies elimination program launched by the Pan American Health Organization (PAHO), the WHO Regional Office for the Americas. The number of reported human rabies cases decreased from 252 in 1990 to 74 in 1998. An impressive and continuously increasing number of dog vaccinations are performed every year in these countries. About 32 million dogs were vaccinated in 1997, including 25 million of them in Brazil and Mexico. In addition, approximately 800,000 dogs a year were captured and eliminated within the framework of this program in 1996 and 1997 (P. Arambulo III, Bogota, Colombia, 1999, personal communication). Many of the capital cities in Latin America are today free of canine rabies as a result of these activities. Progress is especially noticeable in Chile and in Argentina, where the disease has been almost eliminated in humans and dogs. In Argentina, cases of rabies in dogs have been decreasing markedly since 1993 (PAHO, 1997).

In other continents, temporary successes only were recorded in Tunisia (WHO, 1998b) and Sri Lanka where rabies in humans and animals was brought under control after many years of mass vaccination campaigns over most of the national territory (Goonaratna, 1997; Harishandra, 1997). In Tunisia, dog rabies vaccination activities were launched in 1983 in a small pilot area and progressively extended over 4 years to all rabies-affected areas of the country. From 1983 to 1987, a total of 900,000 dogs were immunized with vaccines protecting for a least 2 years. An average of 180,000 dogs were, therefore, vaccinated annually. This would represent only 20% of the estimated national dog population. Dog population reduction activities were only performed in the vicinity of the major urban centres and remain very marginal with 20,000 to 40,000 dogs eliminated each year. The impact of dog vaccination on human cases was remarkable and immediately noticeable, as from an average of 16 cases per year before the program started a total of 19 cases were notified from 1983 to 1987, with no cases reported in 1985 and only one in 1987. A decrease in the intensity of the campaigns was noted from 1988 to 1990 with only 65,000 dogs being vaccinated annually. This led to an immediate upsurge of the number of human cases, with 15 cases in 1991 and 25 cases in 1992, the highest annual number ever recorded in the country. This upsurge was accompanied by a concomitant dramatic increase of cases in animals (454 cases in 1991 and 515 in 1992) against an average of 270 per year before 1983 and 125 during the period 1983-1987. In spite of the increased number of dogs vaccinated annually, the number of human deaths reported from 1993 to 1997 (five cases per year on average) has not decreased to the level observed during the initial period 1983-1987 (Anonymous, 1993; S. Hammami, WHO, Geneva, 1998, personal communication).

In Sri Lanka, a dog rabies control program was initiated in the 1970s. The program was strengthened in 1984 by receiving external support and further WHO technical assistance. In spite of regularly (on an annual or biannual rhythm) carrying out dog mass-vaccination campaigns involving an increasing number of dogs (the number of dogs vaccinated increased from 200,000 in 1984 to about

600,000 a year in 1996, 1997 and 1998), no significant and durable reduction in the number of dog rabies cases and human rabies cases has been observed during the past 15 years. Dog population reduction operations were also conducted, but reached a relatively small proportion of the estimated overall population with about 100,000 dogs eliminated each year (Harishandra, 1997).

Strategies for dog rabies control and elimination

Control of dog rabies is carried out with different levels of intensity, both in developing and developed countries. In many countries where the dog is the reservoir of the virus, there are few activities underway to prevent rabies in humans and to control rabies in dogs. This occurs even in countries where the number of human deaths is high. This is the case in, for example, Bangladesh, Cambodia, India, Laos, Nepal, and Pakistan, as well as in most African and eastern Mediterranean Arabic peninsula countries (WHO, 1997, 1998a). On the other hand, some countries report having improved their post-exposure treatment delivery systems together with conducting significant activities for dog rabies control. In some countries, these activities have led to a sustainable reduction of dog rabies as previously reported for China and Thailand. This is the case in South Africa, Iran and most Latin American countries. In this latter region, especially in Brazil and Mexico, millions of dogs are vaccinated during swift campaigns of short duration (Belotto, 1988). In some other countries (e.g. Morocco, Tunisia, Sri Lanka), as described above, these activities have led to the temporary containment of the rabies situation, although rabies elimination is still a long way in the future.

Dog ownership can have very different meanings in different cultures (see Chapters 2 and 3). As a consequence, in most developing countries the owned dog population is usually only temporarily subject to movement restrictions by their owners. Under these conditions, dog accessibility to health measures whether vaccination, neutering or under certain circumstances removal, usually carried out by public services, is very restricted unless the active co-operation of owners has first been ensured.

Parenteral vaccination and dog accessibility

Globally, many dogs receive rabies shots. The total reported number of dogs vaccinated in countries, which responded to the World Survey of Rabies in 1992, was approximately 50 million. From this and other sources it can be estimated that between 35-40 million of them were vaccinated in dog rabies infected countries either in private practices or during national campaigns organized by ministries of health and/or agriculture. In many parts of Asia and Africa, the estimated overall vaccination coverage established in the dog population is not high enough (34% for Africa and 46% for Asia) to break the transmission cycle of the disease, especially since the total size of the dog populations living in these areas is usually underestimated (WHO, 1998c). Vaccination coverage following mass vaccination campaigns rarely reaches 75% (Matter *et al.*, 2000) which is considered necessary to break the transmission cycle.

In 1985, to collect data in a scientific way on the size and other parameters of dog populations in infected areas, WHO initiated field and research projects in three countries with different socio-cultural backgrounds: Tunisia, Sri Lanka and Ecuador (Ben Osman and Haddad, 1988; Beran and Frith, 1988; Wandeler and Budde, 1988; Matter, 1989). Additional research projects were conducted under WHO aegis in Morocco, Nepal (Bögel and Joshi, 1990), Zambia (De Balogh *et al.*, 1993) and Turkey (WHO, 1992a). The results of these studies were reviewed in various articles (Wandeler *et al.*, 1993; Meslin *et al.*, 1994). Although characteristics of these populations were found to vary greatly both between and within countries the major lessons learned from these studies were that:

- contrarily to what was usually perceived by local officers in most countries, dogs were either owned by an individual, a family or by the community so that only a relatively small proportion of the total dog population could be considered ownerless and as corollaries most of the so-called stray dogs and many of the dogs caught and eliminated were in fact owned dogs;
- the size of the dog populations was usually underestimated and as a result the immunized dog population coverage was overestimated. In most dog population reduction activities an even smaller proportion of the total was reached;
- dog vaccination at permanent vaccination centers was reaching a very small proportion of the owned dog population whereas vaccination from mobile centres could lead to coverage ranging from 40 to 85%. In addition, because of the high turnover of the dog population there was a need in a given area to maintain regular vaccination campaigns organized on an annual or biannual (in highly infected areas) basis.

Dog population management

As described in Chapter 11, dog population management is a rather new concept involving different approaches including dog movement restrictions, removal, reproduction and habitat control (WHO, 1992a, b; 1993a). It requires an appropriate regulatory framework as well as the involvement and co-operation of the public for its effective implementation. Only dog removal and dog movement restrictions have been extensively and successfully applied, particularly at the end of the 19th century and the first half of the 20th century. Considering the recent past, however, dog removal operations have usually been of limited magnitude in most countries where dog elimination has reached smaller numbers than vaccination and usually remained below 10% of the estimated total dog population. For example, in Sri Lanka during the period 1990-1998 the proportion of dogs that were caught and euthanized represented about 21% of the number of dogs vaccinated during the same period and about 6% of the estimated total dog population (P. Arishandra, WHO, Geneva, 1998, personal communication).

In Tunisia, about 60,000 dogs were eliminated annually in 1992 and 1993 when the national dog rabies control program was intensified after the upsurge of cases reported in both humans and animals in 1992. This number represents 4-6%

of an estimated total Tunisian dog population of 1 to 1.5 million dogs (Anomynous, 1993).

Exceptions were noted in China and certain Latin American countries where considerably greater numbers of dogs were eliminated than were immunized during the same period. Chile eliminated 196,000 dogs over 2 years; a number which represented about a third and more than half of the numbers of dogs vaccinated in 1996 and 1997, respectively (PAHO, 1997). From 1984 to 1994 in the Sichuan Province of China, more than 1.4 million dogs where killed each year whereas a total of 26 million were immunized against rabies over 11 years. During the same period, the number of human rabies cases per million inhabitants decreased drastically in Sichuan from 12.5 to 0.1 human cases (Qing Tang *et al.*, 1997). The relative roles played by dog removal, dog immunization and the increase in the number of human post-exposure treatments using cell-culture rabies vaccine in improving the overall rabies situation are difficult to analyze. Attempts to assess the efficacy of dog removal on dog population dynamics were made using results of the dog ecology studies carried out within the framework of the WHO co-ordinated project on dog ecology and rabies control. In Guayaquil, Ecuador, dog removal operations were intensified with 24% of the estimated dog population removed in a single year (1981-1982). There was no significant long-term effect on the size of the population nor on rabies incidence in the city (WHO, 1988a).

Reproduction control is far more complex in its execution and has been implemented in only a small number of developing countries such as India and Thailand. Thailand is leading in this area. Reproduction control activities have become an integral part of the Thai dog rabies control program as the general population as well as decision-makers considered dog removal less and less acceptable. More than 660,000 bitches received hormonal injections in 1996 and about 55,000 were spayed during the same year (Srisonmuang, 1997). None of these projects has been carried out for long enough periods and at a level that allows assessment of the effectiveness of the strategy. It is clear, however, that reproduction control by surgical sterilization and hormonal control by injection reach an even smaller proportion of the dogs than does rabies vaccination. It is unlikely at this level of implementation that this method has an impact on the overall reproduction rate of this population. Unless new technologies become available, such as anti-fertility vaccines, these approaches will not be able to limit the size of the dog population. Habitat control is only attainable over years of continuing efforts and may accompany economic development in these countries (Meslin *et al.*, 1994).

Oral vaccination of dogs: the key to dog rabies elimination?

Attractive oral vaccine baits and efficient bait delivery systems are available for foxes and racoons and considerable progress has been achieved in fox rabies infected areas, particularly in western Europe and Canada. A limited number of trials with vaccines, administered directly in the oral cavity, have been shown to protect dogs against a virulent challenge (WHO, 1988a, 1991, 1992a, 1993b, c, 1994) including two trials to protect most dogs after the ingestion of one bait

(WHO, 1998c). Further studies are required to design safe and cost-effective bait delivery systems for dogs. This technique is still experimental although the first field experiments using vaccine loaded baits have been conducted in Turkey, South Africa (G.C. Bishop, San Diego, USA, 1999, personal communication), Sri Lanka and in Thailand with the Vaccinia Rabies G protein (VRG) recombinant vaccine (P. Saragaseranee, Geneva, Switzerland, personal communication, 1998). Prior to this, baiting trials using mostly placebo baits were carried out in Zimbabwe (Perry *et al.*, 1988), in Mexico (Frontini *et al.*, 1992), in Tunisia (Kharmachi *et al.*, 1992; Matter *et al.*, 1995, 1998; Ben Youssef *et al.,* 1998) and in Turkey within the framework of the WHO co-ordinated activities on the oral vaccination technique (WHO, 1992a).

Three oral vaccine bait delivery systems can be envisaged (H. Matter, Mexico, City, 1992, personal communication) (WHO, 1993b). These are: (1) the distribution of the baits to owned dogs via their owner who would collect the bait at a central location; (2) the placement of baits in selected spots where they can be picked up by free roaming dogs (so called "wildlife immunization model"); and (3) distribution of baits to dogs encountered in the streets (so called 'hand-out' model). The technique could be used alone or in association with parenteral vaccination. Studies in Tunisia (Matter *et al.*, 1995) suggest that an 85 to 90% bait uptake coverage could be achieved in the owned dog population by distributing placebo baits to dog owners at temporary delivery sites. The average cost per bait accepting dog was estimated at US$1.6 assuming a cost of US$1 per vaccine bait. This cost is comparable to that of parenteral immunization (Bögel and Meslin, 1990). Such inexpensive and voluntary vaccine delivery systems involving the community itself or community leaders should be promoted to reduce costs further and thereby open new opportunities for the initiation of large scale vaccination programs. This method would, however, necessitate modifications of regulation in the delivery and application of veterinary rabies vaccines currently enforced in many countries. According to another study also carried out in Tunisia (Matter *et al.*, 1998), door to door vaccination of owned dogs carried out by special teams, associating parenteral and oral vaccination according to dog accessibility to the former, would seem to be the best combination in terms of both expected coverage and costs. This would, in addition, minimize the possibility of contact of household members with vaccine bait. For certain segments of the dog population (owned, free roaming, or ownerless dogs), immunization by handing out baits to dogs encountered on roads/streets should be considered to reduce both vaccine costs associated with the Wildlife Immunization Model and eliminate possible environmental contamination through systematic recovery of the bait in case of non-acceptance. Investigating economics of the oral vaccination of dogs (OVD) is essential since it is very unlikely that all resources required for dog rabies elimination would suddenly become available (Perry and Wandeler, 1993).

Impact on human rabies of dog rabies control/elimination strategies

Dog vaccination campaigns may have a rapid impact on the number of cases occurring in animals and humans even if the immunization blanket is not high enough to stop the transmission of the disease. In Tunisia, after 3 years of implementation of a step-wise national program the number of human deaths was reduced considerably. The average annual number of deaths during the period 1974-1981 was 19. It declined to an average of four during the period 1982-1990. When the number of dogs vaccinated decreased during the years 1987, 1988 and 1989 the number of cases in animals increased progressively to explode in 1992 with the highest figure ever reported in Tunisia. An upsurge of the number of human deaths was also reported during this year reaching 25 cases (Anomynous, 1993).

In Sri Lanka, dog rabies control activities have been carried out continuously since 1973. A clear improvement was recorded after the first 10 years of the program implementation, as the number of human deaths fell from 377 in 1973 to about 200 annually during the early 1980s (P. Harishandra, Colombo, Sri Lanka, 1990, personal communication). Since 1984, no sustainable decrease in the number of human cases has been recorded in spite of a continuous increase in the annual number of dogs vaccinated against rabies (this number almost tripled over the period 1984-1998).

On the other hand, sharp declines of human death numbers have been reported in China and Thailand by about 90% within 15 to 20 years. In China, rabies was highly endemic in many provinces until the end of the 1980s, with a total of 38,000 human cases reported during the period 1984-1995. Since then, the number of rabies cases has been drastically reduced from approximately 3,500 cases in the year 1990 to only 208 cases in 1998 (WHO, 2000a, b). The availability of cell-culture vaccines for human rabies post-exposure treatment was improved at the beginning of the 1990s with the increase in the production of a primary hamster kidney cells (PHKC) rabies vaccine. Today about five million post-exposure treatments are provided annually with this vaccine. In addition, intensive dog rabies control activities were carried out throughout the 1980s at least some of the most affected provinces such as Sichuan where, as previously mentioned, millions of dogs were eliminated or immunized against rabies (Qing Tang *et al.*, 1997). In Thailand, human rabies has been steadily brought down from 370 deaths in 1980, to 74 in 1995 and 58 in 1998. In Thailand, there has been an increasing demand of post-exposure treatments (PET) by 10-15% each year, resulting in more than 220,000 PETs in 1998 (350 treatments per 100,000 inhabitants) (Kingnate *et al.*, 1997; WHO, 1998b). In both China and Thailand, an improved post-exposure treatment and a vaccine delivery system, associated with a major shift in the type of vaccine produced from brain tissue towards cell culture based products, played a major role in drastically and durably reducing the number of human deaths due to rabies.

Future strategies

Future international activities should be focused on rabies control in its canine reservoir and prevention of human rabies in those countries/regions with the highest death toll due to rabies (Africa and Asia). Technical cooperation with these regions and countries should be further strengthened to improve: (1) rabies surveillance and the collection and processing of data at the national, regional and global levels; (2) intersectoral collaborative efforts for the control of rabies in its animal host at the national and regional levels; and (3) new tools under development particularly an oral vaccine for dogs and techniques for effective and humane dog population control. Rabies is a vaccine preventable disease and in the human health area the development and implementation with all necessary partners including the pharmaceutical sector, of a "WHO coordinated Rabies Vaccine Initiative 2000" is very much needed. Its overall objective is to identify means to overcome the current lack in many rabies infected areas of affordable and safe rabies vaccines for humans. This should greatly contribute to reducing in the medium term the estimated 60,000 rabies deaths that occur annually, and advantageously complement the longer term veterinary and population management activities carried out at the level of the dog.

Canine visceral leishmaniasis control

In most regions where canine visceral leishmaniasis (canine VL) is endemic, such as around the Mediterranean basin, dogs are valued highly as companions, as working or hunting animals and for breeding. Owners who have a comfortable socio-economic status can devote considerable financial resources to their dogs. In such circumstances, the health of the dog is the primary reason for interventions against canine VL. The dog may be given frequent and expensive veterinary examinations and treatments. Repetitive therapies for canine VL may be applied, irrespective of possible long-term repercussions on the transmission dynamics of leishmaniasis.

From a wider perspective the overwhelming impetus for the control of canine VL is its association with human VL (Abranches *et al.*, 1998). However, in regions where *Leishmania donovani* is the agent of human VL, there is no such association. Thus in India, the dog has no role as the disease is considered to be entirely an anthroponosis: cyclical epidemics are thought to be sustained by reservoir infections of human post kala azar dermal leishmaniasis, in conjunction with abundant sandflies and an immunologically naïve human population. In contrast, where human VL is caused by *L. infantum* (*Leishmania chagasi*, see below) the dog is generally thought to be the most important source of infection for sandflies. This zoonotic form of VL occurs in southern Europe, North Africa, the eastern Mediterranean, China, Central and South America. The view that the dog is the primary reservoir host for human VL due to *L. infantum* is based on several types of evidence, as follows:

- Dogs are readily susceptible to infection with *L. infantum* (although asymptomatic infections are also common).
- Parasitemias in dogs may be very high, particularly in the skin.
- Infections in dogs may be prolonged, for months or years, with sustained parasitemias.
- Dogs are fed on avidly by the same sandfly species that bite humans.
- Infected dogs are highly infective to sandflies even when asymptomatic.

- Vector borne human VL due to *L. infantum* is inevitably sympatric with canine VL (although canine VL is endemic in some regions where human cases of VL are rare or unknown and more than 1000 cases are known of canine VL imported to non-endemic areas) (Paranhos-Silva *et al.*, 1996, Slappendel and Teske, 1999; Zaffaroni *et al.*, 1999).
- The same *L. infantum* phenotypes and genotypes occur sympatrically in dogs and humans (Dereure *et al.*, 1999; Martin-Sanchez *et al.*, 1999).
- Dogs have a close domestic and peridomestic association with humans.

Nevertheless, it has been difficult to prove unequivocally, for example by mapping acute cases of human VL and the distribution of dogs, that there is a significant correlation between dog ownership and risk of human VL (Evans *et al.*, 1992; Cunha *et al.*, 1995; Costa *et al.*, 1999). This is not perhaps surprising as there are many potential confounding factors, such as: (1) the focal abundance of sandfly vectors; (2) the range of clinical presentation in dogs, from asymptomatic to fulminating infections, which may in part be dependent on the breed of the dog; (3) the predominance of asymptomatic human infections; (4) the role of age and nutritional status in susceptibility to human VL; (5) the time lag between exposure to infection and appearance of symptoms; and (6) and the mobility of humans, dogs and the sandfly vector. Transmission of *L. infantum* from human to human via the sandfly vector cannot entirely be excluded, but studies on transmissibility of *L. infantum* suggest this is a relatively rare occurrence (see below). Other mammals, especially canines such as foxes in the Old and New World (Courtenay *et al.*, 1996) and jackals, or the opossum (*Didelphis* sp.) (Corredor *et al.*, 1989) might be important link hosts between sylvatic and domestic transmission cycles.

There is increasing evidence that the dog is also a very important host of *Leishmania braziliensis*, the agent of human cutaneous and mucocutaneous leishmaniasis in Latin America. The establishment of canine *L. braziliensis* infections in periurban and urban areas may have led to outbreaks of human cutaneous leishmaniasis in Latin American cities. As a result, it has become relevant to consider common approaches to the control of *L. infantum* and *L. braziliensis* (Momen, 1995; Santos *et al.*, 1998; Reithinger and Davies, 1999).

A review of the known global distribution of VL and cutaneous leishmaniasis is given by Desjeux (1991). This justifies the WHO selection of leishmaniasis as a major public health problem and one of its health priorities. VL is endemic in at least 61 countries, 11 in Central and South America, 15 in Europe, 10 in south western Asia, 20 in Africa and 5 in Asia (Arias *et al.*, 1996).

Note that some authors retain the name *L. chagasi* for *L. infantum* in the Americas (Lainson and Shaw, 1998). Recent molecular comparisons, however, confirm the view that *L. chagasi* is indistinguishable from *L. infantum* (Mauricio *et al.*, 1999, 2000). Thus, a DNA probe (Lmet 9) recognizes all Old World species of *Leishmania,* but only *L. chagasi* among the New World species. Phylogenetic analysis based on restriction length polymorphisms and DNA sequence comparisons, group *L. chagasi* and *L. infantum* as a single entity. Hence only the species name *L. infantum* is used here.

Current control strategies

The same three fundamental strategies have been adopted, albeit with different emphasis, for interventions against both human VL and canine VL. They are:

- Treatment of clinical cases, usually passively detected (that is patients referred to physicians, or dogs referred to veterinary surgeons);
- Actively surveying dog populations, usually immunologically, to diagnose *L. infantum* infections and to cull putatively infected animals;
- Destruction of vector sandfly species by the application of insecticides.

Treatment

The first-line drugs recommended for treatment of human VL are the pentavalent antimonials, in the form of sodium stibogluconate (Pentostam®), meglumine antimonate (Glucantime®) or sodium antimony gluconate, at 20 mg per kg per day for 30 days (Arias *et al.*, 1996). Alternative drugs are amphotericin B, pentamidine or, more recently, aminosidine (paromomycin) and amphotericin B included in liposomes (Ambisome®). A new drug, a phosphocholine analog (Miltefosine®), is under clinical trial (phase 3). Aminosidine is an old antibiotic remedy, which, through WHO support, will soon be newly available for treatment of human VL. Combination therapy of pentavalent antimonials and aminosidine can reduce treatment schedules from 30 to 17 days and this can be a great advantage in treating epidemic outbreaks of human VL.

Unfortunately, pentavalent antimonials are considered to be less effective for the treatment of dogs. The pharmacokinetic or other reasons for this are imprecisely known but antimonials are rapidly excreted and the abundance of dermal amastigotes in canine infections may be a factor. Nevertheless, in privileged circumstances dogs are treated with antimonials. Such treatment may suppress parasitemia and give clinical improvement, but not necessarily eliminate the organism or prevent relapse. Treatment may be used repeatedly. This practise carries a risk in that it may generate drug resistant strains of *L. infantum*, which could spread among the dog and human population. Such repeated therapy is commonplace in Europe but rare elsewhere, partly due to the high cost involved, and resistant strains are already considered to occur among European dogs. Allopurinol is often given *per os* with antimonials for treatment of canine VL in Europe and then given as a maintenance treatment, sometimes for life. Lamothe (1999) should be consulted for a detailed review of the status of therapy for canine VL, and for alternative drug administration schedules.

Aminosidine treatment of dogs produces dramatic clinical improvement and occasionally clinical cure, however, most dogs relapse 2 to 4 months after the end of therapy (Vexenat *et al.*, 1998). Thus, there is no satisfactory effective chemotherapy for canine VL. Development of new drugs for canine VL would seem to be of considerable veterinary research interest and may yield new compounds for treatment of human leishmaniasis.

Detection and removal of Leishmania infantum-*infected dogs*

Reliable clinical signs of canine VL are not obvious until late in the disease. Surveillance of dog populations to remove infected animals has thus depended on mass serological surveys, usually with blood samples collected onto filter paper. Serological tests commonly used are the indirect fluorescent antibody test (IFAT) or some form of ELISA. The IFAT requires a fluorescence microscope. The plate ELISA results are best read by optical density with a spectrophotometer but positive and negatives can be recorded visually from the plate. Modified ELISAs include the dot-ELISA, (Vercammen *et al.*, 1998), which is performed on membranes instead of plates and the FAST-ELISA, which uses whole blood as an adaptation for rapid field use. A direct agglutination test (DAT) that is virtually 100% specific for human VL, is also applicable to dogs if lower minimum positive titers are used. The DAT test depends on whole organisms as antigen, which is thus difficult to obtain in quantity; DAT antigen batches may also differ in reproducibility. A lyophilized DAT antigen is now available from the Royal Tropical Institute, Amsterdam. A new "bedside" test (Dipstick k 39) has become available for serological diagnosis of visceral leishmaniasis in humans and animals. It is based on a recombinant *Leishmania* surface antigen (k 39), and is highly specific for visceral leishmaniasis. The cost of the currently available test is US$1 (Sundar *et al.*, 1998). It gives immediate results and can be used to make a rapid decision when a dog is found positive.

In Latin America, it is often recommended that seropositive animals are destroyed as part of control campaigns but, without supportive legislation, it is impossible to get full compliance from owners. Furthermore, some seropositive dogs might be false positives or have self-cured. In a veterinary clinic parasitological examination, for example by microscopy of giemsa stained sternal aspirates, can be routine and helpful, but it is not practical or sufficiently sensitive for mass surveys.

As serological surveys have been adopted as the cornerstone of many control campaigns for canine VL, the validity of this strategy is discussed in more detail below.

Controlling sandfly populations with insecticides

In the absence of resistance, sandflies are exquisitely sensitive to insecticides. DDT is effective, as are the synthetic pyrethroids (deltamethrin, permethrin, cypermethrin and others) which have low toxicity and high residual activity. In localities where malaria and VL are sympatric, spraying against mosquito vectors of malaria can have a dramatic effect on abundance of sandflies and the prevalence of VL. Insecticides are used residually against sandflies, and applied to domestic and peridomestic resting sites. Occasionally ultra low volume spraying into the air (fogging) can help to stem epidemic outbreaks of VL. However, this blanket approach only reaches adult sandflies at the time of spraying. For long-term effect, ultra low volume spraying must be applied repeatedly, with high coverage of the affected area, and at seasonal peaks of sandfly abundance. Insecticide impregnated bed nets offer protection against sandflies at night.

Few studies have attempted to assess the relative values of the treatment of clinical cases, the removal of infected dogs, and spraying against sandflies as components of a VL control campaign.

Withholding treatment for overt clinical human VL, which is usually fatal if not treated, is clearly not an ethical option as part of comparisons of interventions. Comparative studies in which treatment of human VL is specifically withheld to assess its epidemiological impact are thus not available.

Deane and Deane (1962) thought that outbreaks of human VL in Brazil depended on the abundance of the vector, *Lutzomyia longipalpis*, but believed that small sandfly populations could maintain endemic canine VL. Alencar (1961) assessed the impact of sandfly control with insecticides in a comparative study of interventions against human VL. With two groups of communities, he found that the incidence of human VL decreased only when insecticides were used in addition to the treatment of human cases and the removal of seropositive dogs (Table 12.1). This supported Deane and Deane's view of the significance of sandfly abundance and the importance of vector control.

Table 12.1. Comparison of number of cases of human VL in communities with treatment of patients and culling of seropositive dogs, with or without insecticide spraying against sandflies (from Alencar, 1961).

| | Number of cases of human VL | | |
Periods	1953-1956	1957-1960	% change
Localities not sprayed (12 municipalities)	89	101	Up 12%
Sprayed (12 municipalities)	765	320	Down 58%

Studies of the impact of serological screening and removal of seropositive dogs are few and limited. The total removal of the dog population has been reported to be an effective control measure in China (Ashford, 1999).

Ashford *et al.* (1998) were able to show a decrease in both the incidence of human VL and seropositivity rates in dogs when 69% of seropositive dogs were removed promptly by using the FAST-ELISA for serology (Table 12.2). Failure of compliance did not allow removal of all the seropositive dogs.

Akhavan (1996) considered whether control of VL based on the three strategies of treatment of cases, culling of seropositive dogs and spraying against sandflies, had been effective in northeastern Brazil. He assumed that epidemics with increasing levels of incidence occurred every 10 years. The total cost of control campaigns was estimated at US$95,000,000. It was further estimated that 68,000 disability adjusted human life years (DALYs) had been gained at a cost of US$139 for each DALY recovered. The control campaign in northeastern Brazil has been difficult to sustain continuously. Nevertheless, Akhavan concluded that the campaign had been cost-effective. It is not clear, however, what contribution to the campaign is attributable to the culling of seropositive dogs.

Table 12.2. Numbers of paediatric VL cases per 1000 inhabitants per year in areas with or without removal of seropositive dogs (initiated in the second half of 1989) (from Ashford *et al.*, 1998).

	1986	1987	1988	1989	1990	1991	1992	1993
Invention	12	5	14	10	3	2	2	2
No invention	6	2	2	12	8	12	4	2
Total	18	7	16	22	11	14	6	4

A workshop jointly sponsored by the Department for International Development (DFID, UK), the World Health Organization (WHO) and the Pan American Health Organization (PAHO) has produced a guide to the control of VL. The manual is freely available upon request from WHO and includes protocols for the treatment of human cases, for serological and parasitological diagnosis, for insecticide spraying and impregnation of bed nets. Co-ordinating control activities across organizations responsible for human and veterinary health or the management of VL is imperative and various models have been proposed (Arias *et al.*, 1996). Primary health care workers in the community, as well as veterinary surgeons, need to be able to recognize the clinical symptoms of canine VL and to know how to report the presence of canine VL through local health channels. Veterinary surgeons and Zoonosis Centers or similar organizations need to be equipped to make serological and parasitological diagnoses and require clear guidelines on how to manage canine VL. Effective liaison between veterinary health authorities and human health authorities is essential even if human VL has not yet been reported in the locality. This is because sporadic infant cases may go unrecognized, and be fatal. Informed higher level public health authorities will need to decide whether epidemiological survey for human and canine VL is justified, and if further cases are found whether to begin a co-ordinated and integrated control campaign.

Transmissibility, diagnosis and the validity of culling seropositive dogs

The ease with which canine VL is transmissible to sandflies is indisputable. In pioneering studies, Deane (1956) and Deane and Deane (1962) compared dogs and humans as a source of *L. infantum* infection to *Lu. longipalpis* (Table 12.3). Dermal amastigote infections were prolific in dogs but scanty in symptomatic, untreated human VL. It was much easier to infect sandflies by feeding them on the dogs than by feeding them on the human cases. No infections were acquired by *Lu. longipalpis* fed on treated human cases. In more recent studies (Miles *et al.*, 1999), the high transmissibility of canine VL to *Lu. longipalpis* has been confirmed by examining wild-caught sandflies. Up to 67% of engorged female sandflies collected from a kennel housing a dog with disseminated dermal VL were shown to be infected by dissection 5 and 7 days after collection. Infection rates in fed sandflies captured less discriminatory, with a CDC light-trap, were much lower; as well as dogs, alternative hosts such as chickens or pigs were abundant in the endemic area. Similarly, our xenodiagnosis experiments have demonstrated that infection rates of 70% to 90% were common when sandflies were fed on symptomatic dogs, and overall infection rates were greater than 20% even when flies were fed on the normal skin of such animals. Furthermore, like Molina *et al.*, (1994), we found that asymptomatic dogs can also be highly infective to sandflies (Vexenat *et al.*, 1993, 1994; unpublished data, Miles *et al.*, 1999).

Table 12.3. Dermal infections and transmissibility of *L. infantum* from dogs and humans.

	Dogs positive	Humans positive*
Amastigotes (by microscopy)	78% (of 49)	16% (of 43)
	Abundant	Scanty
Xenodiagnoses	75% (of 16)	29% (of 14)
Sandflies positive	23% (of 238)	15% (of 81)

* Clinical VL prior to chemotherapy (from Deane and Deane, 1962).

Diagnosis of canine VL is not straightforward (Ferrer, 1999). A comparison of clinical diagnosis, parasitological diagnosis and serology for the detection of *L. infantum* infection among naturally infected dogs in Teresina, Piaui State, northeastern Brazil confirmed that symptomology was not sufficiently sensitive to diagnose infection. Parasitology, although more sensitive than symptomology, was not as sensitive as serology, and none of several parasitological tests showed more than 60% sensitivity. Although the probability of demonstrating the presence of infection increased with serological titer, it was consistently found that a proportion of serologically negative dogs were parasitologically positive, even though three different serological tests were applied (IFAT, ELISA, DAT). This failure of serology to diagnose all infections is a severe constraint on the effectiveness of serological surveys as part of a control strategy (Vexenat *et al.*, unpublished; Miles *et al.*, 1999).

Furthermore, in a series of experimental dogs infected by sandfly bite, a proportion of the animals were able to transmit infection from early cutaneous lesions and in the absence of seroconversion (Vexenat *et al.*, unpublished; Miles *et al.*, 1999). There are as yet no practical more-sensitive alternatives to serology. A recombinant antigen is said to detect only active disease in serological tests, but presumably also misses some incipient infections and has not been adopted for surveys (Nieto *et al.*, 1999; Rhalem *et al.*, 1999). Experimental trials with polymerase chain reaction (PCR) (Roura *et al.*, 1999) confirm that the sensitivity of serological tests is not optimal. By PCR, Ashford *et al.* (1995) detected infections in more than 30% of dogs that were apparently seronegative.

Thus, field and experimental observations indicate that the basic case reproduction ratio (Ro) for canine VL is likely to be high in endemic areas, implying each case is likely to give rise to several new cases. The high Ro has been supported by careful population studies and mathematical models (Dye *et al.*, 1992), despite assumptions (Hasibeder *et al.*, 1992) that: (1) there is a latent period after an infective bite when the dog is not infective, but serologically positive; and (2) that the asymptomatic and non-infective periods are identical, neither of which assumptions accords with biological observations. The limited sensitivity of serology indicates that a reduced Ro is likely to maintain endemic canine VL even during serological surveillance and the killing of seropositive dogs. In addition, low examination rates, slow response times (Braga *et al.*, 1998) and compliance failures are likely to prejudice the outcome of the serological survey and culling strategy.

There is evidence that both human and canine VL are controlled by a cell mediated immune response, in humans identified as predominantly the Th1 arm of the immune response. In humans, positive skin tests (Montenegro or leishmanin tests) are an indicator of cure but not of the presence of active infection. Thus skin tests are not likely to be an alternative diagnostic procedure for determining the presence of infection but they might be useful for assessing exposure rates or cure rates in canine VL, as they are in human VL (Pinelli *et al.*, 1994, 1999; Cardoso *et al.*, 1998; Santos *et al.*, 1998).

Although in principle epidemiological surveys and removal of infected dogs has high validity, in practice with present methods its efficacy is questionable and requires re-evaluation. Their application in Tunisia only had a temporary effect (Ben Ismail, Tunis, Tunisia, 1998, personal communication).

Vasconcelos *et al.* (1993) confirmed the original observations of Deane and Deane (1962) that amastigotes could be recovered from symptomatic human VL. They isolated *Leishmania* from 7 of 18 patients by culture of skin biopsy samples. Some symptomatic human *L. infantum* infections, prior to treatment, may thus be infective to sandflies and propagate further human infections. Asymptomatic human VL is thought to be much more abundant than symptomatic VL in endemic areas of *L. infantum*. Dermal infections in such asymptomatic infections are thought to be rare and presumed not to be a significant source of infection to sandflies.

Future control strategies

Treatment for canine VL is clearly unsatisfactory. The last-resort methods in Europe of antimonial treatment followed by prolonged or lifelong allopurinol administration cannot be advocated for widespread use elsewhere, or as a control strategy especially in view of the very real risk of generating drug-resistant isolates and sustaining endemicity. There is an urgent need for a cheap, highly effective drug for the treatment of canine VL. The drug should be simple to administer either orally or by few doses given by inoculation. There is a strong case for encouraging veterinary companies to take a research interest in this objective, which is likely to benefit therapy of human VL. In Europe, 50% of human *L. infantum* infections are associated with HIV coinfection (Alvar *et al.*,

1996) and most of these cases will receive prolonged anti leishmanial therapy. In endemic areas in developing countries, some HIV/*L. infantum* coinfections in the community might provide a new reservoir of infection for sandflies, especially in areas where HIV and VL are increasingly sympatric (WHO and UNAIDS 1998). This may shift the pattern of epidemiology of VL due to *L. infantum*.

Epidemiological screening for *L. infantum*-infected dogs should not be entirely abandoned. Nevertheless, considerable improvements are essential if this method is to be effective. In particular, a reliable, specific, highly sensitive, rapid diagnostic test suitable for field use is essential. Such a test maybe beyond reach, although new antigens and new formats are still being sought. Some thought could also be devoted to strategies for increasing dog examination rates and compliance with public health recommendations. Were a new treatment suitable for mass therapy to be found, this could virtually eliminate difficulties with compliance.

Vaccination has to remain a research priority (Dye, 1996). Although there are promising candidate antigens, a proven vaccine whether based on whole organisms, purified antigens, recombinant antigens, peptides or DNA vaccines has yet to be developed. We have proposed that incorporation of *Leishmania* antigens into the vaccine strain of rabies virus should be explored as a delivery system to provide simultaneous rabies and *Leishmania* vaccine coverage (Miles and Mauricio, unpublished).

As described above, attention is repeatedly drawn to sandfly abundance as one of the most important factors in transmission of VL. Thousands of sandflies may be caught in a single CDC trap during a single night. Pyrethroid insecticides are very effective against sandflies. A promising approach is to use pyrethroids in new ways, such as by dipping hosts to diminish sandfly attack and to kill biting sandflies (Xiong *et al.*, 1995). Similar systems are effective against other insect vectors, for example in the form of ear tags on cattle. One of the most promising developments in this context is the use of pyrethroid-impregnated protective bands for dogs, which slowly release insecticide that spreads over the host. Preliminary trials show great promise (Killick-Kendrick *et al.*, 1997; Killick-Kendrick 1999; Lucientes, 1999).

Cystic echinococcosis control

Two species of parasitic organisms of the genus *Echinococcus* are particularly important for public health, namely *Echinococcus granulosus* causing cystic echinococcosis (CE) and *Echinococcus multilocularis* causing alveolar echinococcosis (AE). Final hosts of both parasites are carnivores. However, the cycle of *E. granulosus* involves primarily dogs as final hosts and sheep, goats, camels, cattle, pigs and horses as intermediate hosts. Conversely, the cycle of *E. multilocularis* is predominantly sylvatic (see Chapter 7). Thus, this section will deal with cystic echinococcosis control only.

E. granulosus is very widely distributed, involving the sheep-rearing countries of Australia and South America, including Argentina, Chile, Brazil, Peru and Uruguay (Rausch, 1995; 1997). In the Commonwealth of Independent States (CIS) and parts of Eurasia, vast endemic areas exist. It also occurs throughout Western Europe with transmission at its highest level in the countries bordering the Mediterranean and on the Iberian Peninsula. In Africa, two major areas exist, including countries of the Maghreb (Kachani *et al.*, 1997) and in East Africa (Macpherson *et al.*, 1989). It has been recorded in 21 of China's 51 provinces and is one of the important human diseases in northwest China (Schantz *et al.*, 1995).

Major risk factors for contracting cystic echinococcosis are represented by direct and indirect contacts of humans with feces from dogs. Children are often found infected, because of their close contacts with dogs or with environments/food polluted by dog feces. In endemic areas, such as Mediterranean countries, northern and eastern-central Africa, South America, northern India, Bangladesh and Nepal, and western and central China, cysts may be found in 1-40% of cattle and 1-80% of sheep, and from 0.2-50% of the dogs are infected. In humans, the parasite occurs as a benign tumor, unique or multiple, in the liver or lungs, in most cases. However, any tissue or organ may be involved, including brain, bone, spleen and kidney. After a silent asymptomatic period, various symptoms and signs are observed, depending on the primary location of the cyst(s). Rupture of the cyst may lead to life-threatening anaphylactic shock and to dissemination to many tissues and organs. Treatment is represented by surgery, interventional radiology (puncture and sterilization of the cysts), and benzimidazole drugs. Depending on the area considered, annual incidence of CE human surgical cases in endemic countries ranges from 1 to 20 per 100,000 inhabitants. However, in hyperendemic foci of some countries, mass screenings with ultrasound have shown a prevalence of up to 12% in adults (Macpherson *et al.*, 1989).

Concepts of parasite stability and steady states in control planning

Stability is an essential part of the description of host/parasite systems. It describes the ability of biological systems in equilibrium to withstand perturbation, such as can be expected in a control program, and after that has ceased to return to the previous equilibrium or reach a new one. Factors that contribute to stability include: (1) density-dependent factors, such as the biotic potential of the parasite in the definitive host; (2) immunity acquired by the intermediate host; and (3) density-independent constraints, such as environmental factors. These should be taken into account, particularly when planning the force needed to drive the system towards extinction (Gemmell and Roberts 1995, 1998; Gemmell, 1997; Gemmell and Schantz, 1997). The ratio of the number of adult parasites in the next generation to the number of parasites in this generation defines the basic reproduction ratio (Ro). A mathematical model for quantifying Ro has been developed (Roberts and Gemmell, 1994). If a parasite population is neither increasing nor decreasing with time then it is in a steady state: an endemic steady state if the population size is constant ($R = 1$) and the effects of density-dependent constraints (e.g. immunity) are negligible ($Ro > 1$); and in an hyperendemic steady state when Ro >> 1 and these constraints (e.g. immunity) are effective. The extinction steady state exists when no parasite is present.

Field investigations quantifying the behavior of endemic *E. granulosus* and hyperendemic *E. multilocularis* when perturbated, have been compared. In the first trial, *E. granulosus* was destabilized by using a 3-monthly dog-testing program with arecoline hydrobromide on farm dogs in an endemic area of New Zealand (Gemmell, 1968). In the second, dosing of Eskimo dogs with praziquantel every 4 weeks was used to destabilize hyperendemic *E. multilocularis* in a village on St Lawrence Island, Alaska (Rausch *et al.*, 1990). The results showed that the weak force used against *E. granulosus* in dogs was sufficient as an educational tool to drive it from the endemic state to extinction. With *E. multilocularis*, the strong force drove it from the hyperendemic state to extinction status, but when discontinued it rapidly reverted towards its original status (Gemmell and Schantz, 1997).

Implementing control and elimination programs

Control describes the active implementation of a program by a recognized authority on an instruction from the legislature to limit prevalence of a specific disease. Eradication describes its purposeful reduction to the point of continued absence of transmission within a specified area by means of a time-limited campaign. Many factors may influence a priority for control. These include: (1) prevalence of disease; (2) morbidity or severity of disability; (3) risk of mortality; (4) feasibility of control or eradication; (5) absence of adverse ecological factors; (6) adequate administration, operational and financial resources; (7) availability of effective tools; (8) favourable epidemiological features; and (9) socioeconomic importance (Lawson *et al.*, 1988; Gemmell and Schantz, 1997; Nonnemaker and Schantz, 1997; Gemmell and Roberts, 1998).

Administration, legislation and funding

There are two main administration models. The first, funded mainly by dog owners, involves through specific legislation, a national or regional executive authority (Council or Commission). The second involves a government funding authority, such as a Ministry of Agriculture or Health. Legislation needed includes that for: (1) effective meat inspection and disposal of offal; (2) prohibition of illegal slaughtering; (3) dog registration, testing and treatment of infected owned dogs; (4) control of strays and elimination of ownerless dogs; (5) quarantine of premises with infected livestock; and (6) control of movements of food animals and dogs between infected and "free" areas. CE is theoretically an eradicable disease, but numerous factors are involved in the maintenance of the cycle, including behavioral and cultural factors that are resistant to regulations. Educational campaigns to reach slaughterhouse personnel, farmers, and dog owners are especially needed.

Control options

Five options can be discerned.

1   Deciding not to proceed with any specific measures either because: (1) there is a recognizable health problem, but no suitable infrastructure or funding for control; or (2) an insufficient infection level compared to other concurrent disease problems to warrant applying control.
2   Introducing a permanent horizontal approach with the application of education, particularly for schools. This may include specific health promotion plans to limit CE by routine use of, for example, portable diagnostic screening devices, such as ultrasound.
3   A formal control program in a vertical approach with the adoption of arecoline hydrobromide, or in the future, the newer coproantigen test (yet unproven in a control setting) to detect dogs infected with *E. granulosus* in an educational approach to control with a relatively slow track to complete the attack phase.
4   A fast-track option by including a positive euthanasia policy for dogs.
5   Another fast-track option is to treat all dogs with praziquantel at specified I intervals.

Phases of a control program

Four phases can be recognized using options 3, 4, and 5 listed above. These are "preparatory" or "planning" phase; "attack", "consolidation" and where appropriate "maintenance of eradication" phase. Operational research in the "planning" phase is concerned with quantifying the magnitude of parasite transmission and estimating the costs of and losses from echinococcosis to the community and benefits from control. During the "attack" phase, methods, such as stray dog control, dosing of owned dogs and registration are applied to the entire dog population. When the prevalence of *E. granulosus* reaches a low level, it becomes cost-effective to target control through intermediate hosts in the "consolidation" phase. Here, identification is made of infected food animals at meat inspection with subsequent quarantine of affected premises. Where eradication is potentially feasible, the "maintenance of eradication" phase may be entered if no parasites can be observed during meat inspection. Here, all specific control activities, such as dog dosing, are disbanded, and vigilance is permanently maintained through meat inspection with measures also taken to prevent re-entry of infected animals (Lawson *et al.*, 1988; Roberts and Gemmell, 1994; Gemmell and Roberts, 1995, 1998; Gemmell, 1997; Gemmell and Schantz, 1997; Nonnemaker and Schantz, 1997).

Control technology (veterinary aspects)

In the past, major emphasis in the "attack" phase was placed on detecting the parasite in the dog by using arecoline hydrobromide or arecoline acetarsol as a purgative in a diagnostic approach to control (refer Options 3 and 4). More recently, this technology has been replaced in the "attack" phase in some control programs by killing the worms *in situ* using frequent dosing with praziquantel (see below and Option 5).

Taeniafuges

Arecoline is the chief alkaloid of the areca nut, the seed of *Areca catechu*. Synthetic arecoline was introduced against tapeworms in dogs in the early part of the 20th century. The drug causes increased tone and motility of smooth muscle resulting in purgation. It also has an action on the parasite itself, causing it to relax its hold on the intestinal wall. The subsequent purgation carries the worms out with the feces. Under field conditions, it has been shown that about 20% of dogs may fail to be purged at a dose rate of 1.75 mg per kg to 3.5 mg per kg within 1 hour. A second dose may be given when that occurs. Treatment is regarded as a safe procedure, but some untoward reactions may occur, particularly in hot weather. This may include prolonged stimulation of mucus secretions, excessive salivation and severe dehydration and very occasionally death. Arecoline hydrobromide was successfully used as a diagnostic agent in the control programs of New Zealand, Tasmania and Cyprus (Gemmell, 1973).

Taeniacides

During the past half century, several drugs were tested for efficacy and some, such as the bunamidine salts, niclosamide and nitroscanate, were applied for short periods. However, praziquantel with its very high efficacy at a safe dose rate was evaluated in the 1970s and found to be highly effective by the oral and intramuscular routes against *E. granulosus* at a single dose ED90, with 95% confidence intervals ranging between 2.3 (1.5-3.7), 2.7(2.1-3.5) and 3.2 (1.5-5.6) mg/kg with a recommended dose rate of 5.0 mg per kg for both *E. granulosus* and *E. multilocularis* (Gemmell and Johnstone, 1981).

Immunodiagnosis

Circulating antibodies (serum) can be detected in dogs infected with *E. granulosus* and *E. multilocularis*. An extensive program involving ELISA has been successfully developed (e.g. coproantigens) for use in detecting *Echinococcus* spp. in fecal material. The sensitivity and specificity of the test has been estimated at 67.5%. and 96.5%, respectively. Evidence of successful diagnosis has been obtained, but its practical contribution to control yet remains to be determined (Allan *et al.*, 1992; Deplazes *et al.*, 1992; Lightowlers and Gottstein, 1995; Craig, 1997; Eckert, 1998).

Immunization

A vaccine to protect sheep and goats from echinococcosis, based on a polypeptide antigen, derived from oncospheres and prepared as a recombinant fusion protein expressed as inclusion bodies in *Escherichia coli*, has been developed and successfully applied in field trials. Its role in control has yet to be fully defined (Heath, 1991, 1995; Lightowlers *et al.*, 1992; Heath *et al.*, 1999).

Overview of successful and ongoing island control programs for *Echinococcus granulosus*

Iceland (1869-1979)

Prior to control, about 1/5th of the community harbored hydatid cysts. In that period cattle, sheep, dogs and humans lived in close contact during the winter months, sometimes under the same roof. Following the introduction of control in 1869, transmission from dogs to humans rapidly declined and remained at a very low level for about 90 years and that between dog and sheep for about 110 years. The control structure and funding involved Ministries of Health and of Agriculture with Local Authorities for dog control. The successful "attack" phase, reviewed in detail by Beard (1973b), mainly involved: (1) health education among a literate community, particularly Krabbe's 16-page booklet on the life cycle written in the Icelandic tongue in 1864; (2) meat inspection and restrictions to the size of the dog population. This may have been assisted by a tax on dogs in 1869 and three epizootics of distemper (1870, 1888 and 1892); in addition and most important, (3) changes were made from 1870 from wool to fat lamb production and export of adult sheep. Initially an annual treatment of dogs with areca nut and from 1930 with arecoline hydrobromide was applied. Their impact was not important.

In the 50-year period 1932-1982, 15,888 autopsies were performed and of these 214 were found infected with CE. All but eight of these patients were born before 1900, indicating that considerable control of the parasite in dogs had been achieved before the turn of the century. The last two latent cases of CE were observed in 1984 and 1988. These, however, were born in 1905 and 1920. The last transmission between dogs and humans occurred in a non-latent case in 1960 in a 23-year-old woman: a period of 70-90 years from the beginning of the program. The "maintenance of eradication" phase was probably reached in 1979. From that time, surveillance through meat inspection has been maintained together with an annual treatment of dogs with praziquantel and the application of strict importation regulations (Dungal, 1957; Beard, 1973a, b; Palsson, 1984).

New Zealand (1959-1998)

Some of the first sheep to arrive in Australia in the late 18th century were merinos from South Africa originating from Spanish stock. Further introductions originating from North Africa were procured via Portugal after an embargo was placed on exports from Spain. Sheep were first introduced into New Zealand from Australia in 1814. From that time, numerous opportunities existed for fresh introductions into Australia from Europe and South Africa. Indeed, from 1862, when refrigeration was introduced, an entirely new sheep industry (from wool to meat) was generated in New Zealand with exports of lamb to Europe. This contributed to the serious and largely undocumented human rural health problem, particularly among Maoris that resulted from the feeding of aged sheep to dogs during the latter part of the 19th century. It was made a notifiable disease in 1873. Indeed, about 30 years after control had been initiated in Iceland, specific control was recommended in 1898 by the Department of Agriculture in New Zealand. Then it was considered that all dogs should be dosed with extract of male fern or areca nut.

During the first half of the 20th century, emphasis was placed on health education and on methods that might be applied to reduce prevalence in humans and animals. An amendment was made to the Dog Registration Act (1908) and in 1937 all owners who registered their animals received sufficient arecoline to treat them every 3 months. This was followed in 1940 by a regulation under the Meat Act making it illegal to feed raw offal to dogs. These regulations were unsuccessful and the prevalence of echinococcosis in adult sheep exceeded 50% during this period.

During the 1950s, following the application of a strong educational program involving "Community Participation" (Begg, 1961), it was found that from 0.2 to 37.3% of farm dogs were infected with *E. granulosus*, indicating that owners were unwilling or unable to prevent dogs becoming infected and that control to be successful must be undertaken as a formal program. As a result, a National Hydatids Eradication Council (Hydatid Act 1959) was formed with local authorities applying the day to day control measures, funded through a local dog tax added to the normal dog license fee. The "attack" phase, which lasted about 32 years, involved supervision of formal dog registration and the application of arecoline hydrobromide by technicians to detect and penalize owners of dogs infected with *E. granulosus* or *Taenia hydatigena* up to four times yearly (13 years). During this period, transmission of *E. granulosus* from dogs to humans virtually ceased. Treatment of dogs, however, was continued partly in an unsuccessful attempt from 1972 to eliminate *Taenia ovis* as an economic problem for sheep exports and from 1976, a 6-weekly dog-dosing program with praziquantel was introduced.

A structural change from a Council to the Ministry of Agriculture (Biosecurity Act 1993) was needed to remove dog-dosing and enter the "consolidation" phase and apply surveillance and quarantine of premises with infected livestock. The "maintenance of eradication" phase was reached in about 1998 and consisted of permanent surveillance of livestock at meat inspection together with restrictions to re-entry of the parasite (Anon, 1961-1989; Gemmell and Lawson, 1986; Gemmell, 1990).

Tasmania (1964-1997)

In about 1960, medical and veterinary authorities became fully aware of the need to control echinococcosis. A "Community Participation" educational program was generated along similar lines to that in New Zealand (Beard, 1984). Control was applied and funded by the State Department of Agriculture (now Primary Industry), supported by a voluntary national advisory committee (Tasmanian Hydatid Eradication Council-THEC), with local authorities assuming responsibility for dog registration.

The "attack" phase lasted about 11 years and involved education using arecoline testing of farm dogs voluntarily from 1965 and compulsorily from 1966 with quarantine and supervision of premises for at least 6 months. Transmission to humans ceased within 8 years. By 1975, the program was transformed to the "consolidation" phase to include supervision of farms with infected sheep detected at meat inspection. This lasted for about 22 years. Altogether, the "maintenance of eradication" phase was reached in about 33 years (1996/1997) and involved permanent surveillance of food animals through meat inspection and parasite re-entry restrictions (Anon, 1964-1988; Bramble, 1978; McConnell and Green, 1979; Beard, 1987; McConnell, 1987).

Falkland Islands (1965-1997)

Both cattle and sheep were introduced into the Falkland Islands before 1800. No records have indicated that *E. granulosus* was present during the 19th century, despite introductions of animals from regions of South America. It was first recorded in sheep in 1941, possibly from importations of stud sheep from New Zealand and/or Tasmania and became common during the decade 1950-1959.

Control was introduced in 1965 (Tapeworm Eradication Dogs Order). This order made provision for: (1) the appointment of dog inspectors; (2) the purging of dogs with arecoline acetarsol (Tenoban); and (3) prohibited the feeding of raw offal to dogs. Within the decade, about 60% of the sheep and cattle were still affected with hydatid cysts and Tenoban had fallen into disrepute. From 1970, under a second Tapeworm Eradication Order, dog-dosing was undertaken every 12 weeks with bunamidine hydrochloride and from 1977 with praziquantel every 6 weeks. Strong reliance was placed on offal disposal and confinement of dogs unless being worked. Only two sheep were detected with *E. granulosus* during an 18-month period 1995-1996. Whilst, as in all programs, it is very difficult to define the point at which *E. granulosus* has been eradicated, it seems possible that this may have occurred in about 1997 or about 32 years after control or 20 years after the 6-weekly dog-dosing program with praziquantel was applied.

The first case of CE was recorded in 1963. From 1965-1975, 11 cases were confirmed. The final survey, carried out in 1988, using ELISA technique, showed 18 with positive reactions of varying degree. All had previously been diagnosed as suffering from CHD, implying, as expected, that transmission to humans had ceased before that in animals (Reichel *et al.*, 1996). To retain an eradication status, several permanent measures remain in place. These include: (1) a national dog registration scheme with notifications of transfer to new owners, births and deaths to the Department of Agriculture; (2) copro-antigen tests applied to dogs for *E. granulosus*; (3) retention of dog treatments, with owners paying for the praziquantel; and (4) retention of safe offal disposal and surveillance through meat inspection and restrictions to parasite re-entry (Sommers, 1997, unpublished).

Similarities and differences between successful CE island programs

All four programs required an educational approach to generate approval for the appointment of a formal control authority. The programs themselves and their duration differed. The Icelandic program required about 110 years. In contrast, those of New Zealand, Tasmania and the Falkland Islands required less than 40 years. This difference may in part be accounted for by the application in the "attack" phase of highly educational dog-testing programs in the case of New Zealand and Tasmania and a highly effective anthelmintic (praziquantel) to treat dogs in the Falkland Islands.

With respect to differences in the duration of the "attack" phase between New Zealand and Tasmania (of 34 and 11 years, respectively), this was due to differences in control structure. The former involved a Council with local authorities employing technicians to dose dogs with a national testing station to identify infected dogs. In contrast, the latter, using livestock officers of the Department of Agriculture, tested dogs directly for infection with mobile laboratories and quarantined farms with infected dogs.

Cyprus (1974-): an ongoing but successful island program

A control program was introduced into the Republic of Cyprus in 1971. Administration and funding was undertaken *ab initio* in the "planning" phase by the Ministry of Agriculture. At the time of introduction, the principal measures applied in the "attack" phase were: (1) stray dog control; (2) spaying of bitches and imposition of high registration fees for unspayed animals; (3) obligatory testing with arecoline hydrobromide using the field diagnostic test every 3 months with euthanasia of all positive dogs; (4) a public health educational program; and (5) strict controls at slaughterhouses. This program was successfully pursued throughout the island until the events of 1974 when the island was divided. The campaign was continued only in the area controlled by the Government of the Republic of Cyprus, and comprises some 395 villages. From 1971 to 1985, 85,727 and 13,336 stray dogs were killed and spayed, respectively. Eradication was claimed in 1985 with cessation of activities.

Following a reappraisal, it was found that the parasite was still present and a permanent "consolidation" phase in the Government-controlled area was introduced in 1994. This involves permanent surveillance through meat inspection. A village is designated as an infected area where infected animals are found on any premises. The measures applied include: (1) treatment of all dogs with praziquantel; (2) elimination of stray dogs; (3) movement control of all animals; and (4) prosecution for illegal slaughtering. Release from quarantine is applied after at least 3 years in the absence of *E. granulosus* or *T. hydatigena* at meat inspection (Economides *et al.*, 1998).

Ongoing continental CE control programs

Europe and South America

During the second half of the 20th century, several control programs partially or completely failed. However, countries with active successful control programs, include Spain and Portugal in Europe and several countries in the highly endemic regions of South America, namely the Provinces of Rio Negro, Tierra del Fuego and Chubut in Argentina, Regions 10, 11 and 12 in Chile and all departments of Uruguay (see Gemmell and Roberts, 1998 for review). Control authorities in the South American programs include Ministry of Health (Argentina), Ministry of Agriculture (Chile) and Uruguay (Comision de Lucha Contra La Hidatidosis). By the end of the 20th century, all had reduced the prevalence of the parasite in humans, dogs and sheep, but only in Region 12 in Chile had control reached the stage when transfer from the "attack" to a permanent "consolidation" phase might be considered early in the 21st century.

Africa

In Africa, a pilot control program initiated in 1983 (Macpherson *et al.*, 1984) is still operational in the endemic region of Turkana District in northern Kenya (Macpherson and Wachira, 1997). The preparatory phase ran from 1976 to 1983 and the creation of a control authority, which was modelled after the Peru control authority, involved both governmental and non-governmental agencies (Gemmell and Varela-Diaz, 1975). The attack phase ran from 1983 to 1995. Options 2-5 were all employed with an emphasis on a horizontal educational program in schoolchildren and women: the latter group had almost three times the prevalence of CE due to a closer relationship with dogs. Dosing of dogs was carried out six times a year with only one dosing schedule being carried out in the dry season. This regimen took into account local cultural factors and dogs were treated regularly during the wet season, when large numbers of livestock were slaughtered at wedding ceremonies, etc. Livestock were not killed during the dry season and the people's diet comprised of milk and blood, supplemented with wild berries. Enormous changes in the dog population took place in the pilot control area with the end of the serious drought from 1978 to 1981, when over 70% of the livestock died and dogs had a plentiful food supply. The dog population rose to over 6000 individuals and of these approximately 70% were infected with *E. granulosus* and over 55% of the infected dogs had heavy (> 200 individuals) worm burdens. The dog population crashed to only a few hundred individuals by 1985 and this number has remained relatively constant since then (Macpherson, 1995). The current ongoing drought, which started in 1998, may see a similar trend. Surveillance of the Turkana pilot control program is carried out through annual ultrasound prevalence surveys. Recent data show a decrease in the prevalence of CE in all age groups. Particularly encouraging is that there has been only one new CE case in the under 5-year-old age group since 1987 (Macpherson and Wachira, 1997).

Future control strategies

The first steps for determining the life cycle and applying control of *E.granulosus*were initiated in the late 19th century. Clearly, in the 20th century, it was been shown that by the application of control programs, the "maintenance of eradication" phase could be achieved on islands in a period of less than 40 years. These achievements were made possible by the development of: (1) specific educational programs, such as "community participation"; (2) "arecoline testing" of dogs; and (3) praziquantel to eliminate *E. granulosus* from dogs. Although it has also been shown that the prevalence of *E. granulosus* can be markedly reduced in humans and animals in continental control programs, further research is needed in the 21st century to develop methods for achieving a permanent cost effective "consolidation" phase. Further research on the application of: (1) surveillance through meat inspection; (2) immunodiagnosis of the parasite in dogs; and (3) immunization of intermediate hosts, may contribute towards this end.

Conclusions

These various examples of control reviewed in this chapter clearly show that progress has been achieved in the prevention and control of major canine zoonotic diseases, particularly during the second half of the 20th century. This has resulted from the continuous development during this period of improved methods for disease surveillance and control. Disease occurrence has been avoided in both dogs and people and thus many human lives have been saved. However, the number of countries that have conducted successful elimination programs has remained small. No successful nation-wide rabies elimination program has been reported since Uruguay became rabies free in 1983, and rare are the countries outside the Americas which have during the past 15 to 20 years contained dog rabies in a sustainable manner. For CE, since the first control activities took place in Iceland in 1869, the maintenance of eradication has been achieved in a limited number of countries or territories. Rabies, leishmaniasis and echinococcosis still represent a significant public health problem in most endemic areas. In some of them, they are increasingly reported and this is a cause of major concern for the future if no comprehensive control programs are initiated soon.

Gaining access to dogs is the major factor for the eventual success or failure of any program for the control of a zoonosis in the cycle of which dogs play a central role. The WHO-co-ordinated studies on dog population parameters for rabies control in developing countries carried out in the 1980s showed that under different socio-cultural and economic conditions, at least 65% of the total dog population was accessible to parenteral rabies vaccination without special investments in public educational and motivational campaigns. Experiments also showed that strengthening community involvement through better public information and campaign planning could lead to an even higher coverage. It is likely that health interventions other than vaccination against rabies (e.g. testing and treating for echinococcosis, testing and putting a protective collar into place for CV leishmaniasis) could have been implemented within these dog populations with the same rate of success during these field studies. In spite of the above re-assuring results, many of the examples given show that reaching dogs currently remains a major problem in most countries where rabies, CV leishmaniasis or CE are prevalent. The full collaboration of dog owners is very difficult to obtain especially when coercive measures have to be taken (such as eliminating an excess or putting an animal to death if shown to be infected) or when handling them entails some risks for or requires considerable efforts from the owner himself. This is compounded by reports indicating that unsupervised or insufficiently supervised dog populations are increasing in most developing countries, particularly near urban centres, in view of the increasing availability of food sources. Dog removal is not the solution as it does not have a significant impact on dog population size in the long term and is unacceptable to or counterproductive in many local communities. Comprehensive dog population management policies need to be developed rapidly wherever possible. WHO has initiated joint activities for "dog-borne" zoonoses prevention and control with the World Society for the Protection of Animals (WSPA) and the International Association for Human-Animal Interactions Organizations (IAHAIO) aiming at eveloping a real partnership with dog owners for canine zoonoses control based on the promotion of the concept of "responsible dog ownership".

In addition, a lack of governmental support for canine zoonoses control has been observed in most places. This is a result of: (1) an insufficient appreciation by both the national human and animal health sectors of the burden, which these diseases represent for the their respective sectors and the national economy; and (2) the absence in most countries where these diseases are present, of effective medical-veterinary collaboration for their control. Effective control of these diseases, whether canine or human, demands political will, recognition of cost benefits, co-ordination and integration with other relevant disease control programs. Even if the impact on health and the economy of these diseases receive better recognition at the national and international levels, it is likely that the implementation of canine zoonoses control activities will remain under financial strain as they occur in generally poor economic areas often affecting vulnerable human groups. This situation requires that any new techniques introduced such as a new "bed test" for CV leishmaniasis, an oral rabies vaccination or perhaps the use of a protective dog collar against leishmaniasis be cost effective and that a number of issues, particularly safe vaccine delivery and sustainability of tests, oral vaccines and collar supply be resolved beforehand. If these diseases are not controlled and eventually eliminated in dogs, expenses related to the treatment of existing and prevention of future human cases are likely to increase dramatically in developing countries.

References

Abranches, P., Campino, L. and Santos Gomes, G.M. (1998) Canine leishmaniasis. New concepts of epidemiology and immunopathology: their impact in the control of human visceral leishmaniasis. *Acta Medica Portuguesa* 11, 871-875.

Akhavan, D. (1996) Analise de custo-efetividade do componente de leishmaniose no projeto de controle de doencas endemicas no nordeste do Brasil. *Revista di Patologia Medical* 25, 203-252.

Alencar, J.E. (1961) Profilaxia do calazar no Ceara, Brasil. *Revista do Instituto de Medecina Tropical de Sao Paulo* 3, 175-180.

Allan, J.C., Craig, P.S., Garcia Noval, J., Liu, D., Wang, Y., Wen, H., Zhou, P., Stringer, R., Rogan, M. and Zeyhle, E. (1992) Coproantigen detection for immunodiagnosis of echinococcosis and taeniasis in dogs and humans. *Parasitology* 104, 347-355.

Alvar, J., Gutierrez-Solar, B., Pachon, I., Calbacho, E., Ramirez, M., Valles, R., Guillen, J.L., Canavate, C. and Amela, C. (1996) AIDS and *Leishmania infantum*. New approaches for a new epidemiological problem. *Clinical Dermatology* 14, 541-546.

Anonymous (1961-1989) Annual Reports of the National Hydatids Council, Wellington, New Zealand.

Anonymous (1964-1988) Annual Reports and Accounts of the Tasmanian Hydatids Eradication Council, Hobart, Tasmania.

Anonymous (1993) Ministere de la Sante Publique, Directions de la Sante de Base. Program National de Lutte contre la Rage. Rapport final des travaux du seminaire national d'evaluation Tunis, pp. 24.

Arias, J., Desjeux, P. and Miles, M.A. (1996) *Manual on the Control of Visceral Leishmaniasis.* WHO/ODA.

Ashford, D.A., Bozza, M., Miranda, J.C., Eulalio, C., Freire, M., Miranda, C., Zalis, M.G. and David, J.R. (1995) Comparison of the polymerase chain reaction and serology for the detection of canine visceral leishmaniasis. *American Journal of Tropical Medicine and Hygiene* 53, 251-255.

Ashford, D.A., David, J.R., Freire, M., David, R., Sherlock, I., da Conceicao Eulalio, M., Pedral Sampaio, D. and Badaro, R. (1998) Studies on control of visceral leishmaniasis: impact of dog control on canine and human visceral leishmaniasis in Jacobina, Bahia, Brazil. *American Journal of Tropical Medicine and Hygiene* 59, 53-57.

Ashford, R.W. (1999) Visceral leishmaniasis: epidemiology prevention and control. In: Gilles, H.M. (ed.) *Protozoal Diseases.* Arnold, London, pp. 462-470.

Beard, T.C. (1973a) Observations for Icelanders on hydatids and precautions against them. *Australian Veterinary Journal* 49, 396-401.

Beard, T.C. (1973b) The elimination of echinococcosis from Iceland. *Bulletin of the World Health Organisation* 48, 653-660.

Beard, T.C. (1984) Changing rural behaviour: two campaigns that worked. *Hygie* 111, 9-13.

Beard, T.C. (1987) Human hydatid disease in Tasmania. In: King, H. (ed.) *Epidemiology in Tasmania*. Brolga Press, Canberra, ACT, Australia, pp. 77-88.

Begg, N.C. (1961) The campaign against hydatid disease: an experiment in social medicine. *New Zealand Medical Journal* 60, 229-234.

Belotto, A.J. (1988) Organisation of mass vaccination for dog rabies in Brazil. *Reviews of Infectious Diseases* 10, 693-696.

Ben Osman, F. and Haddad, N. (1988) Experience in field rabies control programs. *Review of Infectious Diseases* 10, 703-706.

Ben Youssef, S., Matter, H.C., Schumacher, C.L., Kharmachi, H., Jemli, J., Mrabet, L., Gharbi, M., Hammami, S., Hicheri, K., Aubert, M. and Meslin F.-X. (1998) Field evaluation of a dog owner participation based bait delivery system for the oral immunization of dogs against rabies in Tunisia. *American Journal of Tropical Medicine and Hygiene* 58, 835-845.

Beran, G. and Frith, M. (1988) Domestic animal rabies control: an overview. *Review of Infectious Diseases* 10, 672-677.

Blancou, J. and Meslin, F.-X. (2000) A brief historical overview of zoonoses. *Office International des Epizooties Scientific and Technical Review* 19, 15-22.

Bögel, K. and Joshi, D.D. (1990) Accessibility of dog populations for rabies control in Kathmandu valley, Nepal. *Bulletin of the World Health Organisation* 68, 611-617.

Bögel, K. and Meslin, F.-X. (1990) Economics of human and canine rabies elimination: guidelines for program orientation. *Bulletin of the World Health Organisation* 68, 281-291.

Braga, M.D., Coelho, I.C., Pompeu, M.M., Evans, T.G., MacAullife, I.T., Teixeira, M.J. and Lima, J.W. (1998) Control of canine visceral leishmaniasis: comparison of results from a rapid elimination program of serum-reactive dogs using an immunoenzyme assay and slower elimination of serum-reactive dogs using filter paper elution indirect immunofluorescence. *Revista da Sociedade Brasileira de Medicina Tropical* 31, 419-424.

Bramble, A.J. (1978) Hydatid disease control in Tasmania. *Tasmanian Journal of Agriculture* 79, 225-228.

Cardoso, L., Neto, F., Sousa, J.C., Rodrigues, M. and Cabral, M. (1998) Use of a leishmanin skin test in the detection of canine *Leishmania*-specific cellular immunity. *Veterinary Parasitology* 79, 213-220.

Corredor, A., Gallego, J.F., Tesh, R.B., Morales, A., de Carrasquilla, C.F., Young, D.G., Kreutzer, R.D., Boshell, J., Palau, M.T., Caceres, E. and Pelaez, D. (1989) Epidemiology of visceral leishmaniasis in Colombia. *American Journal of Tropical Medicine and Hygiene* 40, 480-486.

Costa, C.H.N., Pereira, H.F., Pereira, F.C.A., Tavares, J.P., Araujo, M.V. and Goncalves, M.J.O. (1999) Is the household dog a risk factor for American visceral leishmaniasis in Brazil? *Transactions of the Royal Society of Tropical Medicine and Hygiene* 93, 464.

Courtenay, O., Santana, E.W., Johnson, P.J., Vasconcelos, I.A. and Vasconcelos, A.W. (1996) Visceral leishmaniasis in the hoary zorro *Dusicyon vetulus*: a case of mistaken identity. *Transactions of the Royal Society of Tropical Medicine and Hygiene* 90, 498-502.

Craig, P.S. (1997) Immunodiagnosis of *Echinococcus granulosus* and comparison of techniques for the diagnosis of canine echinococcosis. In: Andersen, F.L., Ouhelli, H. and Kachani, M. (eds) *Compendium on Cystic Echinococcosis in Africa and in Middle Eastern Countries With Special Reference to Morocco.* Brigham Young University, Provo, Utah, USA, pp. 85-118.

Cunha, S., Freire, M., Eulalio, C., Critosvao, J., Netto, E., Johnson, W.D. Jr., Reed, S.G. and Badaro, R. (1995) Visceral leishmaniasis in a new ecological niche near a major metropolitan area of Brazil. *Transactions of the Royal Society of Tropical Medicine and Hygiene* 89, 155-158.

Deane, L.M. (1956) Leishmaniose Visceral no Brasil. Estudos sobre reservatorios e transmisores realizados no Ceara. Thesis de Livre Docencia, Faculdade de Medecina, Universidade de Sao Paulo.

Deane, L.M. and Deane, M.P. (1962) Visceral leishmaniasis in Brazil: geographical distribution and transmission. *Revista do Instituto de Medecina Tropical de Sao Paulo* 4, 198-212.

De Balogh, K.K.I.M., Wandeler, A.I. and Meslin, F.-X. (1993) A dog ecology study in an urban and a semi-urban area of Zambia. *Onderstepoort Journal of Veterinary Research* 60, 437-443.

Deplazes, P., Gottstein, B., Eckert, J., Jenkins, D.J., Ewald, D. and Jimenez Palacios, S. (1992) Detection of *Echinococcus* coproantigens by enzyme-linked immunosorbent assay in dogs, dingoes and foxes. *Parasitology Research* 78, 303-308.

Dereure, J., Pratlong, F. and Dedet, J.-P. (1999) Geographical distribution and the identification of parasites causing canine leishmaniasis in the Mediterranean Basin. In: Killick-Kendrick, R. (ed.) *Canine Leishmaniasis: an Update. Proceedings of the International Canine Leishmaniasis Forum*, Barcelona, Spain. Hoechst Roussel Vet, Germany, pp. 18-25.

Desjeux, P. (1991) Information on the epidemiology and control of the leishmaniases by country and territory. *Report Number WHO/Leish/91.30*, WHO, Geneva, pp. 47.

Dungal, N. (1957) Eradication of hydatid disease in Iceland. *New Zealand Medical Journal* 56, 213-222.

Dye, C. (1996) The logic of visceral leishmaniasis control. *American Journal of Tropical Medicine and Hygiene* 55, 125-130.

Dye, C., Killick-Kendrick, R., Vitutia, M.M., Walton, R., Killick-Kendrick, M., Harith, A.E., Guy, M.W., Canavate, M.C. and Hasibeder, G. (1992) Epidemiology of canine leishmaniasis: prevalence, incidence and basic reproduction number calculated from a cross-sectional serological survey on the island of Gozo, Malta. *Parasitology* 105, 35-41.

Eckert, J. (1998) Alveolar echinococcosis (*Echinococcus multilocularis*) and other forms of echinococcosis (*Echinococcus vogeli* and *Echinococcus oligarthrus*). In: Palmer, S.R., Lord Soulsby and Simpson, D.I.H. (eds) *Zoonoses.* Oxford University Press, Oxford, New York, Tokyo, pp. 689-716.

Economides, P., Christofi, G. and Gemmell, M.A. (1998) Control of *Echinococcus granulosus* in Cyprus and comparison with other island models. *Veterinary Parasitology* 79, 151-163.

Evans, T.G., Teixeira, M.J., McAuliffe, I.T., de Alencar Barros Vasconcelos, I., Wilson Vasconcelos, A., de Queiroz Sousa, A., Wellington de Oliveira Lima, J. and Pearson, R.D. (1992) Epidemiology of visceral leishmaniasis in Northeast Brazil. *Journal of Infectious Diseases* 166, 1124-1132.

Ferrer, L.M. (1999) Clinical aspects of canine leishmaniasis. In: Killick-Kendrick, R. (ed.) *Canine Leishmaniasis: an Update. Proceedings of the International Canine Leishmaniasis Forum*, Barcelona, Spain. Hoechst Roussel Vet, Germany, pp. 6-10.

Frontini, M.G., Fishbein, D.B., Garza Ramos, J., Flores Collins, E., Balderas Torres, J.M., Quiroz Huerta, G., Games Rodrigues, J.J., Belotto, A.J., Dobbins, J.G., Linhart, S.B. and Baer G.M. (1992) A field evaluation in Mexico of four baits for oral vaccination of dogs. *American Journal of Tropical Medicine and Hygiene* 47, 310-316.

Gemmell, M.A. (1968) The Styx Field-Trial. A study on the application of control measures against hydatid disease caused by *Echinococcus granulosus. Bulletin of the World Health Organisation* 39, 73-100.

Gemmell, M.A. (1973) Surveillance of *Echinococcus granulosus* in dogs with arecoline hydrobromide. *Bulletin of the World Health Organisation* 48, 649-652.

Gemmell, M.A. (1990) Australian contributions to understanding of the epidemiology and control of hydatid disease caused by *Echinococcus granulosus* - past, present and future. *International Journal of Parasitology* 20, 431-456.

Gemmell, M.A. (1997) Quantifying the transmission dynamics of the family Taeniidae with particular reference to *Echinococcus* spp. An update. In: Andersen, F.L., Ouhelli, H. and Kachani, M. (eds) *Compendium on Cystic Echinococcosis in Africa and in Middle Eastern Countries With Special Reference to Morocco.* Brigham Young University, Provo, Utah, pp. 54-71.

Gemmell, M.A. and Johnstone, P.D. (1981) Cestodes. *Antibiotics and Chemotherapy* 30, 54-114.

Gemmell, M.A. and Lawson, J.R. (1986) Epidemiology and control of hydatid disease. In: Thompson, R.C.A. (ed.) *The Biology of* Echinococcus *and Hydatid Disease.* George Allen and Unwin, London, pp. 189-216.

Gemmell, M.A. and Roberts, M.G. (1995) Modelling *Echinococcus* life cycles. In: Thompson, R.C.A. and Lymbery, A.J. (eds) Echinococcus *and Hydatid Disease.* CAB International, Wallingford, pp. 333-354.

Gemmell, M.A. and Roberts, M.G. (1998) Cystic echinococcosis (*Echinococcus granulosus*). In: Palmer, S.R., Lord Soulsby and Simpson, D.I.H. (eds) *Zoonoses.* Oxford University Press, Oxford, New York and Tokyo, pp. 666-688.

Gemmell, M.A. and Schantz, P.M. (1997) Formulating policies for control of *Echinococcus granulosus*. An overview of planning, implementation and evaluation. In: Andersen, F.L., Ouhelli, H. and Kachani, M. (eds) *Compendium on Cystic Echinococcosis in Africa and in Middle Eastern*

Countries With Special Reference to Morocco. Brigham Young University, Provo, Utah, pp. 329-345.

Gemmell, M.A. and Varela-Diaz, V.M. (1975) *Review of Programs for the Control of Hydatidosis/Echinococcosis.* Series of Scientific and Technical Monographs, CPZ-8. Pan American Zoonoses Centre, PAHO/WHO Buenos Aires, Argentina.

Goonaratna, C. (1997) Sri Lanka: Human rabies. In: Dodet, B. and Meslin, F.-X. (eds) *Rabies Control in Asia.* Elsevier, Paris, pp. 188-190.

Harishandra, P. (1997) Sri Lanka: Veterinary aspects of rabies. In: Dodet, B. and Meslin, F.-X. (eds) *Rabies Control in Asia.* Elsevier, Paris, pp. 191-193.

Hasibeder, G., Dye, C. and Carpenter, J. (1992) Mathematical modelling and theory for estimating the basic reproduction number of canine leishmaniasis. *Parasitology* 105, 43-53.

Heath, D.D. (1991) A vaccine to protect grazing animals against hydatid disease. Is there a role for such a vaccine? *Archivos Internacionales de la Hydatidosis* 30, 343-349.

Heath, D.D. (1995) Immunology of *Echinococcus* infections. In: Thompson, R.C.A. and Lymbery, A.J. (eds) Echinococcus *and Hydatid Disease.* CAB International, Wallingford, pp. 183-199.

Heath, D.D., Qi Pusheng, Zang Zhuangzhi, Wang Jincheng, Feng Jinglan and Lightowlers, M.W. (1999) Role of immunsation of the intermediate host in hydatid disease control. *Archivos Internacionales de la Hydatidosis* 33, 14-16.

Hussin, A. (1997) Malaysia: Veterinary aspects of rabies control and prevention. In: Dodet, B. and Meslin, F.-X. (eds) *Rabies Control in Asia.* Elsevier, Paris, pp. 167-170.

Kachani, M., Ouhelli, H., Tabyaoui, H., Bouliskhane, M. and Andersen, F.L. (1997) Preparation and evaluation of educational aids on cystic echinococcosis in Morocco. In: Andersen, F.L., Ouhelli, H. and Kachani, M. (eds) *Compendium on Cystic Echinococcosis in Africa and in Middle Eastern Countries With Special Reference to Morocco.* Brigham Young University, Provo, Utah, pp. 169-183.

Kharmachi, H., Haddad, N. and Matter, H. (1992) Tests of four baits for oral vaccination of dogs against rabies in Tunisia. *Veterinary Record* 130, 494.

Killick-Kendrick, R. (1999) Anti-feeding effects of synthetic pyrethroids against phlebotomine sand flies and mosquitoes and the prospects of controlling canine leishmaniasis with deltamethrin-impregnated ProtectorBands (Scalibor®). In: Killick-Kendrick, R. (ed.) *Canine Leishmaniasis: an Update. Proceedings of the International Canine Leishmaniasis Forum*, Barcelona, Spain. Hoechst Roussel Vet, Germany, pp. 82-90.

Killick-Kendrick, R., Killick-Kendrick, M., Pinelli, E., del Real, G., Molina, R., Vitutia, M.M., Canavate, M.C. and Nieto, J. (1994) A laboratory model of canine leishmaniasis: the inoculation of dogs with *Leishmania infantum* promastigotes from midguts of experimentally infected phlebotomine sandflies. *Parasite* 1, 311-318.

Killick-Kendrick, R., Killick-Kendrick, M., Focheux, C., Dereure, J., Puech, M.P. and Cadiergues, M.C. (1997) Protection of dogs from bites of phlebotomine sandflies by deltamethrin collars for control of canine leishmaniasis. *Medical and Veterinary Entomology* 11, 105-111.

Kingnate, D., Saragasaeranee, P. and Choomkasien, P. (1997) Thailand: rabies control in humans. In: Dodet, B. and Meslin, F.-X. (eds) *Rabies Control in Asia*. Elsevier, Paris, pp. 194-196.

Lainson, R. and Shaw, J.J. (1998) New World leishmaniasis – the neotropical *Leishmania* species. In: Collier, L., Balows, A. and Sussman, M. (eds) *Topley and Wilson's Microbiology and Microbial infections*.

Lamothe, J. (1999) Treatment of canine leishmaniasis from A (Amphotericin B) to Z (Zyloric®). In: Killick-Kendrick, R. (ed.) *Canine Leishmaniasis: an Update. Proceedings of the International Canine Leishmaniasis Forum*, Barcelona, Spain. Hoechst Roussel Vet, Germany, pp. 12-17.

Lawson, J.R., Roberts, M.G., Gemmell, M.A. and Best, S.J. (1988) Population dynamics in echinococcosis and cysticercosis: economic assessment of control strategies for *Echinococcus granulosus*, *Taenia ovis* and *T. hydatigena*. *Parasitology* 97, 1-15.

Lightowlers, M.W. and Gottstein, B. (1995) Echinococcus/hydatidosis: immunology and molecular diagnosis. In: Thompson, R.C.A. and Lymbery, A.J. (eds) *Echinococcus and Hydatid Disease*. CAB International, Wallingford, pp. 356-410.

Lightowlers, M.W., Gemmell, M.A., Harrison, G.L.B., Heath, D.D., Rickard, M.D. and Roberts, M.G. (1992) Control of tissue parasites. 11 Cestodes. In: Yong, W. (ed.) *Animal Parasite Control Utilizing Biotechnology*. CRC Press, Boca Raton, Florida, pp. 463-487

Lucientes, J. (1999) Laboratory observations on the protection of dogs from the bites of *Phlebotomus perniciosus* with Scalibor® ProtectorBands: preliminary results. In: Killick-Kendrick, R. (ed.) *Canine Leishmaniasis: an Update. Proceedings of the International Canine Leishmaniasis Forum*, Barcelona, Spain. Hoechst Roussel Vet, Germany, pp. 92-94.

Macpherson, C.N.L. (1995) The effect of transhumance on the epidemiology of animal diseases. *Preventive Veterinary Medicine* 25, 213-224.

Macpherson, C.N.L. and Wachira, T.W.M. (1997) Cystic echinococcus in Africa south of the Sahara. In: Andersen, F.L., Ouhelli, H. and Kachani, M. (eds) *Compendium on Cystic Echinococcosis in Africa and in Middle Eastern Countries With Special Reference to Morocco*. Brigham Young University, Provo, Utah, USA, pp. 245-277.

Macpherson, C.N.L., Zeyhle, E. and Romig, T. (1984) An *Echinococcus* pilot control program for north west Turkana, Kenya. *Annals of Tropical Medicine and Parasitology* 78, 188-192.

Macpherson, C.N.L., Spoerry, A., Zeyhle, E., Romig, T. and Gorfe, M. (1989) Pastoralists and hydatid disease: an ultrasound scanning prevalence survey in East Africa. *Transactions of the Royal Society of Tropical Medicine and Hygiene* 84, 243-247.

Manniger, R. (1968) Rabies in Hungary during the past forty years. *Magyar Allatorvosok Lapja* 23, 5-13.

Martin-Sanchez, J., Lepe, J.A., Toledo, A., Ubeda, J.M., Guevara, D.C., Morillas-Marquez, F. and Gramiccia, M. (1999) *Leishmania (Leishmania) infantum* enzymatic variants causing canine leishmaniasis in the Huelva province (south-west Spain). *Transactions of the Royal Society of Tropical Medicine and Hygiene* 93, 495-496.

Matter, H.C. (1989) Populationsbiologische Untersuchungen an Hundepopulationen in Tunesien. PhD thesis, University of Berne, Berne, Switzerland.

Matter, H.C., Kharmachi, H., Haddad, N., Ben Youssef, S., Sghaier, C., Ben Khalifa, R., Jemli, J., Mrabet, L., Meslin, F.-X. and Wandeler, A.I. (1995) Test of three bait types for oral immunization of dogs against rabies in Tunisia. *American Journal of Tropical Medicine and Hygiene* 52, 489-495.

Matter, H.C., Schumacher, C.L., Kharmachi, H., Hammami, S., Tlatli, A., Mrabet, L., Meslin, F.-X., Aubert, M.F.A., Neuenschwander, B.E. and El Hicheri, K. (1998) Field evaluation of 2 bait delivery systems for the oral immunization of dogs against rabies in Tunisia. *Vaccine* 16, 657-665.

Matter, H.C., Wandeler, A.I., Neuenschwander, B.E., Harishandra, L.P.A. and Meslin, F.X. (2000) Study of the dog population and the rabies control activities in the Mirigama area of Sri Lanka. *Acta Tropica* 75, 95-108.

Mauricio, I.L., Howard, M.K., Stothard, J.R. and Miles, M.A. (1999) Genomic diversity in the *Leishmania donovani* complex. *Parasitology* 119, 237-246.

Mauricio, I.L., Stothard, J.R. and Miles, M.A. (2000) The strange case of *Leishmania chagasi*. *Parasitology Today* 16, 188-189.

McConnell, J.D. (1987) Hydatid disease in Tasmania: control in animals. In: King, H. (ed.) *Epidemiology in Tasmania*. Brolga Press, Canberra, pp. 61-75.

McConnell, J.D. and Green, R.J. (1979) The control of hydatid disease in Tasmania. *Australian Veterinary Journal* 55, 140-145.

Meldrum, K.C. (1988) Rabies contingency plans in the United Kingdom. *Parassitologia* 30, 97-103.

Meslin, F.-X., Fishbein, D.B. and Matter, H.C. (1994) Rationale and prospects for dogs. Rabies elimination in developing countries. In: Rupprecht, C.E., Dietzchold, B. and Koprowski, H. (eds) *Lyssavirus*. Springer-Verlag, Berlin-Heidelberg, pp. 1-26.

Miles, M.A., Vexenat, J.A., Furtado Campos, J.H. and Fonseca de Castro, J.A. (1999) Canine leishmaniasis in Latin America: control strategies for visceral leishmaniasis. In: Killick-Kendrick, R. (ed.) *Canine Leishmaniasis: an Update. Proceedings of the International Canine Leishmaniasis Forum*, Barcelona, Spain. Hoechst Roussel Vet, Germany, pp. 46-53.

Molina, R., Amela, C., Nieto, J., San-Andres, M., Gonzalez, F., Castillo, J.A., Lucientes, J. and Alvar, J. (1994) Infectivity of dogs naturally infected with *Leishmania infantum* to colonized *Phlebotomus perniciosus*. *Transactions of the Royal Society of Tropical Medicine and Hygiene* 88, 491-493.

Momen, H. (1995) II National Meeting on Strategic Research in Leishmaniases: Belo Horizonte, MG, Brazil, September 18-22, 1995. *Memorias Instituto Oswaldo Cruz* 90, 775-776.

Nieto, C.G., Garcia Alonso, M., Requena, J.M., Miron, C., Soto, M., Alonso, C. and Navarrete, I. (1999) Analysis of the humoral immune response against total and recombinant antigens of *Leishmania infantum*: correlation with disease progression in canine experimental leishmaniasis. *Veterinary Immunology and Immunopathology* 67, 117-130.

Nonnemaker, J.M. and Schantz, P.M. (1997) Economic evaluation techniques as tools for planning and evaluation of echinococcosis control programs. In: Andersen, F.L., Ouhelli, H. and Kachani, M. (eds) *Compendium on Cystic Echinococcosis in Africa and in Middle Eastern Countries With Special Reference to Morocco.* Brigham Young University, Provo, Utah, pp. 319-328.

PAHO (1997) Epidemiological surveillance of rabies in the Americas. *Bulletin of Epidemiological Surveillance of Rabies in the Americas* 24, INPPAZ, Bueno-Aires, pp. 29.

Palsson, P.A. (1984) Hydatidosis in Iceland: how it was eradicated. In: Euzeby, J. and Gevrey, J. (eds) *Some Important Parasitic Infections in Bovines Considered from Economic and Social (Zoonosis) Points of View.* Parasitological Symposium, Lyons, France. 24-26th October 1983, pp. 121-131.

Paranhos-Silva, M., Freitas, L.A.R., Santos, W.C., Grimaldi, G. Jr., Pontes-de-Carvalho, L.C. and Oliveira-dos-Santos, A.J. (1996) A cross-sectional serodiagnostic survey of canine leishmaniasis due to *Leishmania chagasi. American Journal of Tropical Medicine and Hygiene* 55, 39-44.

Perry, B.D. and Wandeler, A.I. (1993) The delivery of oral rabies vaccine to dogs: an African perspective. *Onderstepoort Journal Of Veterinary Research* 60, 451-457.

Perry, B.D., Brooks, R., Foggins, C.M., Bleakley, J., Johnston, D.H. and Will, F.W.G. (1988) A baiting system suitable for the delivery of oral rabies vaccine to dog population in Zimbabwe. *Veterinary Record* 123, 76-79.

Pinelli, E., Killick-Kendrick, R., Wagenaar, J., Bernadina, W., del Real, G. and Ruitenberg, J. (1994) Cellular and humoral immune responses in dogs experimentally and naturally infected with *Leishmania infantum. Infection and Immunity* 62, 229-235.

Pinelli, E., Rutten, V.P., Bruysters, M., Moore, P.F. and Ruitenberg, E.J. (1999) Compensation for decreased expression of B7 molecules on *Leishmania infantum*-infected canine macrophages results in restoration of parasite-specific T-cell proliferation and gamma interferon production. *Infection and Immunity* 67, 237-243.

Qing Tang, Zhao Xiuqin and Dou Zhi (1997) Human epidemiology and risk factors for rabies in China. In: Dodet, B. and Meslin, F.-X. (eds), *Rabies Control in Asia.* Elsevier, Paris, pp. 130-136.

Rausch, R.L. (1995) Life cycle patterns and geographic distribution of *Echinococcus* species. In: Thompson, R.C.A. and Lymbery, A.J. (eds) Echinococcus *and Hydatid Disease.* CAB International, Wallingford, UK, pp. 89-134.

Rausch, R.L. (1997) *Echinococcus granulosus*: biology and ecology. In: Andersen, F.L., Ouhelli, H. and Kachani, M. (eds) *Compendium on Cystic Echinococcosis in Africa and in Middle Eastern Countries With Special Reference to Morocco.* Brigham Young University, Provo, Utah, pp. 18-53.

Rausch, R.L., Wilson, J.F. and Schantz, P.M. (1990) A program to reduce risk of infection by *Echinococcus multilocularis*: the use of praziquantel to control the cestode in a village in the hyperendemic region of Alaska. *Annals of Tropical Medicine and Parasitology* 84, 239-250.

Reichel, M.P., Baber, D.J., Craig, P.S. and Gasser, R.B. (1996) Cystic echinococcosis in the Falkland Islands. *Preventive Veterinary Medicine* 27, 115-123.

Reithinger, R. and Davies, C.R. (1999) Is the domestic dog (*Canis familiaris*) a reservoir host of American cutaneous leishmaniasis? A critical review of the current evidence. *American Journal of Tropical Medicine and Hygiene* 61, 530-541.

Rhalem, A., Sahibi, H., Guessous-Idrissi, N., Lasri, S., Natami, A., Riyad, M. and Berrag, B. (1999) Immune response against *Leishmania* antigens in dogs naturally and experimentally infected with *Leishmania infantum*. *Veterinary Parasitology* 81, 173-184.

Roberts, M.G. and Gemmell, M.A. (1994) Echinococcosis. In: Scott, M.E. and Smith G. (eds) *Parasitic and Infectious Diseases*. Academic Press, London, Sydney, Tokyo, pp. 249-262.

Roura, X., Sanchez, A. and Ferrer, L. (1999) Diagnosis of canine leishmaniasis by a polymerase chain reaction technique. *Veterinary Record* 144, 262-264.

Santos, E.G., Marzochi, M.C., Conceicao, N.F., Brito, C.M. and Pacheco, R.S. (1998) Epidemiological survey on canine population with the use of immunoleish skin test in endemic areas of human American cutaneous leishmaniasis in the state of Rio de Janeiro, Brazil. *Revista do Instituto de Medicina Tropical de Sao Paulo* 40, 41-47.

Schantz, P.M., Chai, J., Craig, P.S., Eckert, J., Jenkins, D.J., Macpherson, C.N.L. and Thakur, A. (1995) Epidemiology and control of hydatid disease. In: Thompson, R.C.A. and Lymbery, A.J. (eds) *Echinococcus and Hydatid Disease*. CAB International, Wallingford, UK, pp. 233-331.

Slappendel, R.J. and Teske, E. (1999) A review of canine leishmaniasis presenting outside endemic areas. In: Killick-Kendrick, R. (ed.) *Canine Leishmaniasis: an Update. Proceedings of the International Canine Leishmaniasis Forum*, Barcelona, Spain. Hoechst Roussel Vet, Germany, pp. 54-59.

Srisonmuang, W. (1997) Thailand: structure of veterinary services for rabies control. In: Dodet, B. and Meslin, F.-X. (eds) *Rabies Control in Asia*. Elsevier, Paris, pp. 197-199.

Sundar, S., Reed, S.G., Singh, V.P., Kumar, P.C.K. and Murray, H.W. (1998) Rapid accurate field diagnosis of Indian visceral leishmaniasis. *Lancet* 351, 563-565.

Tan, Y. (1988) Rabies in Malaysia. *Southeast Asian Journal of Tropical Medicine and Public Health* 19, 535-536.

Umeno, S. and Doi, Y. (1921) A study in the antirabic inoculation of dogs. *Kitasato Archives of Experimental Medicine* 4, 89.

Vasconcelos, Par I. de A.B., Sousa, A. de Q., Vasconcelos, A.W., Diogenes, M.J.N., Momen, H., Grimaldi, G. Jr., Menezes, D.B. and Sleigh, A.C. (1993) Parasitisme cutane par *Leishmania* (*Leishmania*) *chagasi* au cours de la leishmaniose viscerale sud-Americaine. *Bulletin de la Societe de Pathologie Exotique* 86, 101-105.

Vercammen, F., Berkvens, D., Brandt, J. and Vansteenkiste, W. (1998) A sensitive and specific 30-min Dot-ELISA for the detection of anti-leishmania antibodies in the dog. *Veterinary Parasitology* 79, 221-228.

Vexenat, J.A., Fonseca de Castro, J.A., Cavalcante, R., da Silva, M.R.P., Batista, W.H., Furtado Campos, J.H., Alves Pereira, F.C., Tavares, J.P. and Miles, M.A. (1993) Preliminary observations on the diagnosis and transmissibility of canine visceral leishmaniasis in Teresina, N.E. Brazil. *Archives de l'Institute Pasteur de Tunis* 70, 467-472.

Vexenat, J.A., Fonseca de Castro, J.A., Cavalcante, R., da Silva, M.R.P., Batista, W.H., Furtado Campos, J.H., Alves Pereira, F.C., Tavares, J.P. and Miles, M.A. (1994) Visceral leishmaniasis in Teresina, Piaui State, Brazil: preliminary observations on the detection and transmissibility of canine and sandfly infections. *Memorias do Instituto Oswaldo Cruz* 89, 131-135.

Vexenat, J.A., Olliaro, P.L., Fonseca de Castro, J.A., Cavalcante, R., Furtado Campos, J.H., Tavares, J.P. and Miles, M.A. (1998) Clinical recovery and limited cure in canine visceral leishmaniasis treated with aminosidine (paromomycin). *American Journal of Tropical Medicine and Hygiene* 58, 448-453.

Wandeler, A.I. and Budde, A. (1988) Dog ecology and dog rabies control. *Review of Infectious Diseases* 10, 684-688.

Wandeler, A.I., Matter, H.C., Kapeller, A. and Budde, A. (1993) The ecology of dogs and canine rabies: a selective review. *Review Scientifique et Technique de l'OIE* 12, 51-71.

WHO (1987) *The Canine Rabies Situation in Guidelines for Dog Rabies Control.* WHO, Geneva, pp. 1-44.

WHO (1988a) *Report of a WHO Consultation on Dog Ecology Studies Related to Rabies Control.* WHO, Geneva, pp. 35.

WHO (1988b) *Report of WHO Consultation on Oral Immunization of Dogs Against Rabies.* WHO, Geneva, pp. 11.

WHO (1991) *Report of the 2nd consultation on Oral Immunization of Dogs Against Rabies.* WHO, Geneva, pp. 21.

WHO (1992a) *Report of the 3rd Consultation on Oral Immunization of Dogs Against Rabies.* WHO, Geneva, pp. 14.

WHO (1992b) *WHO Expert Committee on Rabies*, 8th Report. Technical Report Series n° 824, WHO, Geneva, pp. 84.

WHO (1993a) *Report of the WHO Consultation on Feasibility of Global Control and Elimination of Urban Rabies.* WHO, Geneva, pp. 32.

WHO (1993b) *Report of the Fourth Consultation on Oral Immunization of Dogs Against Rabies.* WHO, Geneva, pp. 17.

WHO (1993c) *Suggestions for the Development of a Research Project for the Field Evaluation of Several Vaccine-Bait Delivery Techniques to Vaccinate Dogs Orally Against Rabies.* WHO, Geneva, pp. 11.

WHO (1994) *Report of the Fifth Consultation on Oral Immunization of Dogs Against Rabies.* WHO, Geneva, pp. 24.

WHO (1997) *World Survey of Rabies n°31 for the Year 1995*. WHO, Geneva, pp. 29.

WHO (1998a) *World Survey of Rabies n°32 for the Year 1996*. WHO, Geneva, pp. 27.

WHO (1998b) *Field Application of Oral Rabies Vaccines for Dogs*: report of a WHO Consultation, WHO, Geneva, pp. 24.

WHO (1998c) *Oral Immunization of Dogs Against Rabies*: Report of the Sixth Consultation, WHO, Geneva, pp. 28.

WHO (2000a) *Report of the Informal Meeting on Oral Vaccination of Dogs Against Rabies Held in San Diego, California*. WHO, Geneva (in press).

WHO (2000b) *World Survey of Rabies n°34 for the Year 1998*. WHO Geneva (in press).

WHO and UNAIDS (1998) *Leishmania and HIV in Gridlock*. WHO, Geneva, pp. 28.

Xiong, G., Jin, C., Hong, Y., Su, Z., Xue, P., Xie, W., Zhang, A., Li, G. and Gao, B. (1995) Studies on the deltamethrin-medicated bath of domestic dogs for interrupting visceral leishmaniasis transmission. *Chung Kuo Chi Sheng Chung Hsueh Yu Chi Sheng Chung Ping Tsa Chih* 13, 178-181.

Zaffaroni, E., Rubaudo, L., Lanfranchi, P. and Mignone, W. (1999) Epidemiological patterns of canine leishmaniasis in Western Liguria (Italy). *Veterinary Parasitology* 81, 11-19.

Index

Figures in **bold** indicate major references.
Figures in *italic* refer to diagrams, photographs and tables.